Meenakshi Radiology Cases

In Association with TNPY–IRIA

Part-1

Meenakshi Radiology Cases

In Association with TNPY–IRIA

Part-1

Editors

Shanmuga Jayanthan S DNB MNAMS

Senior Consultant and Head
Department of Radiology and Imaging Sciences
Meenakshi Hospital
Thanjavur, Tamil Nadu, India
EC Member: TNPY IRIA
National Coordinator for Resident Education IRIA—2024

Flora Nelson MD

Professor and Head
Department of Radiology
Government Thoothukudi Medical College
Thoothukudi, Tamil Nadu, India
Secretary, TNPY IRIA, 2023–2024

Chinnadurai Abdullah MD DMRD

Consultant Radiologist
AR Hospital and Rasi Color Scans
Ramanathapuram, Tamil Nadu, India
President, TNPY IRIA, 2024

G Rupesh MD

Consultant Radiologist
Department of Radiology and Imaging Sciences
Meenakshi Hospital
Thanjavur, Tamil Nadu, India

Forewords

C Amarnath
L Murali Krishna
A Anbarasu

JAYPEE

JAYPEE BROTHERS MEDICAL PUBLISHERS

The Health Sciences Publisher

New Delhi | London

Jaypee Brothers Medical Publishers (P) Ltd

Headquarters
EMCA House
23/23-B, Ansari Road, Daryaganj
New Delhi 110 002, India
Landline: +91-11-23272143, +91-11-23272703
+91-11-23282021, +91-11-23245672
E-mail: jaypee@jaypeebrothers.com

Corporate Office
Jaypee Brothers Medical Publishers (P) Ltd.
4838/24, Ansari Road, Daryaganj
New Delhi 110 002, India
Phone: +91-11-43574357
Fax: +91-11-43574314
E-mail: jaypee@jaypeebrothers.com

Overseas Office
JP Medical Ltd.
83, Victoria Street, London
SW1H 0HW (UK)
Phone: +44-20 3170 8910
Fax: +44(0)20 3008 6180
E-mail: info@jpmedpub.com

Website: www.jaypeebrothers.com
Website: www.jaypeedigital.com

Inquiries for bulk sales may be solicited at: jaypee@jaypeebrothers.com

Meenakshi Radiology Cases: In Association with TNPY–IRIA Part-1 / ***Shanmuga Jayanthan S, Chinnadurai Abdullah, Flora Nelson, G Rupesh***

First Edition: **2025**

ISBN: 978-93-6616-650-6

Printed at: Samrat Offset Pvt. Ltd.

From the Desk of Medical Superintendent

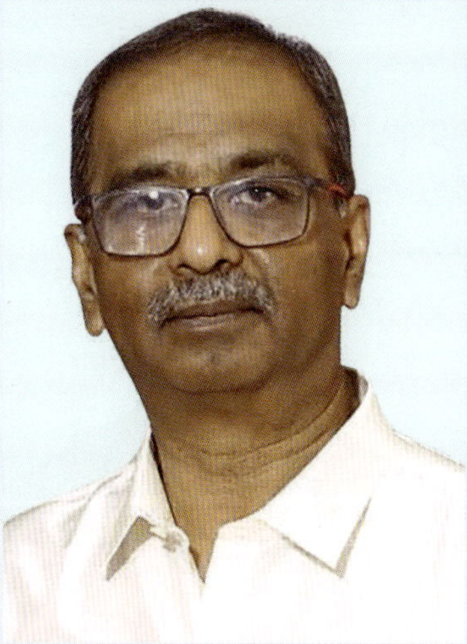

Dr. R Ravichandran MS DNB (Urology)
Medical Superintendent, Sr Consultant and Head
Department of Urology
Meenakshi Hospital
Thanjavur, Tamil Nadu, India

Greetings to all from Meenakshi Family!

A medical professional's goal in life is not only to diagnose and treat his patient's illness. He should also impart, share, and educate, what he has learnt to his colleagues, juniors, and aspiring students in his profession. Keeping this sharing of professional knowledge to their peers, in mind, our Meenakshi Radiologists have come up with an excellent initiative—*"Meenakshi Radiology Cases: In Association with TNPY–IRIA Part-1"*—the First Edition of which covers 100 interesting cases.

This book throws lights upon all aspects—images, clinical correlations, etc., all you wish to know and all you need to know, regarding each case, in a very clear manner.

I am sure that this series would be of great use to many students and I sincerely congratulate our radiologists for coming up with such a useful venture and wish they continue this noble deed, in future.

And, I also request upcoming radiologists and professionals to make use of this and grow in their career confidently.

Best wishes to all !

Author's Note

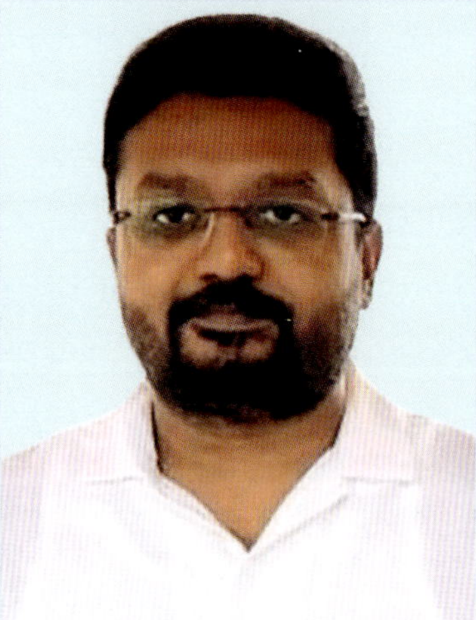

Dr. Shanmuga Jayanthan S DNB MNAMS
Senior Consultant and Head
Department of Radiology and Imaging Sciences
Meenakshi Hospital
Thanjavur, Tamil Nadu, India
EC Member: TNPY IRIA
National coordinator for Resident Education
IRIA—2024

Dr. G Rupesh MD
Consultant Radiologist
Department of Radiology and Imaging Sciences
Meenakshi Hospital
Thanjavur, Tamil Nadu, India

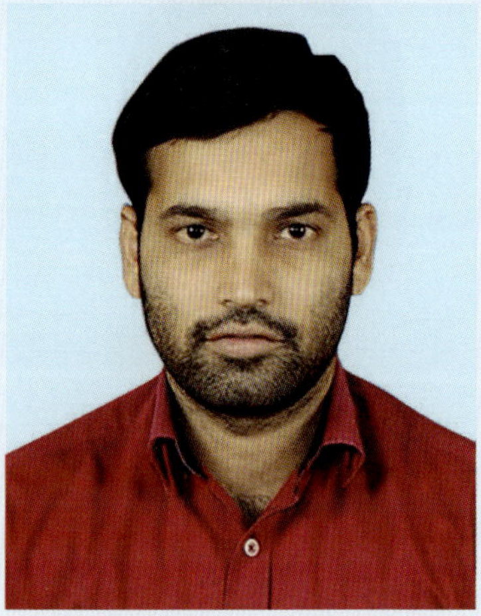

Welcome to *"100 Cases with Clinicoradiological and Pathoradiological Correlation,"* a meticulously curated resource designed to meet the needs of radiology residents, junior consultants, and professionals preparing for important examinations such as DNB, MD, practical examinations, and other Indian and International Board Certifications.

This book presents a unique collection of 100 real-life cases. Our goal is to provide a comprehensive approach to learning, where clinical signs, imaging techniques, and histopathological results are brought together to give a deeper understanding of disease processes. The carefully selected cases aim to reflect the diversity and complexity of scenarios faced by radiologists and clinicians in their practice.

Special emphasis has been placed on offering intraoperative images and follow-up imaging for essential cases. These visuals are invaluable in bridging the gap between diagnostic radiology and surgical outcomes, allowing readers to visualize the entire patient's journey from diagnosis through treatment and follow-up.

Whether you are a resident building a foundation or a junior consultant seeking to refine your expertise, this collection will sharpen your diagnostic acumen by emphasizing the importance of clinicoradiological and pathoradiological correlations. The illustrative nature of the cases, combined with follow-up imaging, will prepare the young radiologists for real-world clinical challenges.

We hope that this compilation becomes a valued companion in your journey toward becoming a skilled, confident, and insightful radiologist.

We would like to express my sincere gratitude to the Tamil Nadu and Pondicherry Chapter of the Indian Radiological and Imaging Association (TN & PY IRIA) for providing a distinguished platform that has greatly contributed to the success of this endeavor. Their continuous support, dedication, and commitment to advancing the field of radiology and imaging have been invaluable in the creation of this work.

Editorial Note

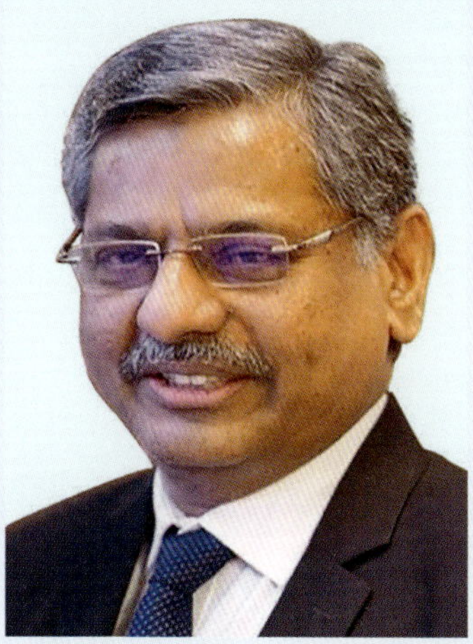

Dr. Chinnadurai Abdullah MD DMRD
Consultant Radiologist
AR Hospital and Rasi Color Scans
Ramanathapuram, Tamil Nadu, India
President, TNPY IRIA, 2024

Prof. Flora Nelson MD
Professor and Head
Department of Radiology
Government Thoothukudi Medical College
Thoothukudi, Tamil Nadu, India
Secretary, TNPY IRIA, 2023–2024

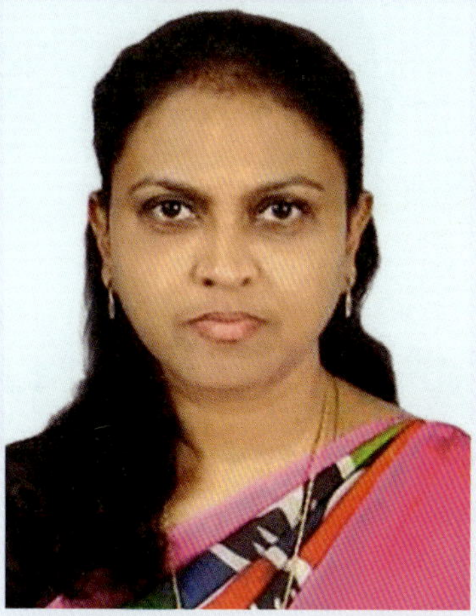

The first edition of the textbook *"Meenakshi Radiology Cases: In Association with TNPY–IRIA Part-1"* gives a concise list of 100 interesting unique radiology cases in the form of case discussions. The most important highlight of the textbook is that the clinical-radiological and radio-pathological correlations are done for all the possible cases, which is very interesting as to get the whole content of a case at one point. The explanations have been written in a cogent manner and without any ambiguity. The sources of the content are mentioned in the references, which the readers are advised to go through for detailed understanding of the content.

We believe that the textbook will be of great satisfaction for the students to read and we will not leave a single stone unturned to satisfy our students.

This textbook will be very useful for all the examination going students (Indian and Foreign Examinations) and junior residents. We feel immense pleasure in conveying our appreciation to the Department of Radiology, Meenakshi Hospital, Thanjavur for coming up with this beautiful concept of the textbook.

Wishing you all the very best future!

Foreword

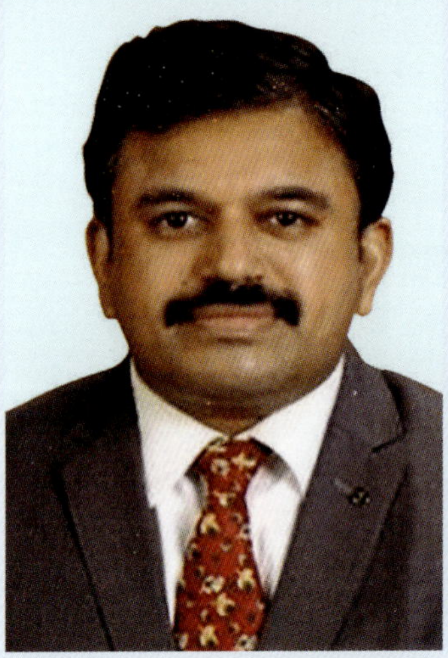

Prof. C Amarnath MD FRCR PhD
Professor and Head
Department of Radiodiagnosis
Stanley Medical College
Senior Consultant
Scans World and Scans Point
Chennai, Tamil Nadu, India

It gives me immense pleasure to write foreword for this book—*"Meenakshi Radiology Cases: In Association with TNPY–IRIA Part-1"* (as a part of Remote Radiology Teaching Program). This pocketbook presents 100 diverse cases, serving as an invaluable resource for embracing your knowledge. Each case is explored in depth, covering clinical history to expert discussion. This structured approach facilitates a thorough understanding of various radiological conditions, enabling examination preparation and professional development.

This resource offers a structured approach to case analysis, combining a broad overview with detailed insights. By applying this systematic methodology, we gain a deeper understanding of each case and develop expertise in handling complex scenarios.

The discussed content, compiled from numerous research articles, provides a comprehensive understanding of evidence-based knowledge grounded in scholarly literature.

Dr Shanmuga Jayanthan S is a distinguished and young and dynamic radiologist who serves as the head of the department at Meenakshi Hospital, Thanjavur. He has earned numerous prestigious awards in recognition of his outstanding contributions and achievements in the field of "Radiology".

I welcome everyone to embark on a journey to radiology mastery with our vast array of instructive cases and structured learning case approach.

Foreword

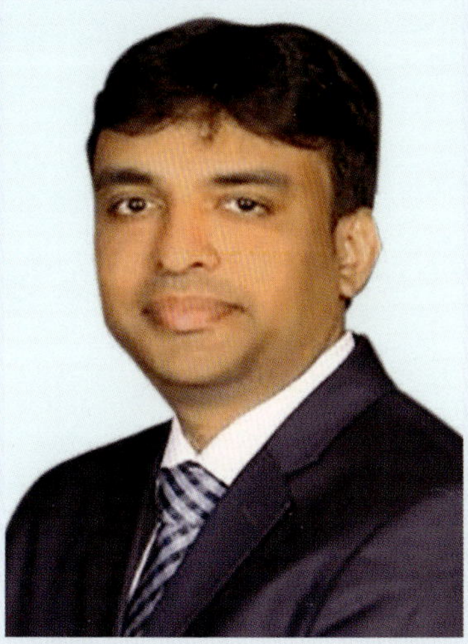

Dr. L Murali Krishna MD
Senior Consultant and Lead
Department of Radiodiagnosis
Kauvery Hospitals, Vadapalani,
Chennai, Tamil Nadu, India
Secretary General, IRIA

Dear Friends,
Season's Greetings!

I am really excited to know that the Tamil Nadu and Puducherry (Pondicherry) Chapter of IRIA in association with Meenakshi Hospital, Thanjavur as a part of its Remote Teaching Program is planning to release a book *"Meenakshi Radiology Cases: In Association with TNPY–IRIA Part-1"*. I understand that this book will be very useful for the postgraduates and the practicing consultants.

I would like to congratulate my dear friend Dr Shanmuga Jayanthan S for taking this wonderful initiate and for starting the *"From the Console Series."* He has been a very enthusiastic teacher and I wish him the very best for all his future endeavors. My gratitude to Dr Chinnadurai Abdullah, President TNPY IRIA and Dr Flora Nelson, a dynamic Secretary TNPY IRIA for providing all the support and guidance for this series. TNPY IRIA has excelled under their zestful leadership. I am sure that this will be another feather in your cap.

Wish the entire team the very best and hope to see you all at the AOCR 2025!

Warm regards!

Foreword

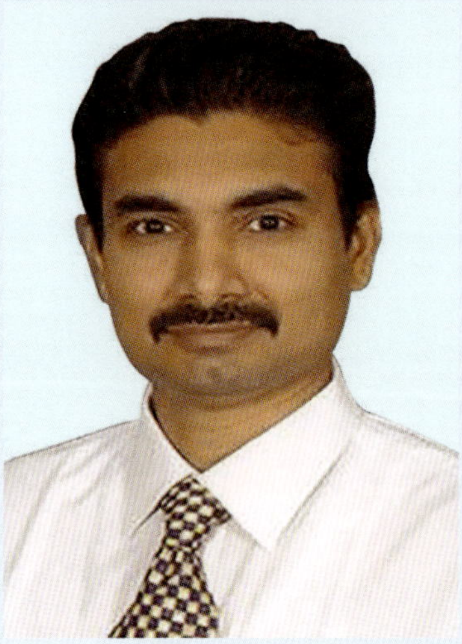

Dr. A Anbarasu MD DNB DMRD (Liverpool) FRCR (London)
Fellowship (Boston) FICR
Consultant Radiologist and Director
Aran Diagnostic Imaging, Coimbatore, Tamil Nadu, India
Chairman, Indian College of Radiology and Imaging
Academic Wing of IRIA Past president, TNPY IRIA

Case reports study is one of the *easy methods* of the learning in medicine especially "Radiology". The significance of case study can be seen at various websites of the world, which are publishing, case of the day/case of the week regularly; there are case reports related to journals too which had increased in the recent past.

Case reports are easy to teach and also easy to learn from because of *focuses on one area* and therefore keeps the attention of the reader to a particular problem. The learning is also made comfortable as it is of short span.

This book *"Meenakshi Radiology Cases: In Association with TNPY–IRIA Part-1"* is a wonderful collection of 100 cases compiled by *Dr Shanmuga Jayanthan S* who is working as a Senior Consultant and Head of the Department, Meenakshi Hospital, Thanjavur. This is done initially as a part of remote radiology teaching program initiated by the *Tamil Nadu and Puducherry (Pondicherry) IRIA;* to take on this responsibility and to collect these cases and consistently delivering to all members of TNPY IRIA every few days, is in itself a *great feat* achieved by Dr Shanmuga Jayanthan S.

First of all, I would like to *congratulate* him for his excellent achievement and his effort to contribute to teaching and education in radiology.

These case reports are one of the few excellent collections of cases which have been compiled in the recent past. They are *across various* systems from head to foot with several important cases of the learning suitable for both for examination and every day practice. This contains *excellent images* with beautiful description and also important learning points.

I have requested Dr Shanmuga Jayanthan S to create one in the *future* more toward the system-based collection such that they could become "Diagnostic Imaging" like casebook series from India.

I am sure that *"this 'first step"* will be a great success and I believe that this is an important milestone of teaching efforts by our Tamil Nadu and Puducherry (Pondicherry) IRIA member.

I also *congratulate* the initiatives taken by the President, Secretary, and Members of Tamil Nadu and Puducherry (Pondicherry) IRIA for such teaching programs and encouraging members to take up on the various teaching initiatives; they have found an excellent teacher in Dr Shanmuga Jayanthan S.

I am sure the reader will enjoy the whole book in hand as a reporting room tool!

I again congratulate Dr Shanmuga Jayanthan S, for his excellent work and hopefully this is the beginning of many *more achievements in academics and education!*

Student Contributors

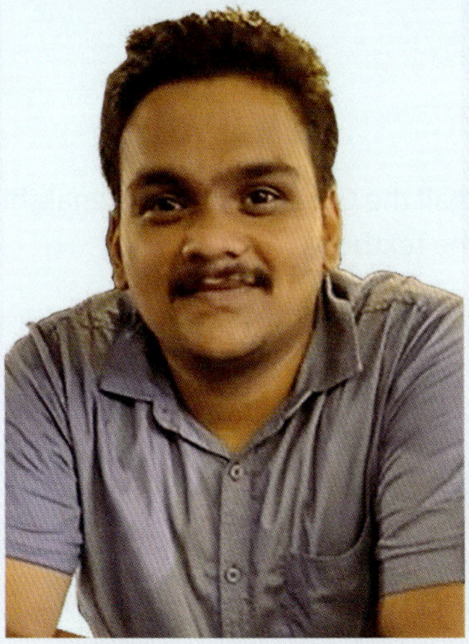

Nadanasadharam K

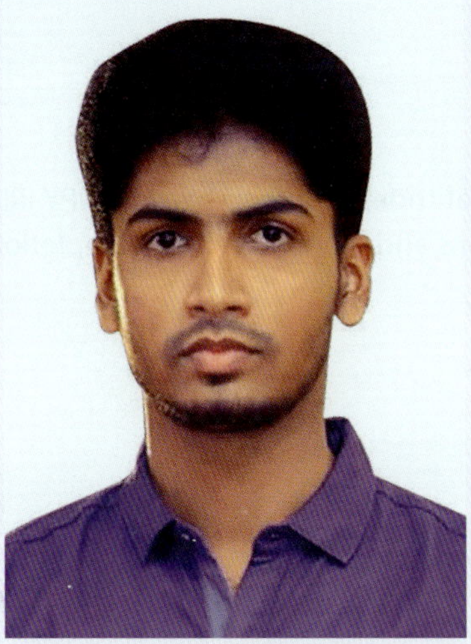

Yuvaraj N

Engaging postgraduates in contributing to textbook chapters offers invaluable experience, as it sharpens their research and writing skills while familiarizing them with the publication process. Participating in such projects provides them with a strong foundation for future academic or professional publications.

This hands-on approach to learning could be instrumental in developing their academic profiles and establishing a track record in research and publication.

My sincere thanks to:

Nadanasadharam K, currently a third-year DNB Radiology Resident in Meenakshi Hospital, began his journey at Mohan Kumaramangalam Medical College, Salem, Tamil Nadu, India. His dedication to learning and hands-on experience in radiology exemplifies the spirit of the next generation of specialists.

Yuvaraj N, an MBBS graduate of Dharmapuri Medical College, Tamil Nadu, is pursuing his second year of DNB Radiology in Meenakshi Hospital. His enthusiasm and drive reflect a strong commitment to mastering the intricacies of radiology.

Acknowledgments

I would like to extend my heartfelt thanks and gratitude to all members of TNPY IRIA and all the Consultants of Meenakshi Hospital, Thanjavur, for their valuable contributions and guidance in the completion of the textbook.

Contents

1 Marchiafava–Bignami Disease

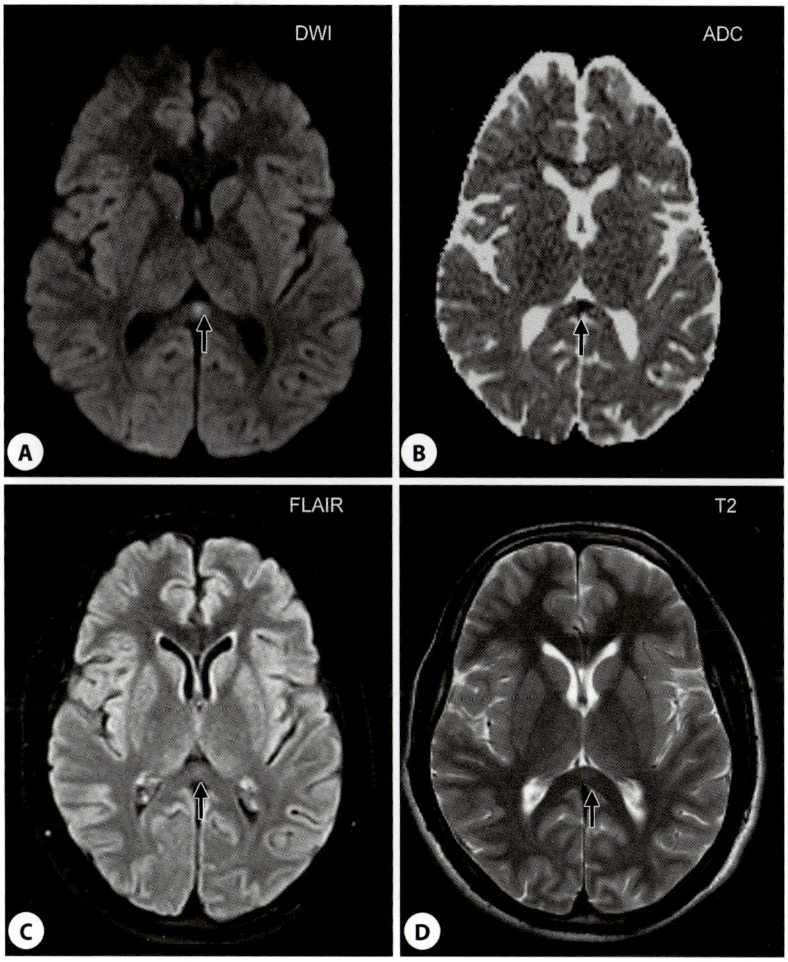

CLINICAL BACKGROUND

A 40-year-old male patient—chronic alcoholic—complaints of acute onset of gait disturbance.

IMAGING FINDINGS

MRI shows small diffusion restriction area in splenium of corpus callosum which appears hyperintense on T2 and FLAIR **(Figs. 1A to D)**.

DISCUSSION

Cytotoxic lesion of the corpus callosum (CLOCC) or the transient hyperintensity of splenium of corpus callosum, is known to be associated with multiple pathological conditions which includes encephalitis, encephalopathy, metabolic disorder (hypoglycemia and hypernatremia), antiepileptic drug withdrawal, alcoholism, infection, and seizure.[1]

Marchiafava-Bignami disease (MBD) is a rare neurological condition which is linked to chronic alcoholism. It is characterized by demyelination and necrosis, that is evidenced as DWI restriction and hyperintensity in T2 FLAIR sequence. These lesions may be subtle in CT and MRI is the imaging modality of choice.[2] This condition does occur in chronically malnourished nonalcoholic patients with vitamin B deficiency.[3]

The pathophysiology of this condition includes cytotoxic edema, blood-brain barrier break, demyelination, and necrosis. The splenium of corpus callosum has more myelin than its other parts and intramyelinic cytotoxic edema is detected as the abnormal signal changes in MRI.[4] Extra-callosal lesions can also occur and are primarily seen in cortical areas, which could be due to Morel's laminar sclerosis.[5]

Wernicke encephalopathy, another acute alcohol related neurological disease, is caused by vitamin B1 deficiency, and can occur together with MBD. But this condition typically involves the medial thalamic nuclei, hypothalamus, mammillary bodies and periaqueductal gray matter.[2]

Important to note that, although corpus callosum is the typical site of involvement in MBD, extra-callosal regions of brain are affected late in this condition and are associated with poor prognosis/severe cognitive impairment. Under appropriate clinical background, early diagnosis of MBD is very important as early diagnosis and intervention results in a favorable outcome.[6]

REFERENCES

1. Toi H, Yagi K, Matsubara S, et al. Clinical Features of Cytotoxic Lesions of the Corpus Callosum Associated with Aneurysmal Subarachnoid Hemorrhage. AJNR Am J Neuroradiol. 2021; 42(6):1046-51.
2. Dong X, Bai C, Nao J. Clinical and radiological features of Marchiafava–Bignami disease. Medicine (Baltimore). 2018;97(5).
3. Kakkar C, Prakashini K, Polnaya A. Acute Marchiafava-Bignami disease: clinical and serial MRI correlation. BMJ Case Rep. 2014;2014:502-4.
4. Yoshizaki T, Hashimoto T, Fujimoto K, et al. Evolution of callosal and cortical lesions on MRI in Marchiafava-Bignami disease. Case Rep Neurol. 2010;2:19-23.
5. Kawarabuki K, Sakakibara T, Hirai M, et al. Marchiafava–Bignami disease: magnetic resonance imaging findings in corpus callosum and subcortical white matter. Eur J Radiol. 2003;48:175-7.
6. Helenius J, Tatlisumak T, Soinne L, et al. Marchiafava–Bignami disease: two cases with favourable outcome. Eur J Neurol. 2001;8:269-72.

2

Herlyn–Werner–Wunderlich Syndrome

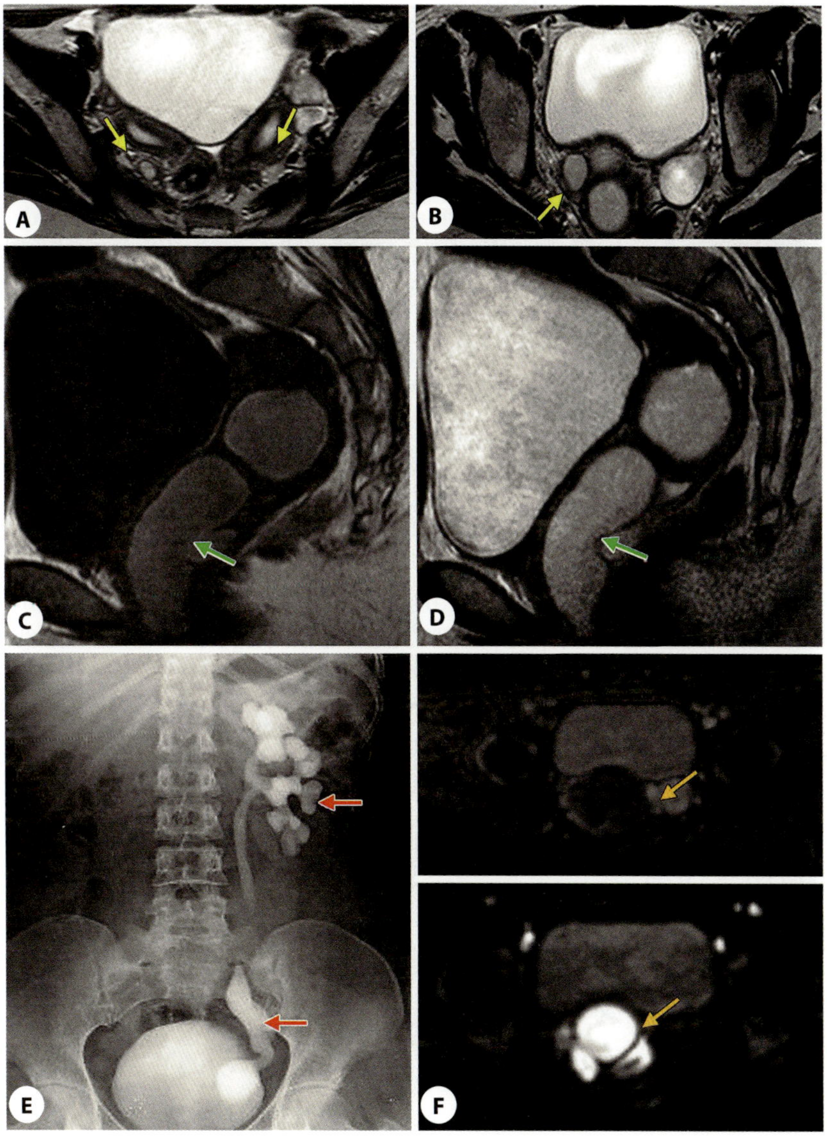

CLINICAL BACKGROUND

A 24-year-old female presented with complaints of cyclical abdominal pain during menstruation for the last 4 months, which aggravated over the past 1 week. She had a normal menstrual cycle 3/28. Physical examination revealed normal external genitalia and clinical examination was unremarkable.

IMAGING FINDINGS

MRI T2 images at the level of pelvis shows didelphic configuration of uterus (yellow arrows). MRI T1 and T2 sagittal images at the level of pelvis showed distended right hemi cervix and vagina with T1 and T2 hyperintense content suggestive of hematometrocolpos (green arrows). ADC and DWI show (orange) areas of diffusion restriction within the right hemi cervix, suggestive of secondary abscess. Agenesis of right kidney and compensatory hypertrophy of left kidney with megaureter, megapolycalycosis and ureterocele which was confirmed with IVP (red arrows) **(Figs. 1A to F)**.

DISCUSSION

The incidence of Müllerian anomaly is estimated about 0.1 to 3.5% among which the incidence of uterine didelphys includes 11%. Renal anomalies are associated with uterine didelphys in approximately 80% of cases. Herlyn–Werner–Wunderlich (HWW) also known as OHVIRA syndrome is a rare complex congenital developmental anomaly is characterized by triad of uterus didelphys, unilateral low vaginal obstruction and ipsilateral renal agenesis (class 3 Müllerian duct anomaly).[1,2]

An early failure of the metanephric diverticulum to develop (around 5 weeks) from the mesonephric duct results in agenesis of the ureteric bud, which leads to agenesis of ipsilateral ureter and kidney. Due to failed positioning of paired paramesonephric duct, the two hemi uterus and hemi cervices fail to unite, resulting in uterus didelphys. Developmental arrest of the distal ipsilateral mesonephric duct results in failure of distal hemivagina to develop, thereby resulting in obstructed hemivagina. Thus in OHVIRA syndrome, all three components are secondary to mesonephric duct-induced Müllerian anomalies. Cyclical dysmenorrhea is the most common complaint.[1-4]

This syndrome has been reported to be associated with high bifurcation of aorta, IVC duplication, ovarian malposition, and intestinal malrotation. Imaging, particularly an MRI plays a major role in diagnosis, which is often missed clinically.[2] Timely surgical intervention and psychological counseling are of utmost importance. Careful consideration must be given to patients with renal malformations to examine the reproductive system given their common embryology.[2-4]

An early correct diagnosis is the goal to relieve the symptoms and prevent complications, caused by retrograde menstruation like endometriosis and, also, preserve sexual and conception abilities.

REFERENCES

1. Acien P. Incidence of Müllerian defects in fertile and infertile women. Hum Reprod. 1997;12:1372-6.
2. Acién P. Embryological observations on the female genital tract. Hum Reprod. 1992;7:437-45.
3. Bajaj SK, Misra R, Thukral BB, et al. OHVIRA: Uterus didelphys, blind hemivagina and ipsilateral renal agenesis: Advantage MRI. J Hum Reprod Sci. 2012;5(1):67-70.
4. Sharma R, Mishra P, Seth S, et al. OHVIRA Syndrome—Diagnostic Dilemmas and Review of Literature. J South Asian Feder Obst Gynae. 2020;12(6):421-6.

3

Glomangioma of Knee

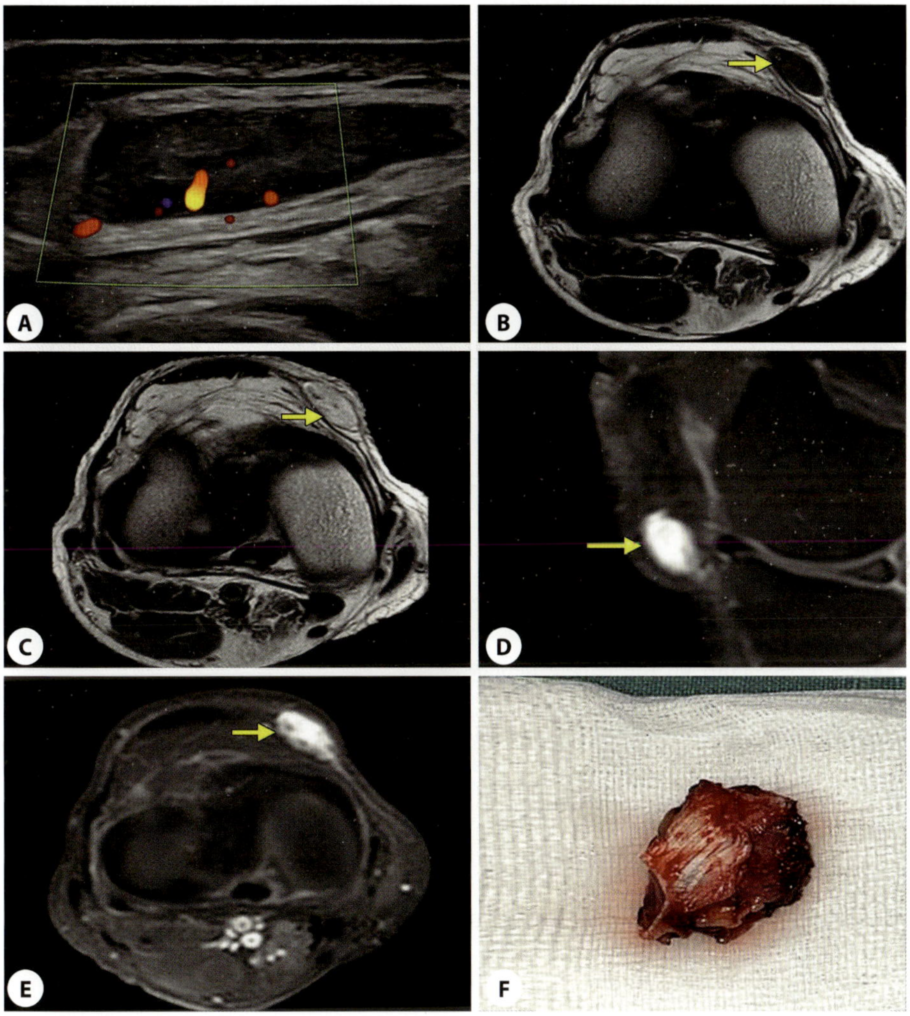

CLINICAL BACKGROUND

A 75-year-old man presented with complaints of knee pain. No history of fever. On examination, a palpable swelling was noticed in anteromedial aspect of right knee.

IMAGING FINDINGS

USG demonstrated a hyper-vascular solid nodule. The lesion was located in anteromedial aspect of knee joint abutting the patellar retinaculum. It was hypointense on T1W sequence and hyperintense on T2W images and showed intense postcontrast enhancement. The lesion was excised en bloc and HPE confirmed it as glomangioma **(Figs. 1A to F)**.

DISCUSSION

Glomangiomas are benign glomus tumors characterized by diffuse angiomatosis and rare malignant potential. They are rare tumor with estimated incidence of 2 in 1,000,000 and accounts for 2–3% of glomus tumors in adults. Both typical glomus tumors and glomangiomas, are painful and typically occur in the extremities.[1]

These tumors occur most frequently in distal extremities, particularly in subungual area.[2] However, atypical extradigital sites, including the head and neck, lungs, mediastinum, stomach, mesentery, bowels, bone and venous system, may be observed.[3] There are reports of multiple possible locations around the knee: subcutaneous, sub-synovial, in patellar ligament, within the fat pad, in the popliteal area or at the fibular head.[4] The preferred methods for diagnosing are MRI and ultrasound. Ultrasound typically show glomangioma as round or ovoid hypoechoic mass which is hyper-vascular. MRI is the most sensitive imaging modality for diagnosis. It appears as low signal intensity on T1-weighted images and show increased signal intensity on T2-weighted images.[4]

In 1924, Masson described histologic variants of glomus tumors. Depending on histologic composition, variations in the MR signals are noted. Three types of variants are described in literature.

1. *Vascular type:* It is comprising vascular lumen, hence exhibiting hyperintensity on T2, and showing avid early arterial enhancement increasing on delayed venous acquisition.
2. *Cellular or solid type:* It is comprising epithelioid cells with a paucity of vascular lumens. Hence exhibiting T2 iso- to hypointense signals with mild postcontrast enhancement.
3. *Mucoid type:* It is characterized by stromal mucoid degeneration. They demonstrate T2 hyperintense signals and very mild enhancement after gadolinium administration.[4] The differentiation of benign from malignant lesions, or uncertain potential malignancy is not absolute in MR or USG and hence warrants tissue diagnosis.[4] Inadequate excision may result in tumor recurrence.

REFERENCES

1. Acien P. Incidence of Müllerian defects in fertile and infertile women. Hum Reprod. 1997;12:1372-6.
2. Acién P. Embryological observations on the female genital tract. Hum Reprod. 1992;7:437-45.
3. Bajaj SK, Misra R, Thukral BB, et al. OHVIRA: Uterus didelphys, blind hemivagina and ipsilateral renal agenesis: Advantage MRI. J Hum Reprod Sci. 2012;5(1):67-70.
4. Sharma R, Mishra P, Seth S, et al. OHVIRA Syndrome—Diagnostic Dilemmas and Review of Literature. J South Asian Feder Obst Gynae. 2020;12(6):421-6.

4 Extragastrointestinal Stromal Tumor

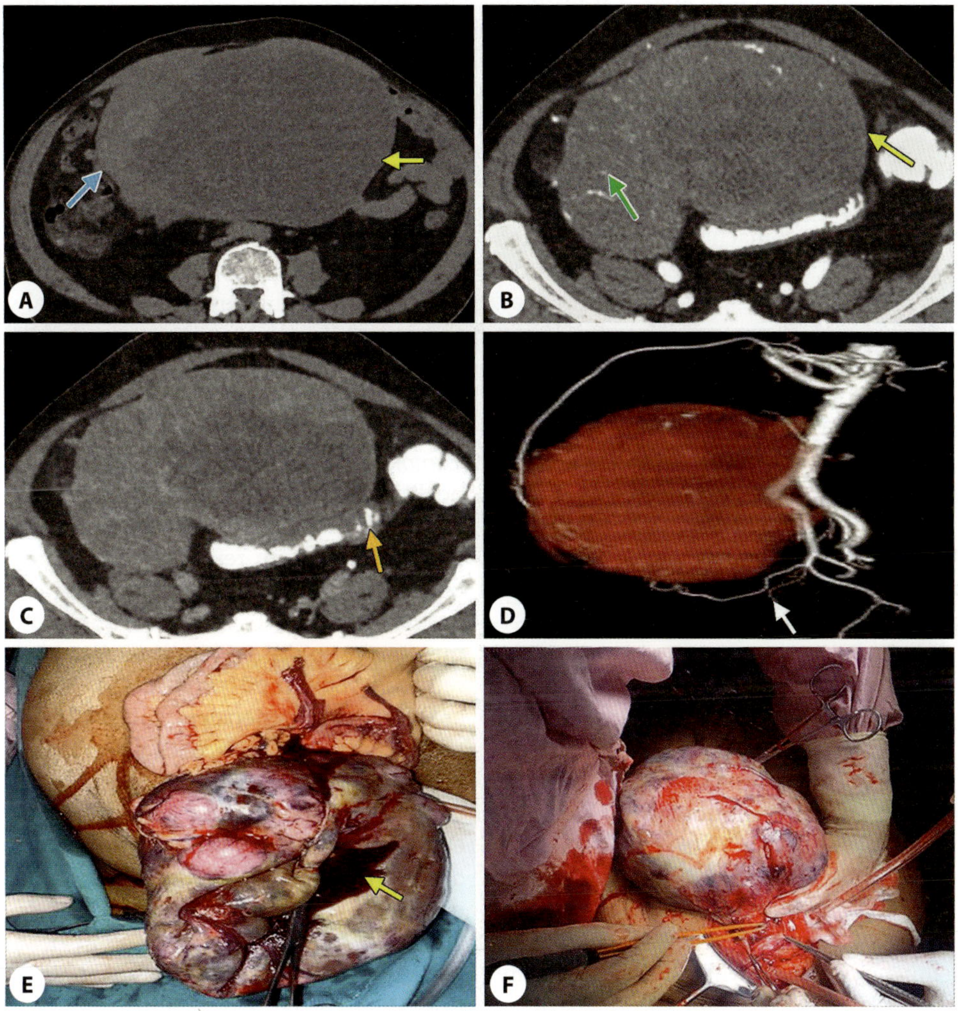

CLINICAL BACKGROUND

A 71-year-old male patient came to the surgery OPD with complaints of mass in abdomen for past 2 months. He had loss of appetite for past 6 months. Known patient of CAD on treatment. On P/A examination mass was palpable on right middle and lower quadrant of abdomen. The patient was advocated for CT-abdomen and pelvis.

IMAGING FINDINGS

CT abdomen plain and contrast studies with VR show a well-defined heterogeneously enhancing mass lesion in mid peritoneal compartment with nonenhancing cystic areas (yellow arrows). The lesion shows internal hyperdense areas likely hemorrhage. No fat components (blue arrows). Multiple dilated intratumoral vessels were seen (green arrows). The lesion causes mass effect and displacement of adjacent small and large bowel loops with no signs of infiltration (orange arrow). Multiple arterial feeders supplying from splenic and internal iliac artery the lesion (white arrow). Intraoperative images showing the large intraperitoneal mass lesion with areas of necrosis (yellow arrows). No attachment with bowel loops was seen **(Figs. 1A to F)**.

DISCUSSION

Gastrointestinal stromal tumors (GISTs) are the most common mesenchymal tumors of the gastrointestinal tract. Most common site is stomach (60–70%) followed by small intestine (25–35%). The colon, rectum, appendix (together 5%) and esophagus (2–3%) are other rare sites. Stromal tumors arising outside the gastrointestinal tract are extremely rare and are known as extragastrointestinal stromal tumor (EGISTs); and account for less than 5% of all GISTs. Approximately 80% of EGISTs are located in the omentum or mesentery, and the remainder develops in the retroperitoneum.[1,2]

The vast majority of GISTs are sporadic; however, a minority (5–10%) occur in the following syndromes, usually as SDH-deficient GISTs.[4-5]

- Carney triad—extra-adrenal paraganglioma, GIST, pulmonary chondroma.
- Carney-Stratakis syndrome rare autosomal dominant condition comprising of familial paraganglioma and GIST
- Neurofibromatosis type 1 (NF1)—rare
- *Familial GISTs:* KIT (more commonly) or PDGFRA germline mutations

Extragastrointestinal GISTs may arise in the omentum, mesentery or retroperitoneum and are unrelated to the gastrointestinal tract. Due to similar histological appearance and immunophenotype compared with GISTs, EGISTs are believed to be representations of either GISTs that have separated from the GI tract wall or independent mesenchymal cell growth. GIST from the primary gastrointestinal tract origin may metastasize to the peritoneum. In these cases, there are usually multiple masses throughout the peritoneal cavity which is uncommon in primary peritoneal GIST.[2,3] CT is the primary modality used for the initial diagnosis of GISTs, surgical planning, postsurgical surveillance, and monitoring therapy response owing to its ability to visualize exophytic and endophytic components and regional/distant metastases.

Tumor vessel sign: Presence of conspicuous vessels that can be directly traced from tumor margin to the named vessels, is helpful in identifying the origin of hypervascular tumors.[4] Early venous return-return of contrast media in the arterial phase, associated with an enlarged draining vein is common in small bowel GISTs but not in gastric GISTs.[4] GISTs mainly metastasize to the liver and peritoneum and rarely to the retroperitoneum and lymph nodes. Pediatric wild type GIST are SDH-complex deficient upon genetic evaluation. These tumors occur almost exclusively in the stomach manifest at younger ages, most common in female patients, and show early lymph node metastasis. Endoscopic USG guided or endoscopic biopsy is preferred than percutaneous biopsy due to the potential risk of primary tumor capsule rupture or spread of metastatic disease.[4,5]

FDG-PET enables visualization of viable tissue with glucose metabolism is helpful for distinguishing GISTs from non-GISTs and stratifying histopathological risk as well as for performing initial disease evaluation and monitoring response to molecularly targeted therapy.

REFERENCES

1. Antonopoulos P, Leonardou P, Barbagiannis N, et al. Gastrointestinal and Extragastrointestinal Stromal Tumors: Report of Two Cases and Review of the Literature. Case Rep Gastroenterol. 2014; 8(1):61-6.
2. Ematteo RP, Lewis JJ, Leung D, et al. Two hundred gastrointestinal tumors: recurrence patterns and prognostic factors for survival. Ann Surg. 2000;231:51-8.
3. Miettinen M, Lasota J. Gastrointestinal stromal tumor: definition, clinical, histological, immunohistochemical, and molecular genetic features and differential diagnosis. Virchows Arch. 2001;438:1-12.
4. Inoue A, Ota S, Yamasaki M, et al. Gastrointestinal stromal tumors: a comprehensive radiological review. Jpn J Radiol. 2022;40(11):1105-20
5. Goldblum J, Tos A, Hornick J, et al. Gastrointestinal stromal tumour. In: WHO Classification of Tumours Editorial Board. Soft tissue and bone tumours. Lyon (France): International Agency for Research on Cancer. 2020. (WHO classification of tumours series, 5th ed.; vol. 3).

5 Hypertrophic Pachymeningitis

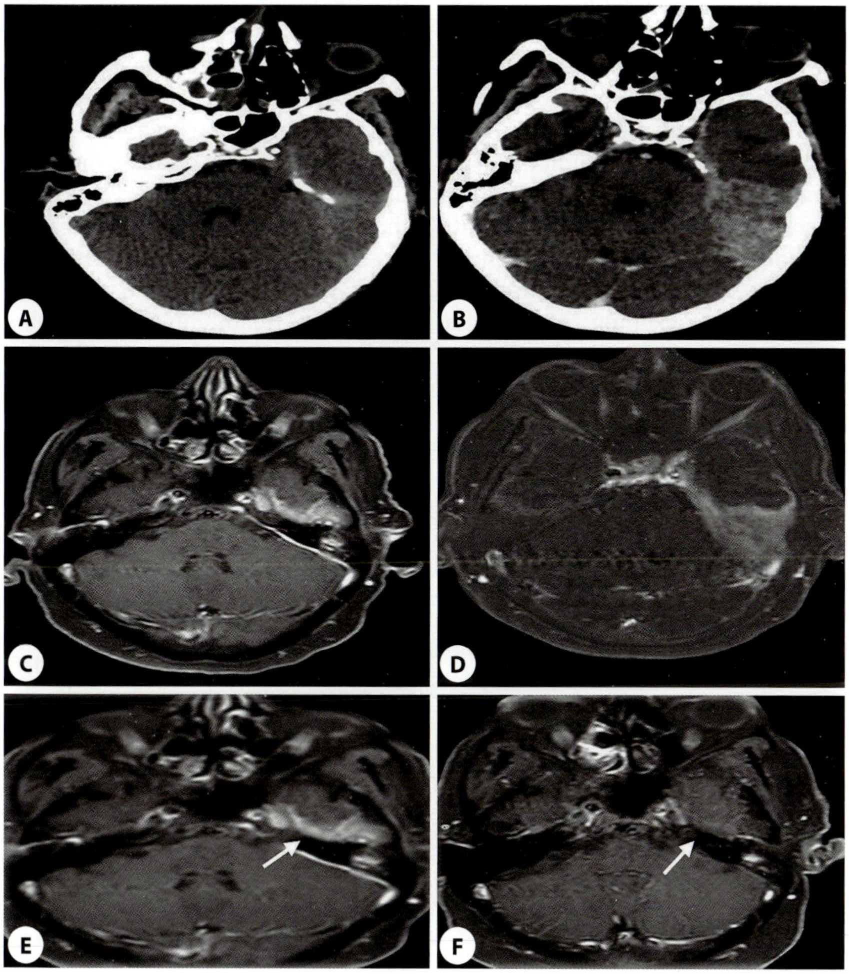

CLINICAL BACKGROUND

A 54-year-old male patient came with the complaints of left sided headache for 4 months on and off which aggravated for past 1 month. He also had the complaints of decreased appetite, nausea for 2 days. No evidence of trauma, fever or seizures. CSF study showed mildly elevated lymphocytes and sugar levels. Total blood count showed mildly elevated white blood cells. The patient was advocated for imaging investigations. Patient was started on ATT and steroids with the clinical suspicion of TB and followed by after 6 months.

IMAGING FINDINGS

CT brain plain/postcontrast and MRI brain T1W postcontrast/subtracted images shows focal abnormal pachymeningeal thickening and enhancement in the left temporal region. Follow up MRI showed near complete disappearance of the meningeal thickening (white arrows) **(Figs. 1A to F)**.

DISCUSSION

Hypertrophic pachymeningitis is a rare form of chronic fibrosing inflammatory disease affecting the cranial or spinal dura matter. It may be either focal or diffuse. It may be idiopathic when primary etiology is unknown or could be secondary to many conditions like infections (TB, syphilis), mastoiditis, and inflammatory conditions like rheumatoid arthritis, sarcoidosis, Wegener's granulomatosis, post radiation, autoimmune disorders.[1]

The most common mechanism of dissemination is lymphatic spread, as there are abundant lymphatic vessels in the dura.[5] Unlike diffuse leptomeningeal thickening or basal exudates which are commonly seen in CNS TB, this condition is characterized by focal thickening of pachymeninges which shows postcontrast enhancement.[1]

MRI brain is the modality of choice for the diagnosis of pachymeningitis. The radiological features of pachymeningitis include dural thickening, dural mass, sinus thrombosis, or venous congestion with white matter changes.[2] Among them dural enhancement is one of the characteristic features of pachymeningitis. Most times, even when radiological features are characteristic of pachymeningitis, the underlying cause may be difficult to be diagnosed. A stepwise workup including CSF analysis and vasculitis panel can be helpful to recognize the precise etiology. Ultimately meningeal biopsy may be essential in few instances when the other diagnostic tests are inconclusive.[3]

The common differential diagnosis includes meningioma en plaque which is characterized by bony changes. Isolated pachymeningitis in tuberculosis is extremely rare and diagnosis of this condition is important to avoid unnecessary surgical interventions. It is important to note that some idiopathic cases of pachymeningitis respond well to antituberculosis therapy, suggesting that a proportion of case is due to undiagnosed tuberculosis.[4,5]

Hence, treatment with antituberculosis medications and steroids should be considered in cases of idiopathic pachymeningitis.[4]

REFERENCES

1. Karthik SN, Bhanu K, Velayutham S, et al. Hypertrophic pachymeningitis. Ann Indian Acad Neurol. 2011;14(3):203-4.
2. Tariq R, Ahmed R. Tuberculous hypertrophic pachymeningitis presenting as visual blurring and headaches. J Pak Med Assoc. 2012;62:966-8.
3. Cordeiro NL, Gupta SS, Kanwar A, et al. Tuberculous Hypertrophic Pachymeningitis. Cureus. 2021 30;13(8).
4. Parney IF, Johnson ES, Allen PB. "Idiopathic" cranial hypertrophic pachymeningitis responsive to antituberculous therapy: case report. Neurosurgery. 1997;41:965-971.
5. Fonseka CL, Kanakkahewa TE, Singhapura SD, et al. Tuberculous pachymeningitis presenting as a diffused dural thickening in a patient with chronic headache and recurrent neurological abnormalities for more than a decade: a case report and a review of the literature. Case Rep Infect Dis. :2018:3012034.

6 Pyogenic Ventriculitis

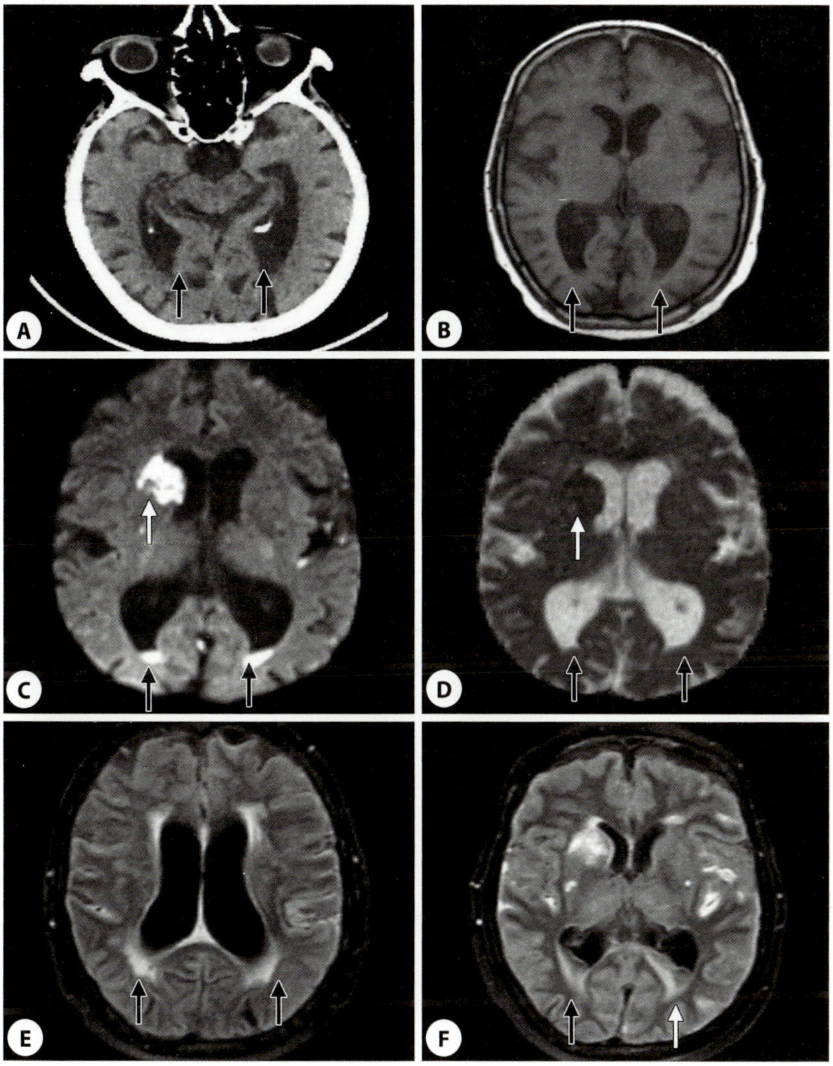

CLINICAL BACKGROUND

A 70-year-old female patient with sudden unconsciousness—history of fever for 3 days.

IMAGING FINDINGS

Intraventricular debris at dependent location in both lateral ventricles in CT. FLAIR hyperintense signals in both lateral ventricles at corresponding location which appear hypointense on T2 and hyperintense on T1 (compared to CSF signals). Also noted is obstructive hydrocephalus with periventricular seepage. Diffusion restriction noted in right anterior capsuloganglionic region **(Figs. 1A to F)**.

DISCUSSION

Pyogenic ventriculitis (PV), also known as ependymitis, ventricular empyema, pyocephalus, and ventriculitis. It is an uncommon complication of intracranial infection.[1] In adults with primary PV, clinical signs of meningeal irritation are seen in only 76% cases.[2] Only nine cases of PV are reported till date in adults.[3]

CT and MRI are the important imaging modalities used in the diagnosis. MRI is more sensitive. The features that are specific for ventriculitis include intraventricular debris, hydrocephalus, periventricular hyperintense signals, and ependymal enhancement.[1-3]

Among the above MRI findings, irregular ventricular debris is seen commonly in about 94% and ependymal enhancement manifest less frequently in 60%.[1,2] Absent of blooming in gradient image can exclude blood products.[1,4]

The hyper intense signals/fluid-fluid level within ventricles (especially at dependent locations) on diffusion-weighted images (DWIs) is seen along with diffusion restriction in ADC. The presence of diffusion restriction is suggestive of pus.[4,5]

The hypointense signals on T2-weighted images in ventricles, periventricular FLAIR hyperintensities and ependymal contrast enhancement are other MRI features, highly sensitive for diagnosis of pyogenic ventriculitis.[4,5]

This condition is clinically indolent yet fatal (1). Clinical worsening in a diagnosed case of pyogenic meningitis, could be due to ventriculitis (2). Recognition of MRI features and early initiation of treatment may lead to a favorable outcome.[4,5]

REFERENCES

1. Fukui MB, Williams RL, Mudigonda S. CT and MR imaging features of pyogenic ventriculitis. AJNR Am J Neuroradiol. 2001;22(8).
2. Jayendrakumar CI, Ganesan DB, Thampi SJ, et al. Primary pyogenic ventriculitis caused by Streptococcal pneumoniae in adults. J Family Med Prim Care. 2019;8(11):3745-7.
3. Maheshwarappa HM, Rai AV. A Rare Case of Primary Pyogenic Ventriculitis in a Patient with Community-acquired Meningitis. Indian J Crit Care Med. 2022;26(7):874-6.
4. Hatakeyama M, Kanazawa M, Ishihara A, et al. [Pathognomonic magnetic resonance imaging (MRI) finding of fluid-fluid level in pyogenic ventriculitis: two case reports]. Rinsho Shinkeigaku. 2014;54(9):732-7.
5. Pezzullo JA, Tung GA, Mudigonda S, et al. Diffusion-weighted MR imaging of pyogenic ventriculitis. AJR Am J Roentgenol. 2003;180:71-5.

7 Sinus Tarsi Syndrome

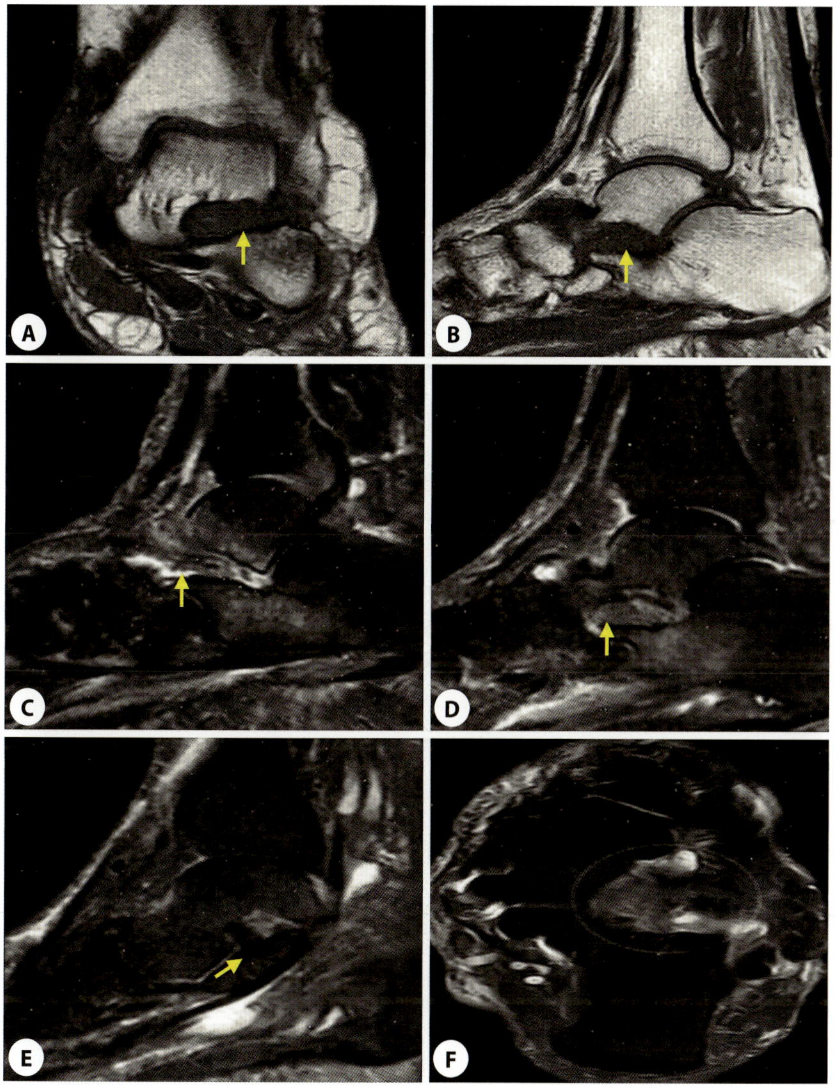

CLINICAL BACKGROUND

History of trauma to ankle followed by pain in lateral aspect of foot 3 months. No history of fever.

IMAGING FINDINGS

Loss of normal T1 hyperintense fat signals in sinus tarsi with STIR/T2 (fat-sat) hyperintense signals. Intact interosseous talocalcaneal ligament with edematous cervical ligament and inferior extensor retinaculum (yellow arrows) **(Figs. 1A to F)**.

DISCUSSION

Anatomically at the junction of mid-foot and hind-foot, is a funnel-shaped space known as sinus tarsi. It contains fat, vessels, nerves and ligaments. Sinus tarsi syndrome is a clinical entity recognized by lateral hind-foot pain which gets worsened on palpation or weight-bearing. It could be the result of either traumatic or nontraumatic etiologies and magnetic resonance imaging (MRI) is the imaging modality of choice.[1]

The medial hindfoot variant is a more severe form characterized by pain in medial aspect of hindfoot along with the typical lateral symptoms, known as canalis tarsi syndrome.[2] The cervical ligament (Fick ligament), interosseous talocalcaneal ligament and the roots of the inferior extensor retinaculum contribute to the stability of sinus tarsi.[3]

While the most common cause for this syndrome trauma (70%), this condition is also noted to be associated with inflammatory or crystal deposition arthritis, foot deformity and chronic hindfoot instability.[4] Concomitant lateral ankle ligament abnormalities are seen in about 80% cases while few of them were also associated with tears in posterior tibial tendon.[5]

In this syndrome, T1-hyperintense fat in the sinus tarsi space is replaced by either fluid or scar tissue. Acute ligament injury is associated with high signals in the ligament with fibers discontinuity, whereas, in sprain the fibers are intact. Acute injuries are also associated with marrow edema in adjacent bones of talus and calcaneum.[1,2]

At chronic stages, the ligaments may appear thickened/hyperintense on T2 or at times hypointense in all sequences, as the result of fibrosis. Early detection of this syndrome by imaging facilitates appropriate patient management.[1,2,4]

REFERENCES

1. Khan I, Peters J, Welck M, et al. Sinus tarsi and sinus tarsi syndrome: An imaging review. Eur J Radiol. 2023;161:110725.
2. Zwipp H, Bemmerl JG, Holch M, et al. Sinus tarsi and canalis tarsi syndromes. A post-traumatic entity, Foot and Ankle Surgery. 1996;2:181-8.
3. Mittlmeier T, Rammelt S. Update on Subtalar Joint Instability. Foot Ankle Clin. 2018;23(3):397-413.
4. Taillard W, Meyer J, Garcia J. et al. The sinus tarsi syndrome. International Orthopaedics. 1981;5:117-30.
5. Lektrakul N, Chung CB, Lai YM, et al. Tarsal sinus: arthrographic, MR imaging, MR arthrographic, and pathologic findings in cadavers and retrospective study data in patients with sinus tarsi syndrome. Radiology. 2001;219(3):802-10.

8

PIPA with Lung Hypoplasia

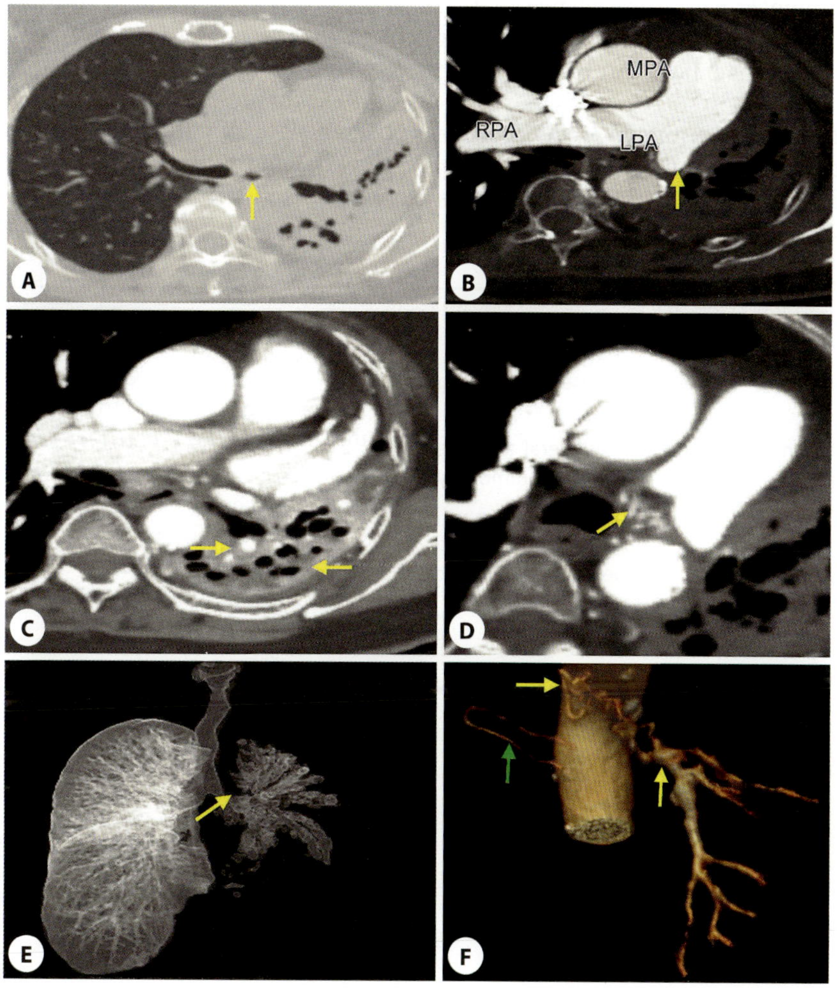

CLINICAL BACKGROUND

A 60-year-old female patient c/o hemoptysis.

IMAGING FINDINGS

Hypoplastic left main bronchus and left lung with bronchiectasis. Absent left pulmonary artery, except for 1 cm from its origin. Bronchial artery hypertrophy on left side supplying the lung (yellow arrows) compared to normal appearance of right bronchial artery **(Figs. 1A to F)**.

DISCUSSION

Unilateral pulmonary hypoplasia has a prevalence of 1-2 per 12,000 births and commonly seen on left side (70%). Primary lung hypoplasia remains silent, due to compensatory hypertrophy of contralateral lung and also due to the absence of associated embryological abnormalities.[1]

Proximal interruption of pulmonary artery (PIPA) is a rare congenital anomaly with a prevalence of 1 in 200,000.[2] It can be an isolated abnormality or can occur in association with many congenital heart diseases, lung hypoplasia etc.[2]

Interruption is the preferred terminology over absence as in this condition, the intrapulmonary vascular network is intact.[3] A well-developed pulmonary arterial tree is present in the lung, with a proximal blind ending at hilum via collaterals.[4]

CECT of thorax is the imaging modality of choice to diagnose above condition. Lung hypoplasia is characterized by the small hemi thorax, ipsilateral mediastinal shift and herniation of hypertrophied contralateral lung.[5] Pulmonary vessel termination may occur at or within 1 cm, of the origin in PIPA with distal collaterals from systemic vessels like bronchial, internal mammary, innominate and subclavian vessels.[5]

PIPA can present with life-threatening hemoptysis and imaging plays an important role to delineate the vascular anatomy before intervention. Associated congenital cardiac anomalies must be excluded.

REFERENCES

1. Kant S. Unilateral pulmonary hypoplasia—a case report. Lung India. 2007;24(2):69-71.
2. Pool PE, Vogel JH, Blount SG. Congenital unilateral absence of the pulmonary artery: Importance of flow in pulmonary hypertension. Am J Card. 1962;10:706-32.
3. Castaner E, Gallardo X, Rimola J, et al. Congenital and Acquired Pulmonary Artery Anomalies in the Adult: Radiologic Overview. Radiographics. 2006;26:349-71.
4. Ten Harkel AD, Blom NA, Ottenkamp J. Isolated Unilateral Absence of a Pulmonary Artery: A Case Report and Review of the Literature. Chest. 2002;122:1471-77.
5. Anand SH, Jasper A, Mani SE, et al. Proximal Interruption of the Pulmonary Artery: A Case Series. J Clin Diagn Res. 2015;9(12):TD04–TD06.

9 Chiari II Malformation

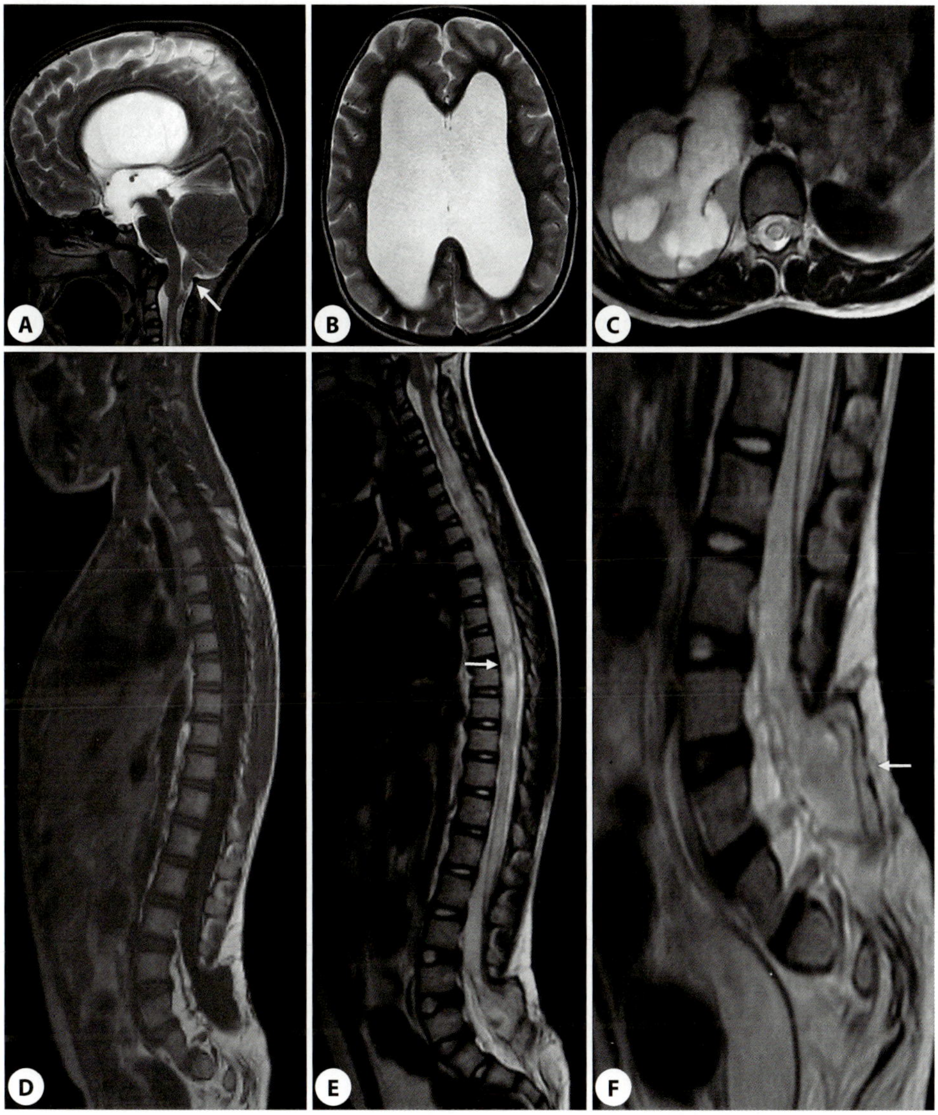

CLINICAL BACKGROUND

A 10-year-old female—known patient for spinal dysraphism

IMAGING FINDINGS

Small posterior fossa with brainstem and cerebellum herniation through foramen of magnum. Associated dilatation of both lateral and third ventricles(hydrocephalus). Long segment syringohydromyelia (T1 hypo and T2 hyper intense signals in spinal cord) and lumbosacral myelomeningocele with posterior element osseous defect. Incidental detection of left renal agenesis and right moderate HUN **(Figs. 1A–F)**.

DISCUSSION

Chiari II malformation is a complex developmental CNS malformation, which is characterized by a small posterior fossa and caudal displacement of the cerebellum and brainstem (hindbrain herniation) through foramen magnum. It is associated with open spinal dysraphism. Approximately 1/3rd. of these patients develop signs and symptoms of brainstem compression with reported mortality 15–35%.[1]

This condition is believed to be due to no closure of the caudal end of the neuropore.[2] It is associated with cerebellar hypoplasia and caudal herniation of the cerebellar tonsils, which wrap around the medulla, i.e., the so-called banana sign, along with towering of the cerebellum. Other cerebellar abnormalities include heterotopic and dysplastic gray matter.[3]

The midbrain is elongated, with the fusion of the colliculi and tectal beaking. There is also elongation and stenosis of the cerebral aqueduct with hypoplasia or aplasia of cranial nerves. In 75–90%, the massa intermedia is enlarged and anteriorly displaced along with elongation of the habenular commissure and pineal gland.[3-5]

Associated hydrocephalus and disproportionate enlargement of the atria and occipital horns of ventricles (colpocephaly) is seen in ~90%. In about 1/3rd. cases, ventricular margins may show a nodular appearance, due to subependymal nodular heterotopia.[3-5] The corpus callosum may show partial or complete agenesis with the absence of the septum pellucidum. The cerebral cortex may show multiple small gyri (stenogyria) with a partial or complete absence of the olfactory bulbs and tracts.[3-5]

In 25–45% of patients, fusiform dilation of the central ependymal canal noted (<2–3 mm prominent central canal and >3 mm syringomyelia). Open spinal dysraphism, i.e., lumbar meningocele and/or myelomeningocele, is associated with CM-2 in >90% cases along with posterior elements defect in lumbosacral vertebrae.[6]

The aim of preoperative imaging is to identify the size and extent of cord involvement. It is also essential to identify the presyrinx state, i.e., an abnormal spinal cord signal intensity adjacent to the syrinx, and the presence of flow voids within the syrinx on T2-weighted MRI because these features are potential predictors of a good response after correction of the CSF obstruction.[6]

REFERENCES

1. Geerdink N, van der Vliet T, Rotteveel JJ, et al. Essential features of Chiari II malformation in MR imaging: an interobserver reliability study--part 1. Childs Nerv Syst. 2012;28(7):977-85.
2. McLone DG, Nakahara S, Knepper PA. Chiari II malformation: pathogenesis and dynamics. Concepts Pediatr Neurosurg. 1991: 1-17.
3. Tubb RS, Pugh JA, Oakes WJ. Chiari Malformations. In: Youmans Neurological Surgery, Winn HR (ed). Elsevier Saunders: Philadelphia. 2011:1918-27.
4. Van den Hof MC, Nicolaides KH, Campbell J, et al. Evaluation of the lemon and banana signs in one hundred thirty fetuses with open spina bifida. Am J Obstet Gynecol. 1990;162:322-27.
5. Soto-Ares G, Delmaire C, Deries B, et al. Cerebellar cortical dysplasia: MR findings in a complex entity. AJNR Am J Neuroradiol. 2000;21:1511-19.
6. Hiremath SB, Fitsiori A, J Boto J, The perplexity surrounding chiari malformations—are we any wiser now? AJNR Am J Neuroradiol. 2020;41(11):1975-81.

10 Colloid Cyst with Obstructive Hydrocephalus

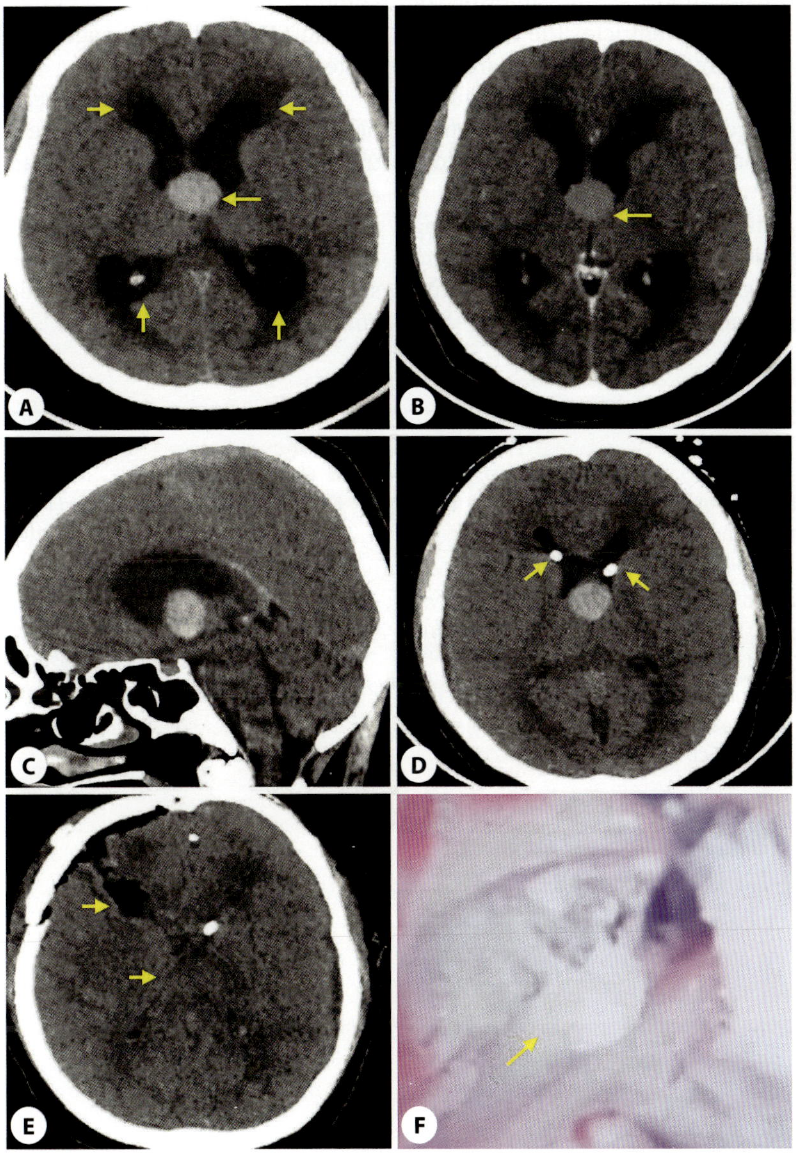

CLINICAL BACKGROUND

A 28-year-old female with acute onset of severe headache and vomiting.

IMAGING FINDINGS

Well defined hyperdense lesion in roof of third ventricle. Moderate dilatation of both lateral ventricles with periventricular seepage. No demonstrable enhancement within the lesion. No evidence of DVT. Emergency ventricular drain was placed followed by excision of the tumor **(Figs. 1A to F)**.

DISCUSSION

Colloid cysts are rare congenital and benign intracranial tumors (2% of all intracranial tumors). Although solitary and sporadic, rare familial forms are described in literature.[1,2] Symptoms vary from incidental detection, related to hydrocephalus such as headache, nausea and vomiting, psychiatric symptoms and even sudden death.[3]

The most common location is the anterior or anterosuperior part of the third ventricle. The incidence of colloid cyst detection is increasing due to extensive use of computed tomography (CT) and magnetic resonance imaging (MRI).[3] Earlier age of detection and a female predominance are common with familial form of colloid cyst.[2]

These cysts have a diverse appearance on imaging due to variable composition (quantity of cholesterol and protein). Cysts with a high content of cholesterol and protein are hyperdense on plain CT, hyperintense on T1- and hypointense on T2 weighted MRI sequences. A higher cholesterol content results in T1 hyperintense cysts. They generally do not show diffusion restriction or post contrast enhancement.[4]

Sometimes, it is difficult to recognize colloid cysts with fluid-attenuated inversion recovery (FLAIR) sequence, which are hypointense on T2W evaluations. Similarly, it could be hard to diagnose cysts that are isointense with CSF on T1W and T2W images, and, sometimes, CT could better show them.[5]

The radiologic appearances of colloid cysts could be helpful in directing these patients to alternative treatment modalities. Cysts that are hypodense on CT and hyperintense on T2W could be treated by aspiration whereas T2 hypointense cysts (highly viscous) may be difficult to be aspirated.[5] To note, minimally invasive surgeries (aspiration) are associated with recurrence compared to surgical excision.[4,5]

REFERENCES

1. Turillazzi E, Bello S, Neri M, et al. Colloid cyst of the third ventricle, hypothalamus, and heart: a dangerous link for sudden death. Diagn Pathol. 2012;7:144.
2. Salaud C, Hamel O, Buffenoir-Billet K, et al. Familial colloid cyst of the third ventricle: Case report and review of the literature. Neurochirurgie. 2013;59(2):81-4.
3. Ravnik J, Bunc G, Grcar A, Zunic M, Velnar T. Colloid cysts of the third ventricle exhibit various clinical presentation: a review of three cases. Bosn J Basic Med Sci. 2014;14(3):132-5.
4. El Khoury C, Brugières P, Decq P, et al. Colloid cysts of the third ventricle: are MR imaging patterns predictive of difficulty with percutaneous treatment? AJNR Am J Neuroradiol. 2000;21(3):489-92.
5. Algin O, Ozmen E, Arslan H. Radiologic manifestations of colloid cysts: a pictorial essay Can. Assoc Radio J. 2013;64(1):56-60.

11 WOPN with Portal Vein Thrombosis

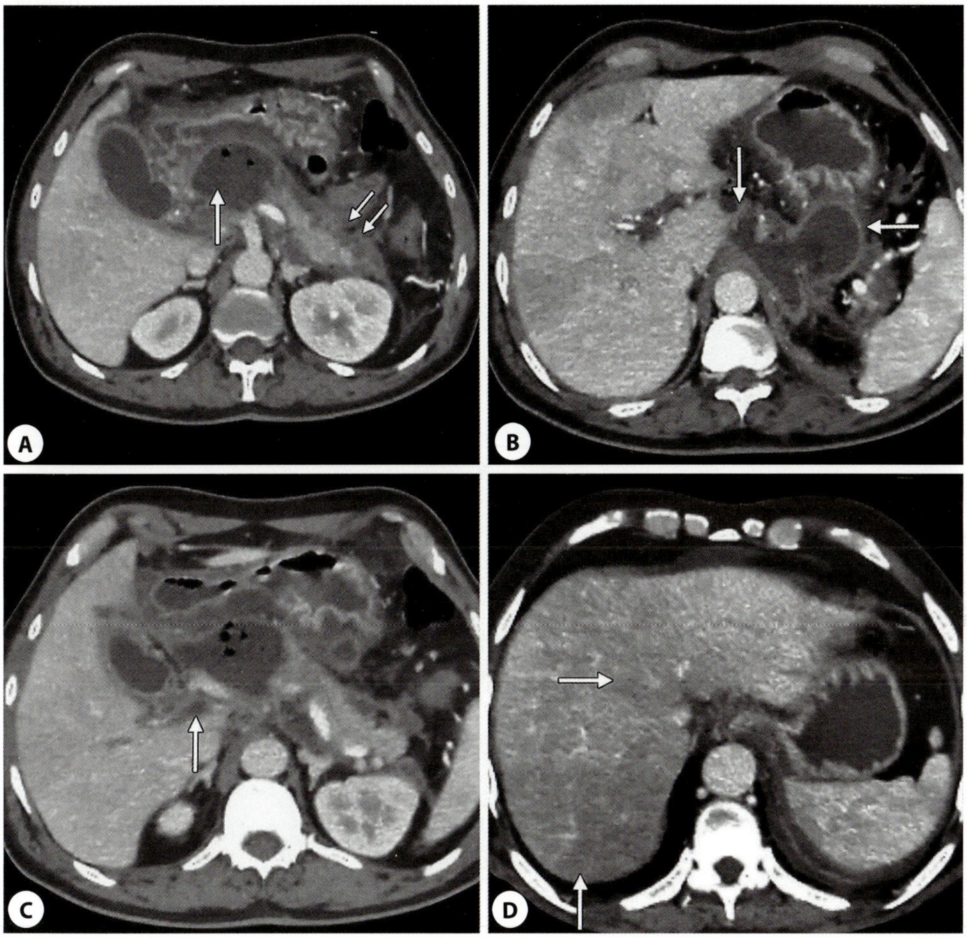

CLINICAL BACKGROUND

A 48-year-old male patient—chronic alcoholic—known patient of necrotizing pancreatitis for 6 weeks, now presented with severe epigastric pain.

IMAGING FINDINGS

Heterogeneously enhancing pancreatic parenchyma with well-defined multiloculated fluid collection with air pockets in neck of pancreas extending into peripancreatic region and lesser sac. Peripancreatic inflammatory fat strandings noted. Main pancreatic duct is not dilated. Filling defects noted in main portal vein with altered liver parenchymal **(Figs. 1A to D)**.

DISCUSSION

Acute pancreatitis is classified into interstitial edematous pancreatitis and necrotizing pancreatitis (NP). The later is a severe form of acute pancreatitis which is defined as the necrosis of the pancreatic parenchyma and peripancreatic fat, associated high morbidity and mortality.[1] The most common complications are thrombosis of portal venous system, hemorrhage related to the arterial erosions and pseudoaneurysm.[2]

The morphological change that occurs later in the course of acute necrotizing pancreatitis (>4 weeks) results in circumscribed area of fluid collection which contain necrotic pancreatic debris replacing pancreatic parenchyma. This is known as "walled-off pancreatic necrosis" (WOPN). It differs from pseudocyst by the fact that the former replaces part of the necrotic pancreatic parenchyma and presents with thick contents (pancreatic necrotic debris), while the later do not contain necrotic debris and most commonly develop in the peripancreatic spaces.[3]

The solid components in WOPN are better identified on USG and T2-weighted MR images than CT. In general, findings that are in favour of WOPN include larger size, extension to the paracolic or retro colic space, an irregular wall definition, the presence of solid or fat attenuation debris, presence of pancreatic parenchymal deformity and discontinuity, and absence of dilatation of the main pancreatic duct.[2,4]

The differentiation is clinically and therapeutically important, as the pseudocyst can be more easily drained by endoscopic means than WOPN. Also the former has a better prognosis. With respect to the peripancreatic fat necrosis, CT cannot reliably diagnose retroperitoneal fat necrosis, and hence it has been suggested that in necrotising pancreatitis, all heterogeneous peripancreatic collections should be considered as areas of fat tissue necrosis unless proven otherwise.[4,5]

REFERENCES

1. Zaheer A, Singh VK, Qureshi RO, Fishman EK. The revised Atlanta classification for acute pancreatitis updates in imaging terminology and guidelines. Abdom Imaging. 2013;38(1): 125-36.
2. Türkvatan A. Erden A. Türkoğlu M.A. et al. maging of acute pancreatitis and its complications. Part 2: complications of acute pancreatitis. Diagn Interv Imaging. 2015;96:161-169
3. Cunha EF, Rocha Mde S, Pereira FP, et al. Walled-off pancreatic necrosis and other current concepts in the radiological assessment of acute pancreatitis. Radiol Bras. 2014;47(3):165-75.
4. Bharwani N, Patel S, Prabhudesai S, et al. Acute pancreatitis: the role of imaging in diagnosis and management. Clin Radiol. 2011;66:164-75.
5. Boškoski I, Costamagna G. Walled-off pancreatic necrosis: where are we? Ann Gastroenterol. 2014;27(2):93-94.

12 Medulloblastoma

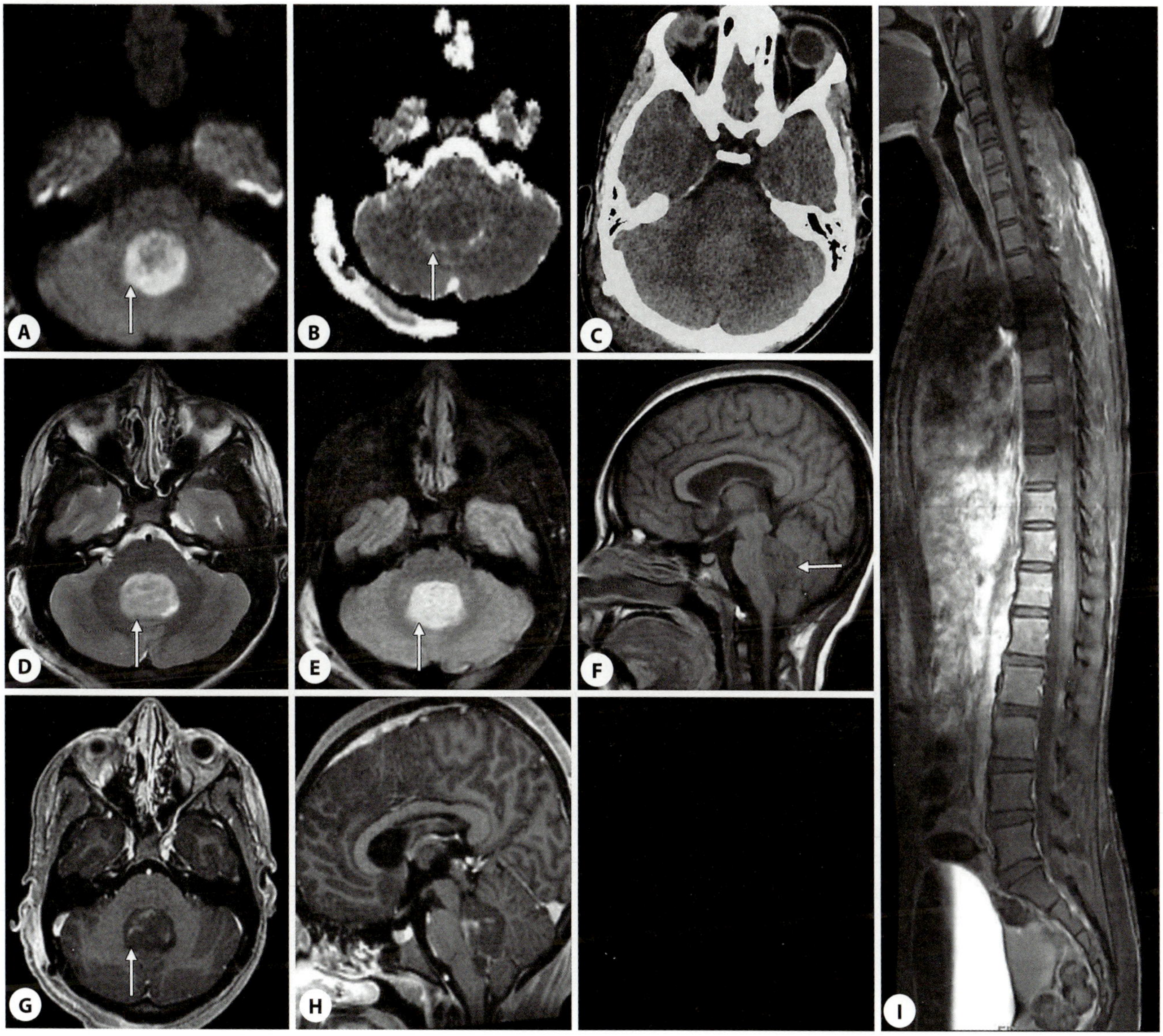

CLINICAL BACKGROUND

A 15-year-old girl presented with complaints of headache.

IMAGING FINDINGS

Well defined hyperdense lesion in posterior fossa on CT causing obstructive hydrocephalus. The lesion is T1 hypo and T2/FLAIR hyperintense with mild diffusion restriction. The lesion shows mild postcontrast enhancement. Effacement of fourth ventricle noted with ventricular drain in situ in right lateral ventricle **(Figs. 1A to I)**.

DISCUSSION

Medulloblastoma is the most common malignant paediatric brain tumor (15–20%) of the central nervous system (CNS) malignancies and 40% of them are located in the posterior fossa.[1] Four distinct molecular subgroups are identified: Wingless (WNT), Sonic Hedgehog (SHH), group 3 and 4 based on genomic profiles and each of them are associated with specific genetic abnormalities, typical age of onset as well as survival prognosis.[2]

Magnetic resonance imaging (MRI) has a key role in the diagnosis, surgical guidance and follow up of patients with medulloblastoma. Recent studies seem to indicate MRI as a promising tool for early detection of medulloblastoma subgroups.[3] The tumor classically appears hyper- or isodense on CT. However, in MRI the signal intensity may be hypo- or isointense on T1- and T2-weighted imaging depending on the tumor cellularity. High tumor cellularity is classical and results in restricted diffusion.[3,4]

They are most commonly situated in the inferior vermis, and often compress the IV ventricle, resulting in obstructive hydrocephalus, but hemispheric location is also possible. About 50% of them has intratumoral cyst/necrosis and calcification is seen in 10–20%. Leptomeningeal dissemination across the cerebrospinal fluid (CSF) pathway can occur commonly at the sylvian fissures, suprasellar subarachnoid space and in posterior fossa cistern. Thoracic and lumbosacral metastases are also relatively common.[4]

Blüml et al. highlighted the role of MRS in genomic categorisation and found that, group 3 and 4 had readily detectable taurine and creatine levels; SHH medulloblastomas also showed prominent choline and lipids peaks, notably low creatinine levels while, WNT medulloblastoma spectroscopic analysis was unreliable.[4]

MR can predict the subgroup and decide treatment option as for example, dynamic susceptibility weighted perfusion MRI and SWI are clinically relevant biomarkers for tumor vascularity and overall survival and could be used to direct the use of antivascular therapies for patients with group 3 medulloblastoma, which express VEGF. The accuracy and feasibility of some MRI features for predicting molecular subgroups suggests that it may be a useful additional and noninvasive tool for subgroup determination and treatment stratification in future.[4]

TABLE 1: Molecular subtypes of medulloblastoma.[4]

WNT	Cerebellar peduncle/CP angle cistern localization (75%). Laterality and the dominantly extra-parenchymal location. Brainstem contact (cuneate nucleus)/intraventricular expansion and an infiltration of fourth ventricle + (90%)
SHH	Cerebellar hemispheres (54%) Contact with the brain-stem or intraventricular expansion (48%)
Group 3	73% vermian localization VEGF expression/brainstem contact (cuneate nucleus)/intraventricular expansion and an infiltration of the fourth ventricle + (100%)
Group 4	70% vermian localization brainstem contact (cochlear nucleus)/intraventricular expansion and an infiltration of fourth ventricle + (100%). Non enhancing tumors in the midline/fourth ventricle site—typical to differentiate from group 3

REFERENCES

1. Ostrom QT, Gittleman H, Fulop J, et al. CBTRUS statistical report: primary brain and central nervous system tumors diagnosed in the United States in 2008–2012. Neuro Oncol. 2015;17:1-62.
2. Taylor MD, Northcott PA, Korshunov A, et al. Molecular subgroups of medulloblastoma: the current consensus. Acta Neuropathol. 2012;123:465-72.
3. Yeom KW, Mobley BC, Lober RM, et al. Distinctive MRI features of pediatric medulloblastoma subtypes. Am J Roentgenol. 2013;200:895-903.
4. Colafati GS, Voicu IP, Carducci C, et al. MRI features as a helpful tool to predict the molecular subgroups of medulloblastoma: state of the art. Ther Adv Neurol Disord. 2018;11:1756286418775375.

13 Spinal Cord Astrocytoma

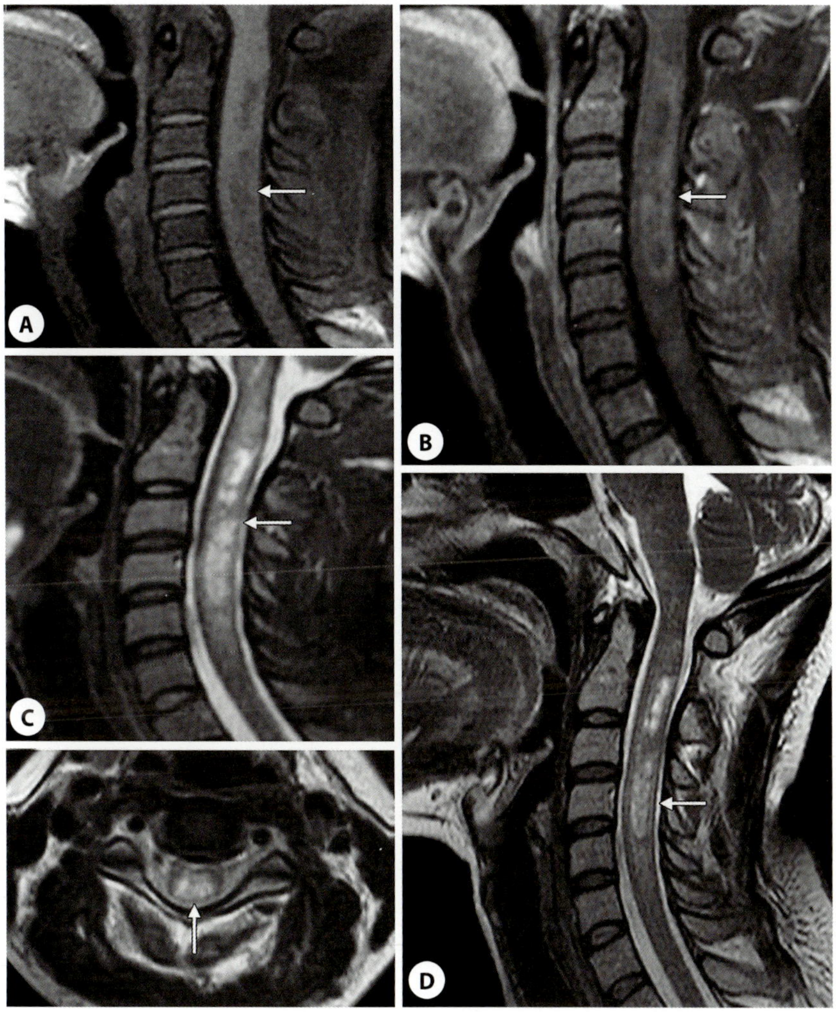

CLINICAL BACKGROUND

A-30-year old female patient presented with complaints of weakness in left upper limb. No history of fever or trauma.

IMAGING FINDINGS

Long segment T1 hypo-, T2/STIR hyperintense lesion noted extending from C2 to C5 vertebral levels with holocord involvement causing expansion of spinal cord. The lesion shows irregular postcontrast patchy pattern of enhancement. No evidence of hemorrhage or perilesional edema or cysts **(Figs. 1A to D)**.

DISCUSSION

Astrocytomas are the tumors arising from astrocytic glial cells. The two most common histologic subtypes are pilocytic astrocytomas (WHO grade I) and fibrillary astrocytomas (WHO grade II). Glioblastoma (WHO grade IV), unlike in brain, rarely occurs in the spinal cord (0.2–1.5%). Pilocytic astrocytomas, unlike fibrillary astrocytomas tend to displace rather than infiltrating the cord.[1]

Astrocytomas usually have a vertical extent less than four vertebral body segments in length. Holocord involvement may occur, especially with pilocytic astrocytomas. The tumor usually involves a portion of the cord with non neoplastic peritumoral cysts. The lesion appears T1 hypo- and T2 hyperintense with irregular post contrast-enhancement, although few lesions (30%) may show lack of enhancement. Of note, the enhancement is less intense and less sharply demarcated than its most common differential diagnosis, the ependymomas.[2]

Astrocytomas may be associated with intratumoral (not seen in ependymoma) and polar cyst (may be seen in ependymoma). they are typically eccentric while ependymomas are central in location. Hemorrhage is an uncommon feature, unlike ependymoma. CSF dissemination may occur and imaging of the entire neuroaxis is indicated. Rim of peripheral T2 low signal, around the lesion is known as the "cap sign" is highly specific for ependymoma.[1,2] Diffusor tensor imaging (DTI) can be used to differentiate ependymoma from astrocytoma, as the former displaces white-matter tracts but the later infiltrate.[3]

REFERENCES

1. Smith B, Soderlund KA, Rushing EJ, et al. Radiologic-pathologic correlation of pediatric and adolescent spinal neoplasms: part 1, intramedullary spinal neoplasms. Am J Roentgenol. 2012;198(1):34-43.
2. Seo HS, Kim JH, Lee DH, et al. Nonenhancing intramedullary astrocytomas and other MR imaging features: a retrospective study and systematic review. AJNR. 2010;31:498-503.
3. Hurnher MM, Law M. Diffusion-weighted imaging, diffusion-tensor imaging, and fiber tractography of the spinal cord. Magn Reson Imaging Clin N Am. 2009;17(2):225–44.

14 Coronary Artery—Pulmonary Artery Fistula

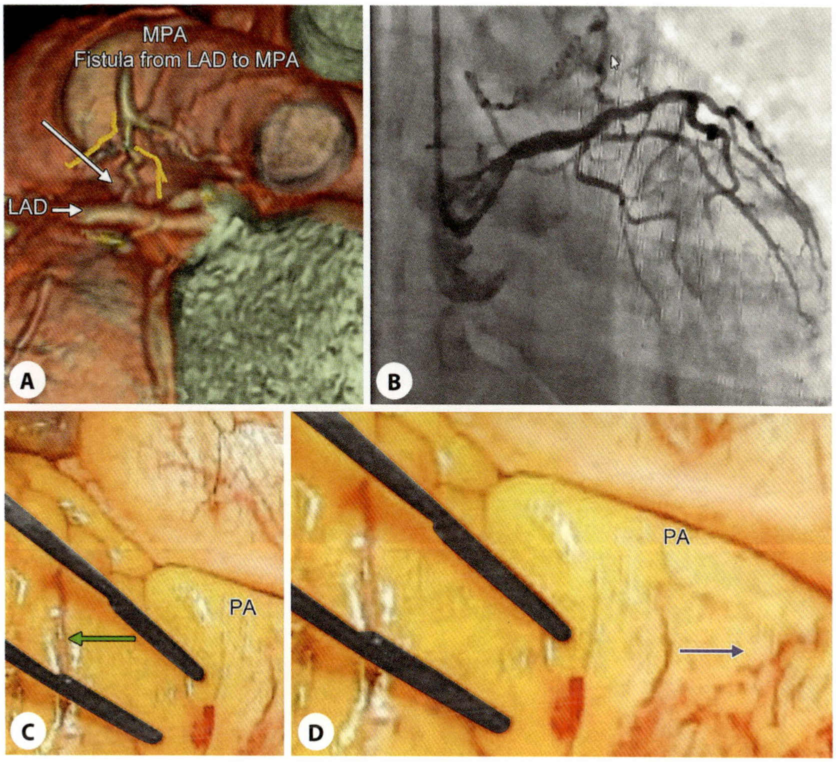

CLINICAL BACKGROUND

A 50-year-old male patient with chest pain under went catheter angiogram of coronary arteries with incidental detection of suspicious coronary artery fistula.

IMAGING FINDINGS

Catheter angiograms showing tortoise vascular communication from LAD to the region of pulmonary artery and CT coronary angiogram confirming the same. Intraoperative images confirming the fistula (green arrow) and also few insignificant capillary networks over the pulmonary artery (blue arrow) **(Figs. 1A to D)**.

DISCUSSION

Coronary artery fistula (CAF) is a rare abnormality that is characterized by an abnormal communication between coronary artery and the heart chamber or the great vessels. It is a rare anomaly with a prevalence rate of 0.002%. The coronary-to-pulmonary artery fistula (CPAF) is the most common type of CAF. When diagnosed incidentally these lesions are generally benign with small shunts that are hemodynamically insignificant.[1,2]

CAFs can originate from any coronary artery, but right coronary artery (RCA) is most commonly involved (50–55%). They are often congenital but can be acquired as a result of trauma, inflammation etc. Most fistulas drain into the venous system-right ventricle (41%) >right atrium

(26%) > pulmonary artery (17%). It is essential to identify cardiac chamber enlargement/features of pulmonary hypertension.[3]

Associated congenital heart anomalies are seen in 20–45% of patients, which include TOF, ASD, VSD, PDA and pulmonary atresia with intact ventricular septum.[3] Invasive coronary angiography however, is still the preferred imaging for diagnosis. However, sometimes it might be difficult to demonstrate the complex and small fistulas due to the limitation of 2D imaging. MR and CT are useful noninvasive imaging techniques in detecting cardiac and coronary artery anomalies, while the later can precisely depict complex fistulas at ease.[4]

LAD-MPA fistula is the most common CPAF. Lee et al.,[5] divided all CPAFs into four categories: Types 1 and 2—single origin without or with aneurysm. Types 3 and 4—multiple origins without or with aneurysm.[4] While surgical closure of fistula is recommended only in symptomatic patients, familiarity with the image features of this rare anomaly (CAF) would help most in diagnosis and treatment.[4]

REFERENCES

1. Lim JJ, Jung JI, Lee BY, et al. Prevalence and types of coronary artery fistulas detected with coronary CT angiography. AJR Am J Roentgenol. 2014;203:W237–W243.
2. Burch GH, Sahn DJ. Congenital coronary artery anomalies: the pediatric perspective. Coron Artery Dis. 2001;12:605-16.
3. Saboo SS, Juan YH, Khandelwal A, et al. MDCT of congenital coronary artery fistulas. AJR 2014;203:[web]W244-W252.
4. Li N, Zhao P, Wu D, et al. Coronary artery fistulas detected with coronary CT angiography: a pictorial review of 73 cases. Br J Radiol. 2020;93(1108).
5. Lee CM, Song SY, Jeon SC, et al. Characteristics of coronary artery to pulmonary artery fistula on coronary computed tomography angiography. J Comput Assist Tomogr. 2016;40: 398-401.

15 Sella Metastasis

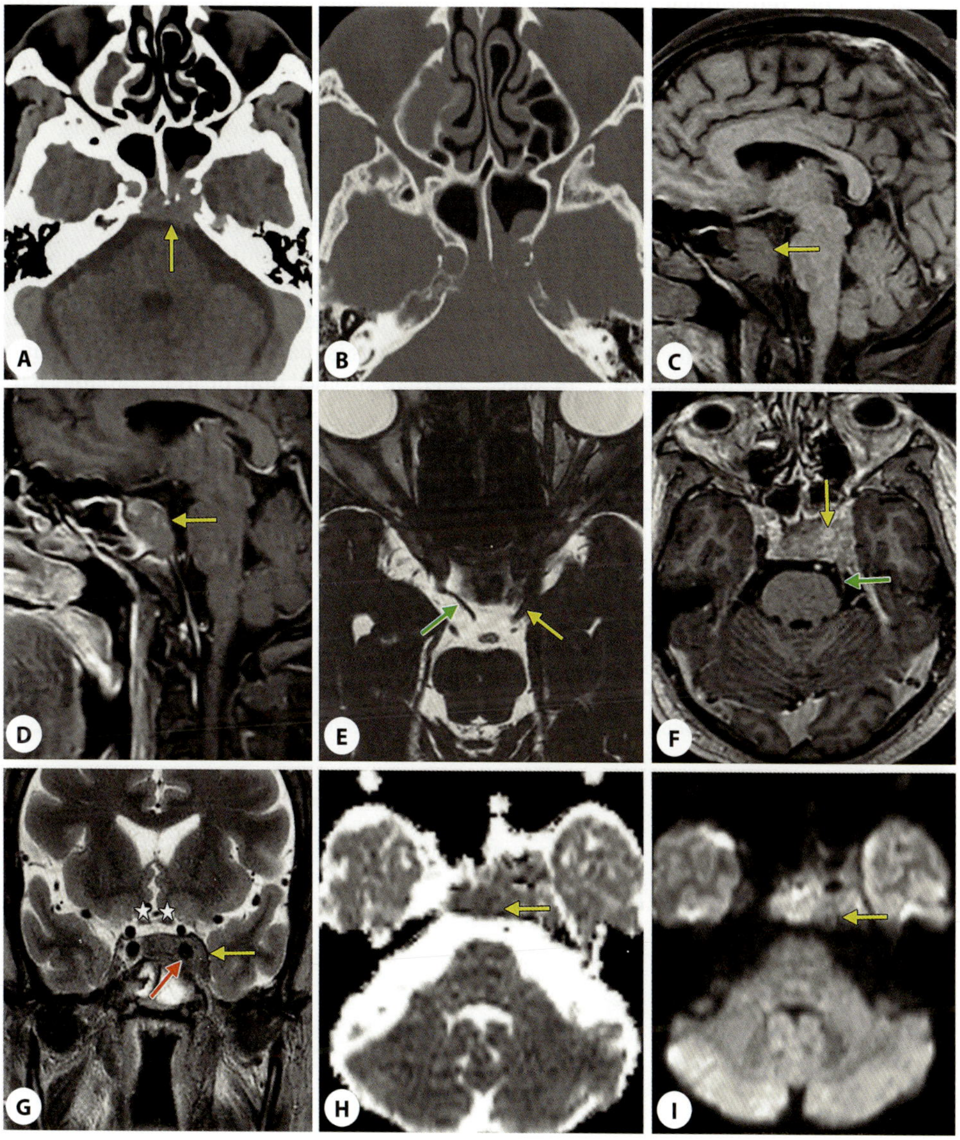

CLINICAL BACKGROUND

A 50-years-old male patient, known case of carcinoma oropharynx—presented with complaints of right ptosis.

IMAGING FINDINGS

Well defined T1-iso and T2-iso- hyperintense lesion noted in sella and left parasellar regions (pituitary gland and infundibulum are not separately visualized from lesion) with left cavernous sinus invasion. The lesion also seen completely encasing the left ICA, III and V cranial nerves. The lesion shows homogenous post contrast enhancement with bone erosions **(Figs. 1A to I)**.

DISCUSSION

Sellar and parasellar metastasis are rare (<1% of all lesions), but it is a vital area as it is rich in neurovascular structures. Breast and lung malignancy are the two most common primary tumors which metastasize to this region. Despite the advancement in the imaging modalities, it is difficult to differentiate metastasis from pituitary adenoma. Ophthalmoplegia, headache, retroorbital or facial pain, diabetes insipidus, and visual field defects are the most commonly reported symptoms.[1]

The diagnostic imaging modalities include both CT and MRI. Although the former is superior in detecting the bone involvement, the latter is preferable to determine the relationship of the lesion to the surrounding neurovascular structures.[2] The proposed mechanisms of spread to the pituitary include, via the hypophyseal arteries of the posterior lobe or the hypophyseal portal system of the anterior lobe. The second-degree nature of the portal system may confer some degree of protection and hence metastases are common in neurohypophysis with only 15% of them involving the anterior lobe alone.[3]

Although nonspecific, the MRI findings of metastasis include T1-iso or hypointense mass lesion which is usually hyperintense on T2-weighted with homogeneous post contrast enhancement. Invasion of the cavernous sinus, sclerotic changes around the sella turcica and clivus, isointense signal on both T1- and T2-weighted imaging, and loss of high-intensity signal in the posterior pituitary have been reported to be helpful in identifying the metastatic lesion. Thickening/enhancement of infundibulum and invasion of the infundibular recess are the other features favoring metastasis.[1]

Because pituitary adenomas (PA) also present with features of invasion, differentiating metastatic lesions from PA is difficult. PAs can also present with increased metabolic uptake and hence, functional imaging with PET-FDG is also limited in distinguishing between adenomas from metastasis. Once histopathological diagnosis of metastasis is made, the prognosis is generally poor with a median survival time of approximately 6 months.[4]

REFERENCES

1. Altay T, Krisht KM, Couldwell WT. Sellar and parasellar metastatic tumors. Int J Surg Oncol. 2012;2012:647256.
2. Hirsch WL, Jr., Hryshko FG, Sekhar LN, et al. Comparison of MR imaging, CT, and angiography in the evaluation of the enlarged cavernous sinus. AJR Am J Roentgenol. 1988;151(5):1015-23.
3. Henry A, Nugent A, Wallace IR, et al. Pituitary metastasis: a clinical overview. Ulster Med J. 2021;90(3):146-50.
4. Kameda-Smith MM, Zhang E, Lannon M, et al. Pituitary metastasis: from pathology to clinical and radiologic considerations. J Clin Neurosci. 2021;93:231-40.

16 Infected Right Para Tracheal Cyst

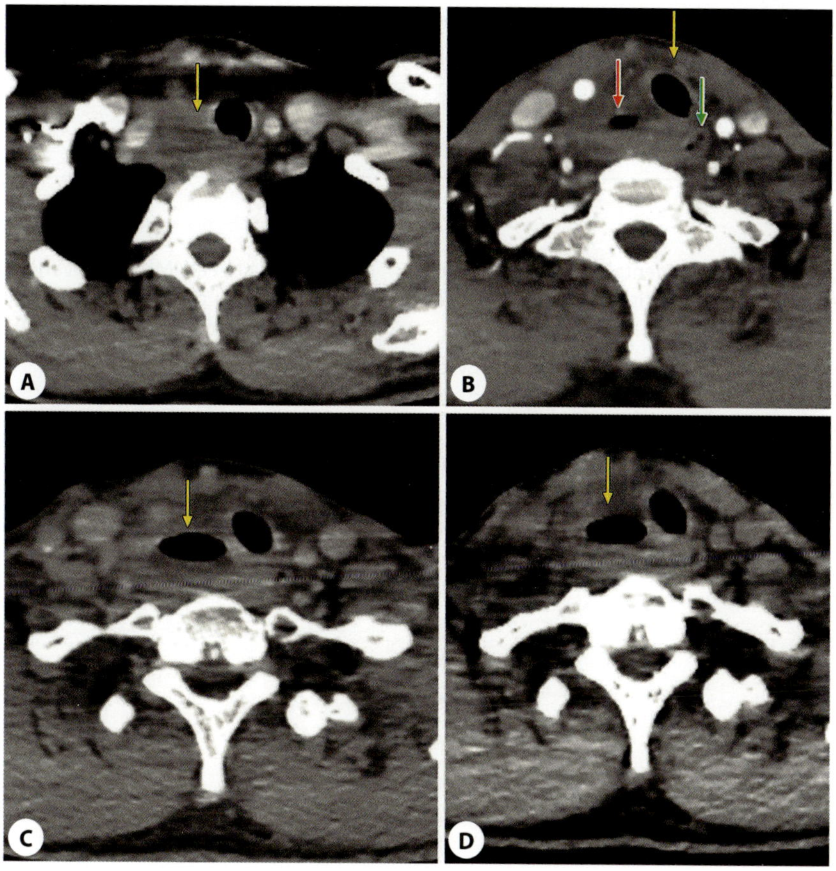

CLINICAL BACKGROUND

A 35-year-old male patient presented with sudden onset of respiratory distress.

IMAGING FINDINGS

Air-filled cystic lesion in right paratracheal region with ill-defined collection and inflammation causing displacement of trachea and esophagus to left side. The lesion shows thin rim of peripheral postcontrast enhancement without demonstrating direct communication with trachea **(Figs. 1A to D)**.

DISCUSSION

Air-filled cysts originating from the trachea are relatively common, with the prevalence rate of 0.75–6.5%. This can be a para tracheal cyst or diverticula.[1] The paratracheal cyst occurs at the thoracic inlet level, more commonly on right side. It has been reported in literature, that these cysts are associated with pulmonary emphysema, chronic obstructive pulmonary disease, inflammatory conditions such as recurrent pneumonia, chronic bronchitis and bronchiectasis.[2]

These paratracheal air cysts can become infected as these are reservoir of respiratory secretions and can cause respiratory symptoms such as cough, sputum, fever, and hemoptysis. However, infected paratracheal air cysts as the focus of respiratory symptoms can be overlooked in practice because of nonspecific symptoms, their small size, and scant knowledge for this entity.[3]

Infected paratracheal cysts are best demonstrated on CECT as an air filled cysts with signs of inflammation like, ill-defined collection, fat stranding and with thin rim of peripheral post contrast enhancement. There may be mild reactive thickening seen involving the posterolateral wall of trachea with Communication between these cysts and trachea was able to be demonstrated only in about 35 and 55% cases.[2,3]

Most infected paratracheal air cysts can be managed conservatively, but few might require surgical intervention especially when there is a potential life threat or those with refractory symptoms. Thoracoscopy may be needed for excision of paratracheal air cysts. Other associated malformations like tracheoesophageal fistula need to be excluded before surgical planning.[2]

REFERENCES

1. Kosehan D, Kayıhan A, Koktener A. Incidental right paratracheal air cyst: significance of 64-detector multislice CT in differential diagnosis. New J Med. 2011;28:62-3.
2. Kim HJ, Jou SS, Kim YT, et al. Infected Paratracheal Air Cyst: A Case Report. J Korean Soc Radiol. 2016;75(1):68-72.
3. Bae K, Jeon KN, Park MJ, et al. Overlooked diagnosis of infected paratracheal air cysts in patients with respiratory symptoms: Case report. Medicine (Baltimore). 2017;96(29):e7536.

17 Testicular Germ Cell Tumors

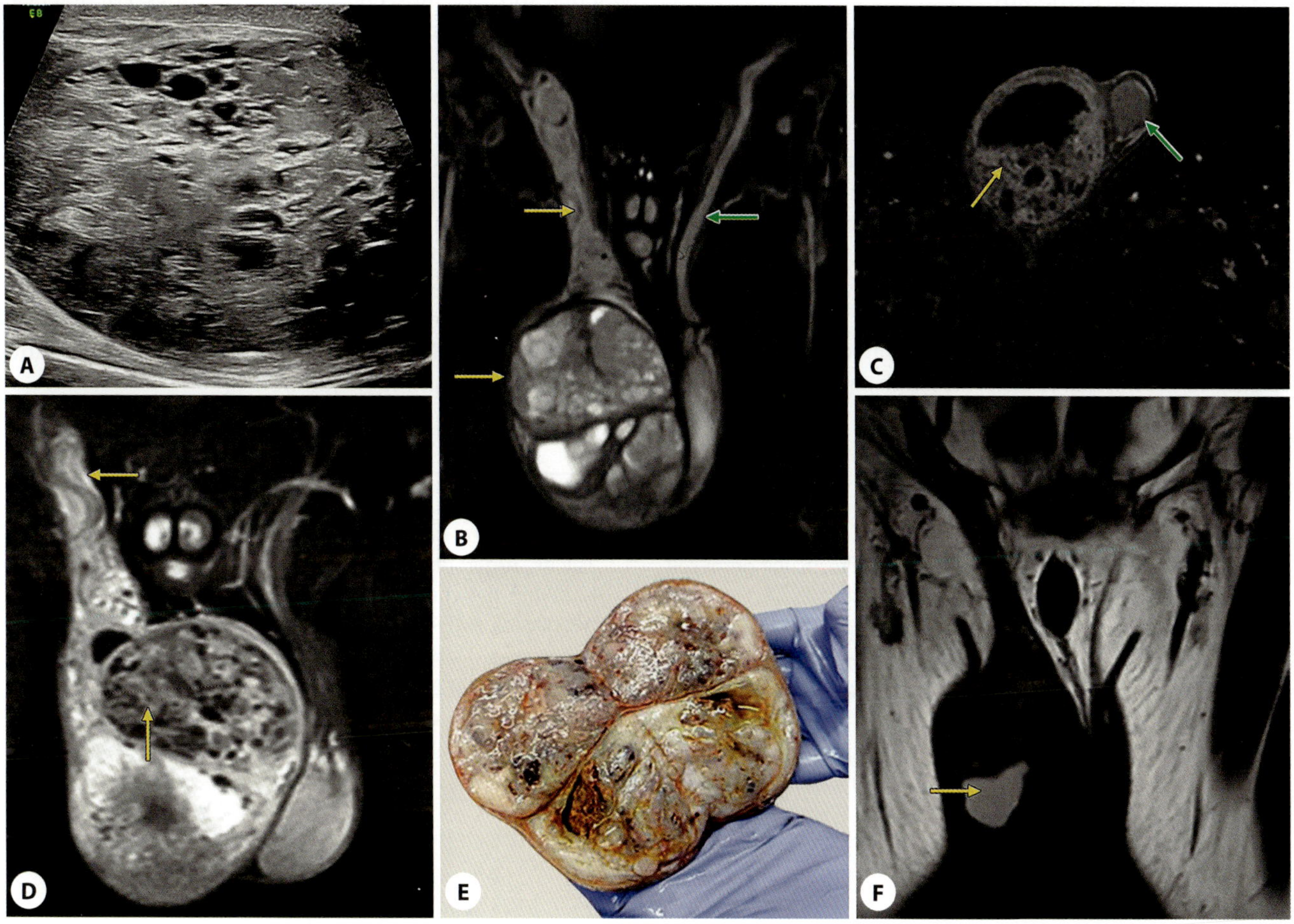

CLINICAL BACKGROUND

A 35-year-old male patient presented with testicular swelling with occasional pain. No history of fever or trauma.

IMAGING FINDINGS

Entire testis is replaced by a large complex solid cystic mass lesion which is T1 hypo and T2 heterogeneous signal intensity. Areas of hemorrhage as T1 hyperintensity and lesion shows heterogeneous postcontrast enhancement. Associated thickening and enhancement of cord structures on right side **(Figs. 1A to F)**.

DISCUSSION

Testicular germ cell tumors (GCTs) are common neoplasms in young males. Serum markers are useful to assess disease activity, but they cannot accurately assess disease bulk or locate sites of tumor spread. Imaging plays an essential role in the tumor bulk assessment, metastases, preoperative surgical planning and also to assess the disease response to therapy.[1]

Serum markers are imperative in screening and diagnosis: Increased levels of AFP are associated with yolk-sac tumors, and elevated β-hCG is found in choriocarcinoma. In patients with seminomatous testicular tumors, LDH may be elevated in 80% of patients, but this tumor marker can also be elevated in up to 60% of NSGCTs. Testicular choriocarcinoma very often has elevated serum β-hCG levels. While, embryonal-cell tumors demonstrate elevation of both AFP and β-hCG.[2]

USG is used in primary assessment of the testicular mass. These tumors are usually well defined and hypoechoic relative to the normal testicle, although some may display a heterogeneous echotexture, calcification or cystic change. Vascularity on Doppler study may vary depending on size of tumor.[2] USG is not routinely used in the staging of disease, for which CT is more commonly used.

Tumor spread occurs via lymphatic channels which pass through the inguinal ring (accompanying the spermatic cord and testicular vessels) to enter retroperitoneal nodes. Vascular spread is most commonly to the lungs. For practical purposes a cut-off of 10 mm is used to differentiate between normal and abnormal lymph nodes. Those measuring between 8 and 10 mm are treated as suspicious.[1,5]

MRI is more efficient than US for detecting local staging of the tumor: Involvement of the tunica albuginea, epididymis, and spermatic cord. It can also differentiate seminomas from NSGCTs, the later demonstrating heterogeneous signal and enhancement characteristics caused by necrosis and hemorrhage, although there may be overlap of findings.[3] MRI with lymphotrophic nanoparticles (LNMRI) can effectively raise sensitivity and specificity in evaluating lymph nodes.[4]

REFERENCES

1. Dalal PU, Sohaib SA, Huddart R. Imaging of testicular germ cell tumours. Cancer Imaging. 2006;6(1):124-34.
2. Marshall C, Enzerra M, Rahnemai-Azar AA, Ramaiya NH. Serum tumor markers and testicular germ cell tumors: a primer for radiologists. Abdom Radiol. 2019;44:1083-90.
3. Horstman WG, Melson GL, Middleton WD, Andriole GL. Testicular tumors: findings with color Doppler US. Radiology. 1992;185:733-7.
4. Tsili AC, Argyropoulou MI, Giannakis D, Sofikitis N, Tsampoulas K. MRI in the characterization and local staging of testicular neoplasms. AJR Am J Roentgenol. 2010;194:682-9.
5. Pandharipande PV, Mora JT, Uppot RN, Goehler A, Braschi M, Halpern EF, et al. Lymphotropic nanoparticle-enhanced MRI for independent prediction of lymph node malignancy: a logistic regression model. AJR Am J Roentgenol. 2009;193(3):W230-7.

18 Renal Lymphangiectasia with Ascites

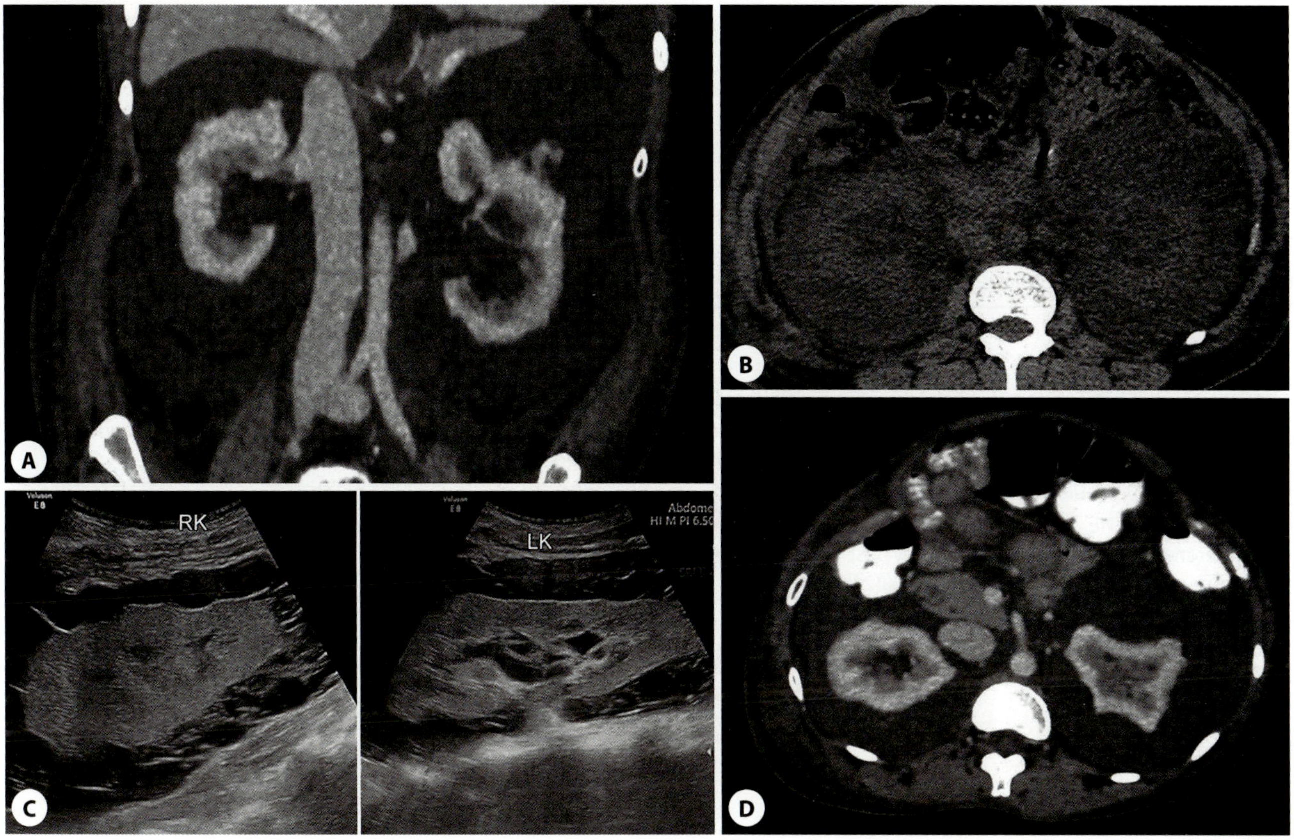

CLINICAL BACKGROUND

A 35-years-old female patient presented with sudden onset of abdomen distension.

IMAGING FINDINGS

Both kidneys show normal parenchymal enhancement and excretion with perinephric multiloculated cysts on both sides indenting renal parenchyma and moderate ascites. No bowel or peritoneal thickening **(Figs. 1A to D)**.

DISCUSSION

Renal lymphangiectasia is a rare benign disorder of renal lymphatics.[1] It is known by different names like renal lymphangiomatosis, lymphangioma, per pelvic multicystic/peripelvic lymphangiectasia, hygroma renale and polycystic disease of the renal sinus.[1,2] It is usually asymptomatic and incidentally diagnosed.[2]

The pathophysiology of this condition is not very clear yet it is attributed to abnormal dilatation of these lymphatic ducts which is a result of failure to communicate with larger retroperitoneal lymphatic channels. It is bilateral in more than 90% of cases with familial association in few cases.[2,3]

The distribution and severity of the lymphatics involved will determine the imaging characteristics. If only small intra-renal lymphatics are involved, it is seen as mild diffuse enlargement of the kidney with no cystic space. These cases show diffusely echogenic renal parenchyma with poor corticomedullary differentiation on US and hyperintense signal in the cortex and hypointense signal in medulla with corticomedullary inversion on T2 weighted sequences of MR due to renal edema.[2,3]

The peripelvic cysts are seen in cases with the involvement of lymphatics in the renal sinus. These peripelvic cysts show thin wall which are well appreciated on US and T2 weighted sequences of MR which may also show enhancement on T1 weighted sequences acquired after gadolinium administration. The larger cysts can cause obstruction of collecting system resulting in hydronephrosis. Capsular lymphatic dilatation leads to septated perinephric fluid collections which show CT attenuation values of 0–10 HU, causing parenchymal indentations.[3]

Ascites may be found, and is a known complication. The imaging features on ultrasound and CT are diagnostic of the condition. This case emphasizes that we have to be familiar with imaging features of this rare condition to allow prompt diagnosis due to its potential complications of renal vein thrombosis and hypertension.[3,4]

REFERENCES

1. Schwarz A, Lenz T, Klaen R, et al. Hygroma renale: pararenal lymphatic cysts associated with renin dependent hypertension (page kidney). Case report on bilateral cysts and successful therapy by marsupialization. J Urol. 1993;150:953-7.
2. Lin QZ, Wang HE, Wei D, et al. Pleural effusion and ascites in extrarenal lymphangiectasia caused by post-biopsy hematoma: A case report. World J Clin Cases. 2020;8(24):6330-6.
3. Arora R. Bilateral renal lymphangiectasia—an unusual cause of abdominal distension and flank pain in a child. Quant Imaging Med Surg. 2016;6(4):466-9
4. Al-Dofri SA. Renal lymphangiectasia presented by pleural effusion and ascites. J Radiol Case Rep. 2009;3(10):5-10.

19 Common Carotid Artery Occlusion with Retrograde Collateral ICA Flow

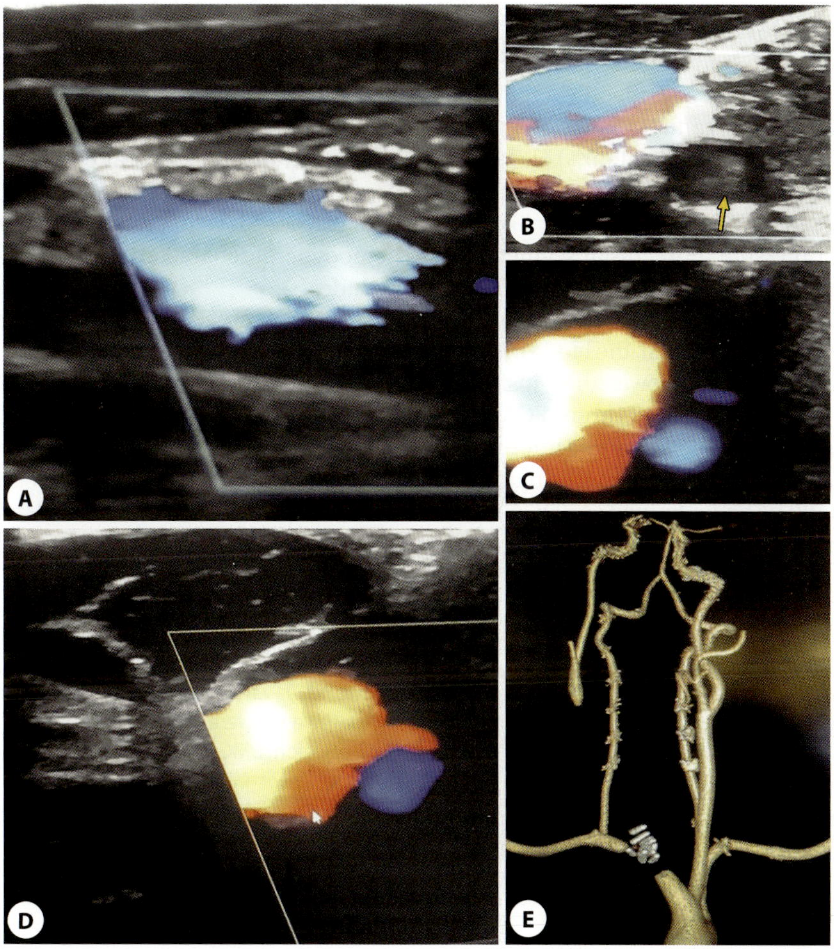

CLINICAL BACKGROUND

A 25-year-old male patient came with history of RTA with right clavicle fracture.

IMAGING FINDINGS

CT angiogram show absent opacification of right common carotid artery with normal opacification of right ICA and ECA. Doppler study shows echogenic thrombus in common carotid artery and retrograde blood flow from ECA to ICA–ICA steal **(Figs. 1A to E)**.

DISCUSSION

Common carotid artery occlusion (CCAO) is a rare condition that may be associated with ischemic cerebral diseases. There is no clear consensus on the role of invasive treatment of CCAO. Owing to collateral circulation, about 61.5% of patients with CCAO have patent ipsilateral ICA and ECA.[1] Riles et al's classifies CCAO into four types:

1. Type 1A with patent ICA and external carotid artery (ECA): Most common (61.5%),
2. Type 1B with occluded ICA and patent ECA (26.6%),
3. Type 1C with patent ICA and occluded ECA (could be theoretical, practically none) and
4. Type 2 with occluded ICA and ECA (11.9%).[2,3]

The reason for formation of collateral circulation is the change in blood pressure. When a main artery like CCA is occluded, the blood pressure in the distal segment gets lower than adjacent arteries and may be drawn reversely to the distal segment. This phenomenon is called "steal" e.g., subclavian steal. When CCA is occluded, the blood pressure in ipsilateral ICA can be obviously lower than ipsilateral ECA. As a result, ICA "steals" blood from ECA. This phenomenon was originally defined as "carotid artery steal" by Anne G Osborn. However, since ECA supplies blood and ICA receives blood, could be better termed as - "ICA steal".[3]

Four collateral circulation pathways of "ICA steal" is identified by DSA and CTA:[3]

1. Ipsilateral vertebral artery, occipital artery, ECA, ICA
2. Ipsilateral thyrocervical trunk or costocervical trunk, ascending cervical artery or deep cervical artery, occipital artery, ECA, ICA
3. Contralateral ECA contralateral superior thyroid artery, ipsilateral superior thyroid artery, ipsilateral ECA, ICA, and
4. Ipsilateral thyrocervical trunk, inferior thyroid artery, superior thyroid artery, ECA, ICA.

The imaging characteristics of ICA steal in CT and MR angiogram include: Absent contrast flow in CCA, normal development of ICA, ECA and carotid bifurcation, and in few case developments of thyrocervical trunk. The hemodynamic characteristics of ICA steal in Color Doppler include:

- No Color uptake in the occluded CCA which may be filled by echogenic thrombus;
- Opposite blood flow colors in ipsilateral ECA and ICA indicative of the possibility of ICA steal.[3]

Hence it is essential to remember that ICA can still be patent due to several collateral circulation pathways as described above even after complete CCAO.

REFERENCES

1. Klonaris C, Kouvelos GN, Kafeza M, et al. Common carotid artery occlusion treatment: revealing a gap in the current guidelines. Eur J Vasc Endovasc Surg. 2013;46(3):291-8.
2. Riles TS, Imparato AM, Posner MP, et al. Common carotid occlusion. Assessment of the distal vessels. Ann Surg. 1984;199(3):363-6.
3. Wang, J, Zheng, C, Hou B, et al. Four collateral circulation pathways were observed after common carotid artery occlusion. BMC Neurol. 2019;19:201.

20 Central Neurocytoma

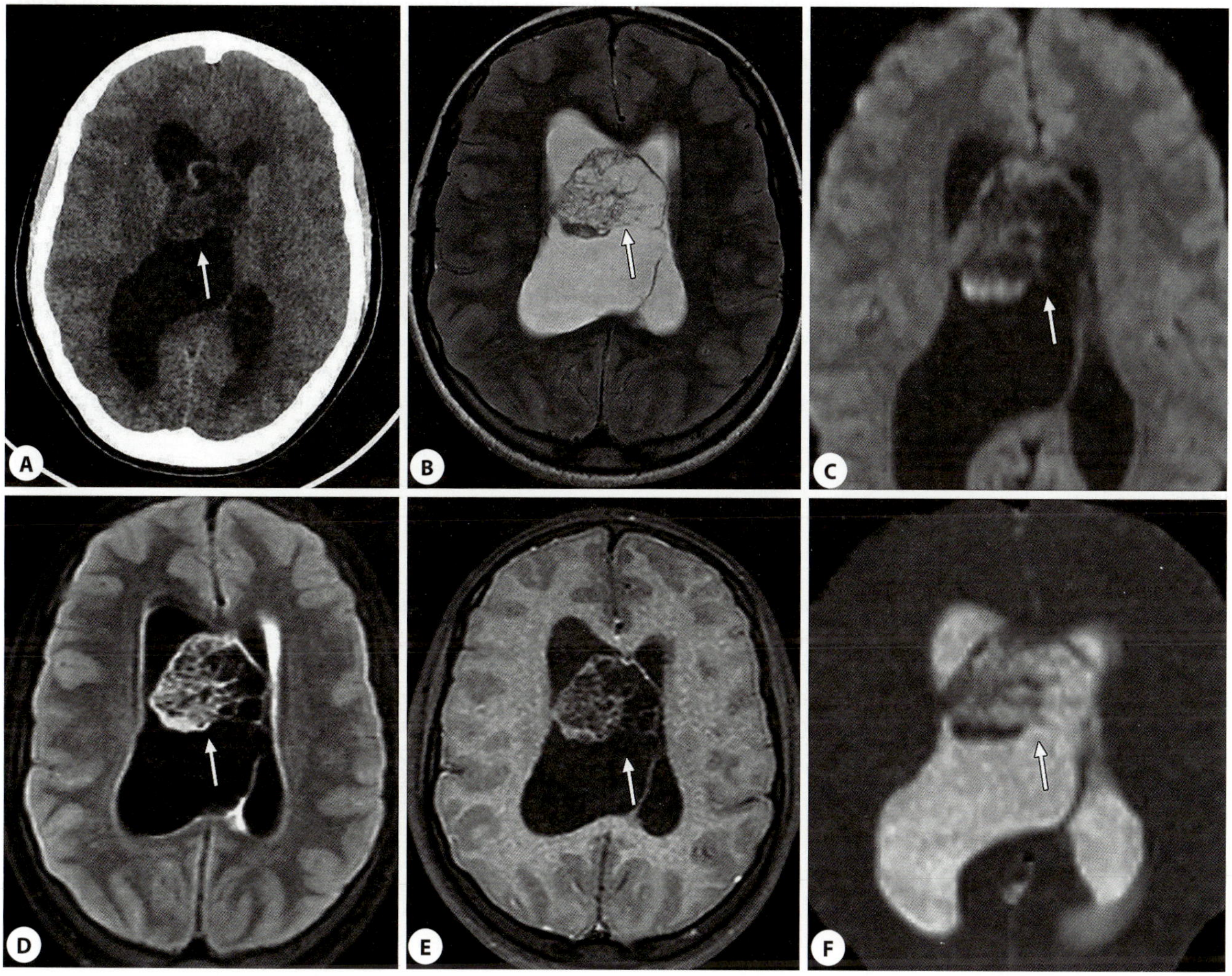

CLINICAL BACKGROUND

A 14-years-old female patient presented with headache.

IMAGING FINDINGS

Well defined cystic lesion attached to septum pellucidum seen in right lateral ventricle with hydrocephalus. The lesion was T2 hyperintense and T1 hypointense. The lesion shows no enhancing solid components or diffusion restriction **(Figs. 1A to F)**.

DISCUSSION

Central neurocytoma (CN) is rare, benign brain tumor (0.1–0.5% of all brain tumors) was first described in the 1980's by Hassoun et al. It occurs commonly within ventricular system and rarely can also occur extraventricularly in the cerebral hemispheres, spinal cord, brainstem, thalamus, pons, amygdala, pineal gland, retina, and cerebellum. The most common site of the tumor is near the foramen of Monro and is usually attached to the septum pellucidum.[1]

The lesion appears as a dense mass in computerized tomography (CT) with patchy and coarse calcifications can be seen in up to 50% of cases. The heterogeneous appearance can be due to cystic degeneration and the lesion shows mild to moderate postcontrast enhancement. On T1-weighted MRI the lesion appears hypointense to iso-intense and iso-intense to hyperintense on T2-weighted MRI. In both T1- and T2W MRI, hypointensity can indicate the presence of a hemorrhage, cyst, or calcification. Typically, moderate postcontrast enhancement is noted.[2]

The "**scalloping sign**" considered as a combination of ventricular wall undulations and spicules of peripheral cysts, was the most specific sign and is better depicted on sagittal views. The "**broad-based attachment**" is another imaging feature with the highest sensitivity. It is related to the origin of this intraventricular tumor, which is explained by its derivation from the small gray nuclei of the septum pellucidum/the bipotential progenitor cells on the periventricular matrix. The "**bubble-soap sign**" consists on a large number of cysts varying in size conferring to the tumor a sponge form appearance of the lesion. The "**fluid-fluid level**" appearance is an infrequent finding, which is the consequence of bleeding. The "**Gemstone**" sign is a recent feature considered as highly specific for CN and consists in one or several well-demarked enhanced areas compared to the surrounding nonenhanced or mildly enhanced tumor.[3,4]

The spectroscopic profile of CN is characterized by the presence of high levels of choline and glycine, low levels of NAA and absent or low level of alanine compared to intraventricular meningioma. The choline/creatinine and NAA/creatinine ratios seem to be significantly higher compared to other intraventricular tumors, including oligodendroglioma, astrocytoma, subependymoma and glioblastoma multiforme.[4]

REFERENCES

1. Lee SJ, Bui TT, Chen CH, et al. Central Neurocytoma: A Review of Clinical Management and Histopathologic Features. Brain Tumor Res Treat. 2016;4(2):49-57.
2. Shin JH, Lee HK, Khang SK, et al. Neuronal tumors of the central nervous system: radiologic findings and pathologic correlation. Radiographics. 2002;22:1177-89.
3. Li X, Guo L, Sheng S, et al. Diagnostic value of six MRI features for central neurocytoma. Eur Radiol 2018;28(10): 4306-13.
4. Andour H, Rostoum S, Cherraqi A, et al. Ech-Cherif El Kettani N, Jiddane M, Touarsa F. Central neurocytoma-positive and differential diagnosis: An example through a case report. SAGE Open Med Case Rep. 2023.

21 Azygos ACA with Saccular Aneurysm

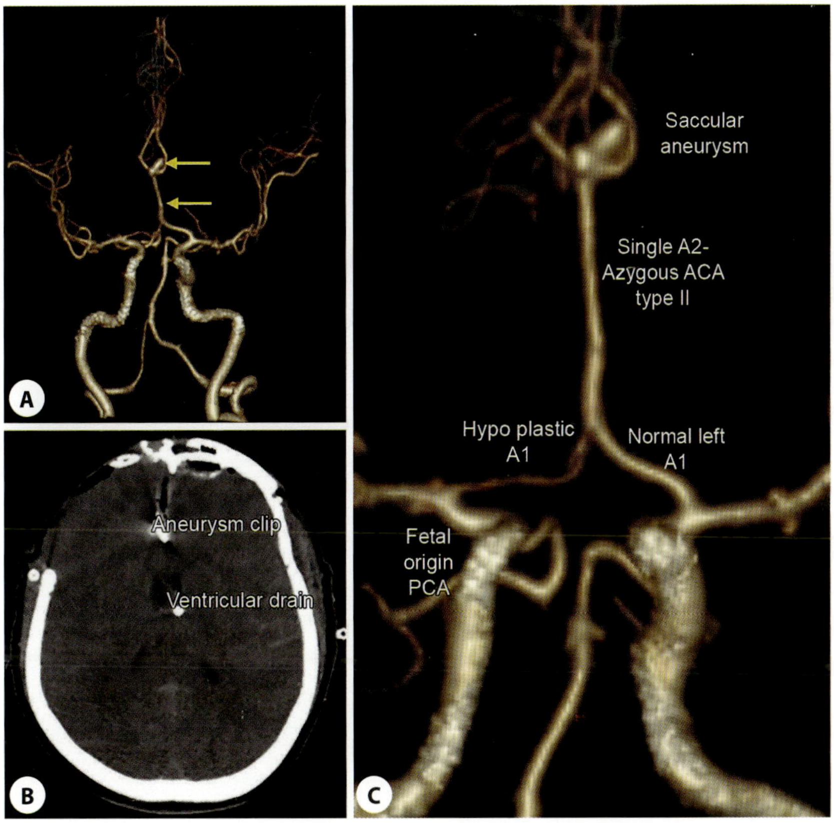

CLINICAL BACKGROUND

A 52-year-old female patient with sudden onset of severe headache and followed by loss of consciousness.

IMAGING FINDINGS

Diffuse subarachnoid hemorrhage with CT angiogram showing single A2 segment of ACA (azygos ACA) with a saccular aneurysm at the level of bifurcation. Hydrocephalus was noted and emergency ventricular drain was done followed by aneurysm clipping **(Figs. 1A to C)**.

DISCUSSION

The azygos anterior cerebral artery (ACA) is a rare anatomical anomaly (<1%) in the circle of Willis. In this vascular anomaly, the distal segments (A2) of both ACAs are represented by a single vessel and aneurysms of the azygos ACA are even rare. Wilder was the first to describe the fusion of both A2 segments of ACA to form a single artery and to introduce the term arteria termatica in 1885.[1]

Baptista defined three ACA variations. In type I anomaly (true azygos ACA), there is only one azygos ACA from which all major branches spread to both the hemispheres. Type II anomaly is bihemispheric ACA, where both right and left ACA are present, but most of the major branches to the bilateral hemispheres arise from one ACA and the other one is rudimentary. In type III anomaly, a third artery (accessory ACA) arises from anterior communicating artery. Among the three types, the azygos, or single unpaired ACA, is the most important.[2,3]

Azygos ACA is also known to be associated with other midline malformations including agenesis of the corpus callosum, porencephalic cysts, holoprosencephaly, and saccular aneurysms. Although saccular aneurysm is more common, Nonsaccular aneurysms of azygos ACA have also been reported, which require complex clip application or multiple clips. Aneurysms of azygos ACA are rare, with only few cases reported in the literature. The mechanism of aneurysm formation in azygos ACA could be due to hemodynamic stress or because of a congenitally anomalous artery.[1]

Management of aneurysms of azygos ACA is by surgical clipping or by endovascular coiling. Most of the reported cases of azygos ACA aneurysms have been managed by surgical clipping. Endovascular coiling of azygos ACA aneurysm has been reported in few cases. Temporary clipping of the proximal A2 (ACA) is an essential adjunct for dissecting the aneurysm neck and final clip application. The temporary clipping can give rise to bilateral infarcts as single A2 ACA supplies bifrontal cortex.[1]

REFERENCES

1. Ghanta RK, Kesanakurthy MV, Vemuri VN. Aneurysm of azygos anterior cerebral artery: A report of two cases. Asian J Neurosurg. 2016;11(3):312.
2. Baptista AG. Studies on the arteries of the brain. II. The anterior cerebral artery: Some anatomic features and their clinical implications. Neurology. 1963;13:825-35.
3. Huh JS, Park SK, Shin JJ, et al. Saccular aneurysm of the azygos anterior cerebral artery: three case reports. J Korean Neurosurg Soc. 2007;42(4):342-5.

22 Submucosal Fibroids

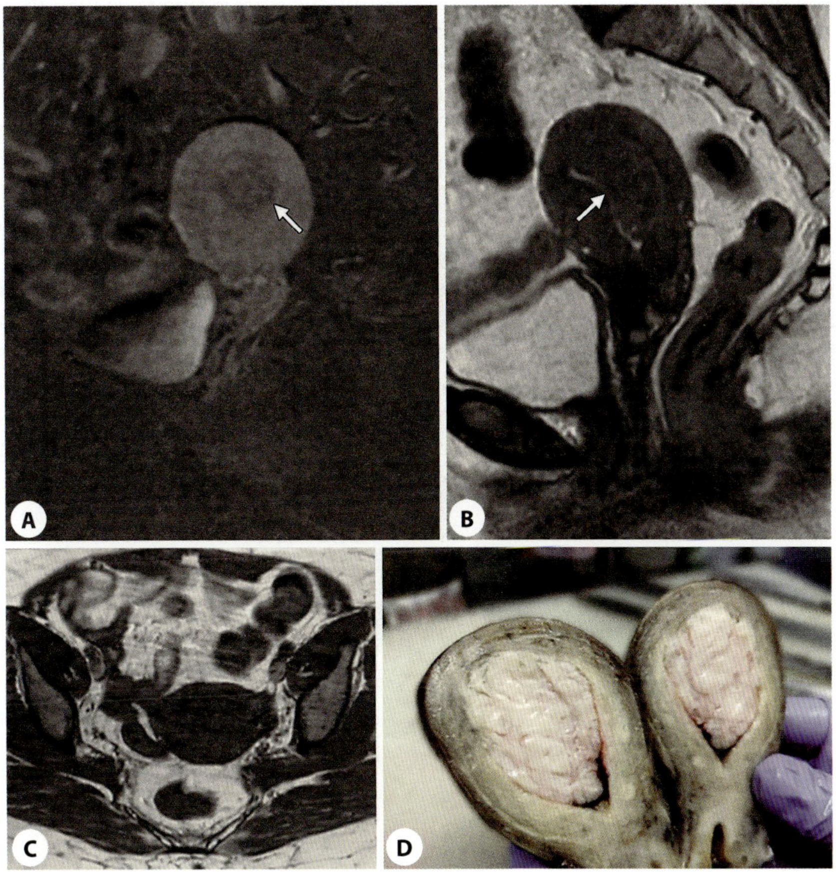

CLINICAL BACKGROUND

Postmenopausal status with incidentally detected mass in USG, referred to MR with deferential diagnosis of submucosal leiomyoma/endometrial CA.

IMAGING FINDINGS

Well defined T1 iso- and T2 hypointense lesion indenting the endometrium without significant postcontrast enhancement of the lesion **(Figs. 1A to D)**.

DISCUSSION

Uterine fibroids are also called as leiomyomas or myomas. They are the commonest uterine neoplasms. They usually arise in the myometrium but may be also located in the cervix, broad ligament or ovaries. These benign lesions are generally asymptomatic; About 20–50% of them might be symptomatic and symptoms include menorrhagia, pelvic pain and infertility or complications during pregnancy. The symptomatic fibroid is the commonest indication for hysterectomy. Also important to remember that it is a rare cause of pseudo-Meigs syndrome and can occasionally present with ascites.[1]

Submucosal fibroids: These are rare type of fibroids (5% of all fibroids) but they are often symptomatic since they protrude into the endometrial cavity. They can occasionally be pedunculated and prolapse into the cervical canal or vagina and sometimes are difficult to be differentiated from endometrial polyps on routine USG.[1]

Sonohysterography is a technique in which sterile saline is instilled into the uterine cavity via a transcervical catheter whilst performing a scan. This method allows better visualization of the endometrium and has been shown to be more accurate than USG in detecting submucous fibroids and in differentiating them from polyps.[2]

On T2W MRI, fibroids appear as well-defined masses of low-signal intensity as compared to uterine myometrium and isointense to the myometrium on T1W sequence. They may have a high-intensity rim on T2W images which has been shown to be secondary to a zone of dilated lymphatic vessels, dilated veins, edema or a combination of these.[2]

Fibroids may show degeneration due to larger size and inadequate blood supply which results in a variable and often heterogeneous appearance, with minimal or irregular enhancement. The commonest type of degeneration is hyaline degeneration (60% of all degeneration) and appears hypo-intense on T2W images and with no enhancement.[2]

MRI is also used to both predict and to assess the response of fibroids to UAE. Fibroids that demonstrate high signal on T1W images prior to embolization are likely to have a poor response to UAE as they may already have outgrown their blood supply and undergone hemorrhagic necrosis. High signal on T2W images prior to embolization has been shown to be a predictor of good response.[2]

REFERENCES

1. Wilde S, Scott-Barrett S. Radiological appearances of uterine fibroids. Indian J Radiol Imaging. 2009;19(3):222-31.
2. Burn PR, McCall JM, Chinn RJ, et al. Uterine fibroleiomyoma: MR imaging appearance before and after embolization of uterine arteries. Radiology. 2000;214:729-34.

23 Wunderlich Syndrome

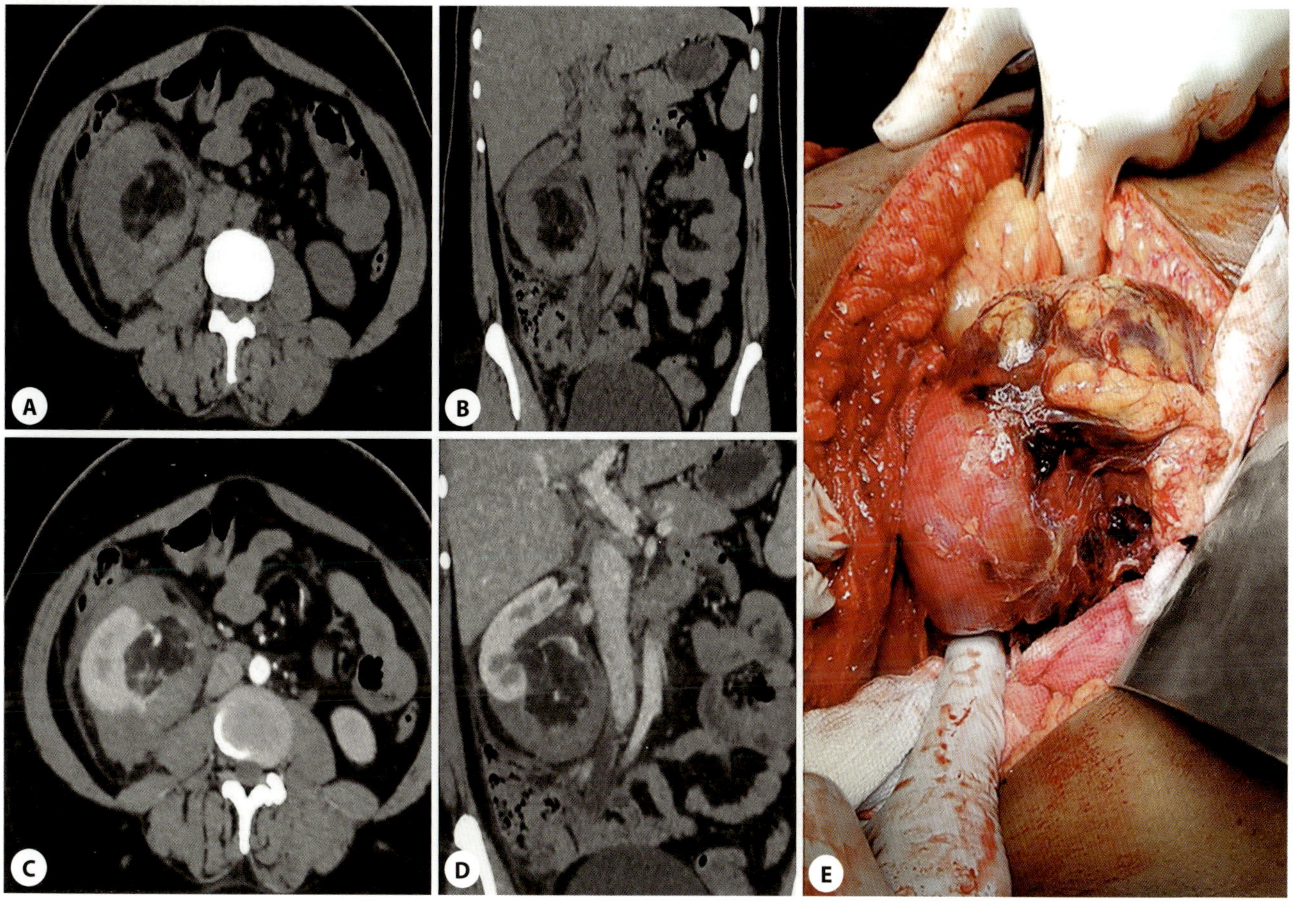

CLINICAL BACKGROUND

A 42-year-old female patient presented with hypovolemic shock.

IMAGING FINDINGS

Large fat dense lesion noted in lower pole of right kidney with perinephric extension and intralesional vascular channels. Associated subcapsular and perinephric hematoma seen **(Figs. 1A to E)**.

DISCUSSION

Wunderlich syndrome (WS) is a rare condition characterized by acute onset of spontaneous/ nontraumatic retroperitoneal hemorrhage. It is characterized by Lenk's triad—acute flank pain, flank mass, and hypovolemic shock. The most common cause for WS, is renal tumors angiomyolipoma (MC benign neoplasm) and renal cell carcinoma (MC malignant neoplasm). The list of non-neoplastic causes includes vasculitis, renal artery aneurysm, arteriovenous malformation, renal vein thrombosis, nephritis, cystic renal disease, and coagulopathy.[1]

Angiomyolipoma (AML) is the most common benign tumor (choristoma tumor composed of tissues not normally occurring within the organ of origin) which is composed of fat, smooth muscle and thick-walled blood vessels. encountered with WS. 80% of AMLs are sporadic in nature while, the remaining 20% are associated with tuberous sclerosis (TS). Sporadic AMLs are generally solitary and unilateral, more common on the right side. AMLs that occur in association with tuberous sclerosis on the other hand, manifest at a younger age, are likely to be larger and bilateral, and are prone to grow requiring surgical treatment.[2]

The presence of fat attenuation in a renal mass on MDCT is highly suggestive of AML. Other renal tumors with intra-lesional fat include clear cell renal cell carcinoma, liposarcomas, atypical Wilms' tumor and teratomas this end, urgent diagnostic imaging is essential. Ultrasonography (USG) is often the first imaging method used in WS. However, due to the known inadequacies and disadvantages of ultrasonography in evaluating the retroperitoneum, a cross-sectional method, such as MRI or CT should also be used for a definitive diagnosis. Triphasic CECT is the most preferred imaging modality and the angiographic phase is essential to identify the active arterial contrast extravasation necessitating immediate surgical interventions.[3]

WS is a urological emergency, CT should be the preferred method for the detection of renal/perirenal bleeding and its underlying cause due to its easier accessibility, shorter examination time during emergencies. To note, the risk of spontaneous tumor (AML) rupture increases with increase in size (> 4 cm in diameter at higher risk). Aneurysm formation due to poor elastic vascular structure could possibly explain tumor rupture during tumor growth. Arteriography with selective embolization represents an increasingly employed treatment in selected cases while surgery is reserved for refractory ones.[3]

REFERENCES

1. Katabathina VS, Katre R, Prasad SR, et al. Wunderlich syndrome: cross-sectional imaging review. J Comput Assist Tomogr. 2011;35(4):425-33.
2. Logue LG, Acker RE, Sienko AE. "Best Cases from the AFIP: Angiomyolipomas in Tuberous Sclerosis". RadioGraphics. 2003; 23(1):241-6.
3. Albi G, del Campo L, Tagarro D. Wünderlich's syndrome: causes, diagnosis and radiological management. Clin Radiol. 2002;57: 840-5.

24 Leriche Syndrome

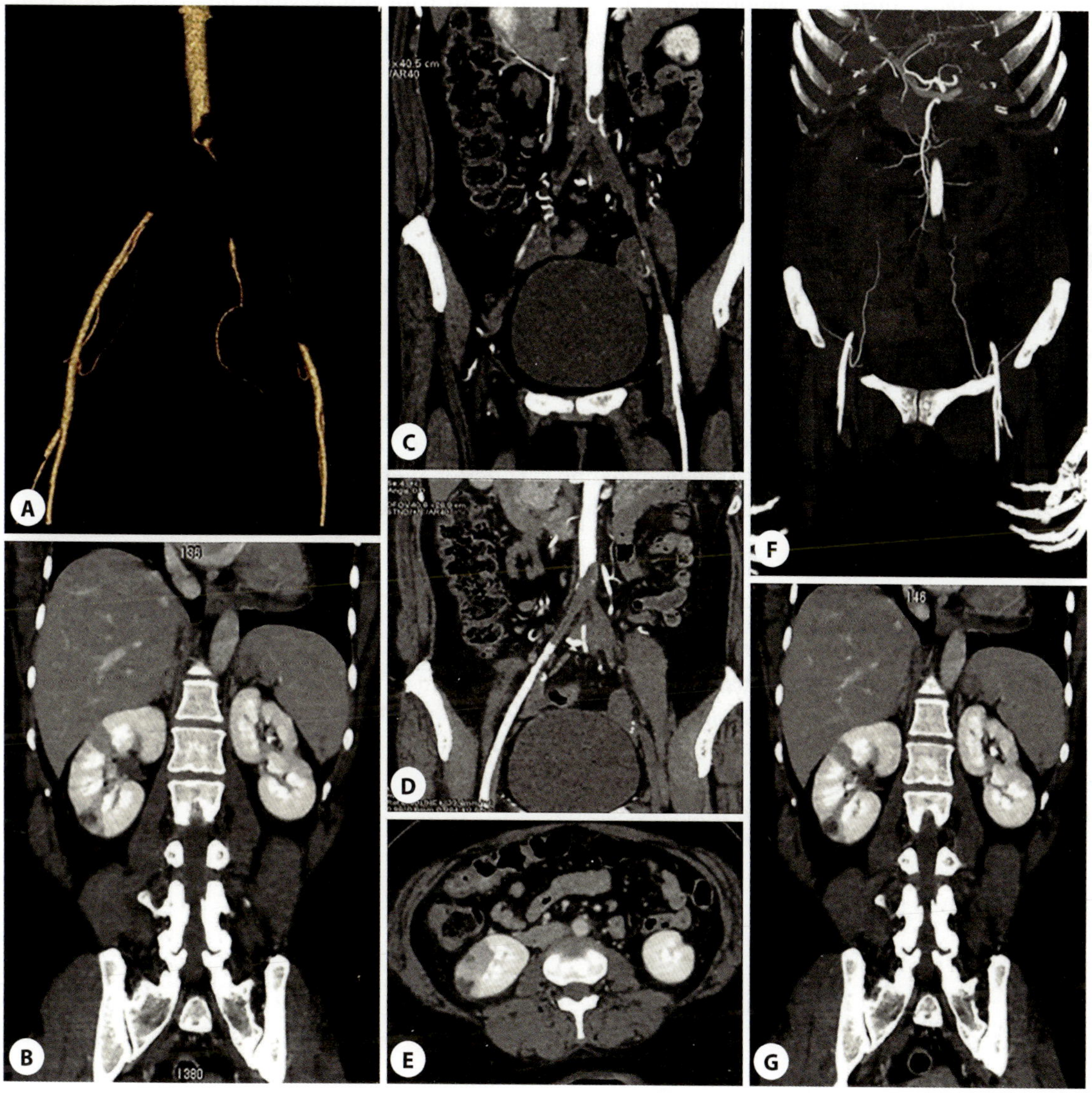

CLINICAL BACKGROUND

A 36-year-old female with complaints of bilateral lower limb pain.

IMAGING FINDINGS

Thrombus in infrarenal portion of aorta extending into bilateral iliac arteries with collateral supply distal to the level of occlusion. Multifocal bilateral renal infarcts noted. Patient tested APLA positive **(Figs. 1A to G)**.

DISCUSSION

Leriche syndrome (LS), also called as aortoiliac occlusive disease (AIOD) is a vascular disease affecting the distal abdominal aorta, iliac arteries, and femoropopliteal vessels. It was first described in 1914 by Robert Graham, but the symptom triad was documented as a syndrome by Henri Leriche, a French surgeon. The triad of clinical symptoms and signs include claudication, erectile dysfunction and decreased distal pulses,[1] classically described in male patients. Herein we report a case of aortoiliac occlusive disease in a female patient.

AIOD, based on the extent and location, is classified into three types.

- Type I: Confined to the distal abdominal aorta and common iliac arteries
- Type II: Predominately distal abdominal aorta with disease extension into common iliac and external iliac arteries and
- Type III: Affecting the aortoiliac segment and femoropopliteal vessels.

Hence, Leriche syndrome can be seen in four variations: a) the primary iliac stenosis, b) the aortic bifurcation stenosis involving only the aortic termination and the origin of the primary iliac, c) the abdominal aorta and iliac stenosis (as in our case), d) complete stenosis of the infrarenal aorta.[1,2]

CT angiography of the abdomen and the lower extremities is the modality of choice for assessing the arteries. It is useful in the management and planning of surgery. Leriche syndrome is associated with other diseases like pancreatic, colon malignancies and can also present with multisystem infarction,[2] as it's in our case with renal infarction. While Leriche syndrome is typically a chronic disease process however, acute cases have also been reported. Concomitant pulmonary embolism and myocardial infarctions were also reported.[2]

The development of systemic and visceral vessels collaterals is an important compensation in this disease process. The patency of the external iliac arteries is reconstituted by the most common systemic pathway which collects flow from iliolumbar, lumbar, sacral, and inferior epigastric artery to supply the ascending branches of the deep circumflex iliac arteries. The visceral pathway helps in shifting the flow from the distal SMA to the branches of the IMA. Sometimes the internal iliac artery is supplied by the development of collaterals from the superior mesenteric artery which may also anastomose with rectal plexus.[3]

REFERENCES

1. Brown KN, Muco E, Gonzalez L. Leriche Syndrome. [Updated 2023 Feb 13]. In: StatPearls [Internet]. Treasure Island (FL): StatPearls Publishing; 2024 Jan-. Available from: https://www.ncbi.nlm.nih.gov/books/NBK538248.
2. Marak JR, Narayan S, Lal NR, et al. Leriche syndrome: Clinical and diagnostic approach of a rare infrarenal aortoiliac occlusive disease Radiol case series. 2024;19(2):540-6.
3. Morotti A, Busso M, Cinardo P, et al. When collateral vessels matter: asymptomatic Leriche syndrome Clin Case Rep. 2015;3 (11):960-1.

25 Isolated Renal Mucormycosis

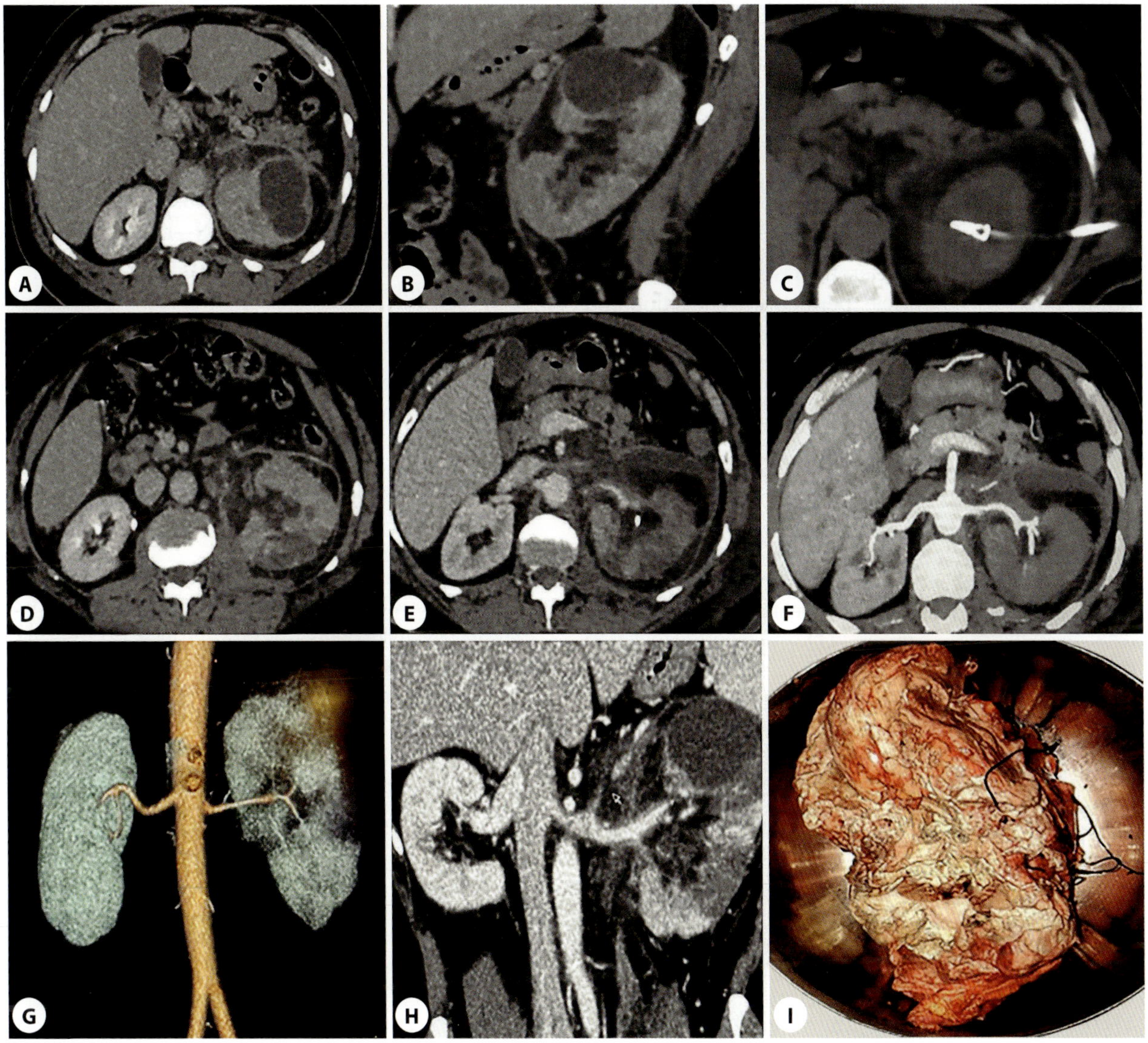

CLINICAL BACKGROUND

A 55-year-old male patient presented with fever and left loin pain. Not a known diabetic or immunocompromised.

IMAGING FINDINGS

Enlarged and edematous left kidney with striated nephrogram and upper pole collection showing peripheral post contrast enhancement consistent with left pyelonephritis and abscess. CT guided pig tail was placed and DJ stenting was also done. Urteroscopic sample showed suspicious fungal components on HPE. Patient underwent nephrectomy as there was no clinical improvement on medical management **(Figs. 1A to I)**.

DISCUSSION

Renal mucormycosis (RM), although has been reported in up to 20–22% of the cases with disseminated forms—isolated RM is a rare presentation of invasive mucormycosis with a high mortality rate. Fever, flank pain, and oliguria are the most common yet nonspecific clinical symptoms. Isolated renal mucormycosis (IRM) is reported rarely in the literature and mainly as unilateral. The early diagnosis of RM is crucial.[1,2]

Imaging findings of IRM on contrast-enhanced CT of the abdomen include enlargement of the kidneys with or without abscess, multiple low attenuations and non-enhancing areas in the parenchyma (infarcts), reduced or absent contrast excretion and rarely hydroureteronephrosis. The CECT imaging findings are referred as 'diffuse patchy nephrogram'. The characteristic extra renal findings on CECT include thickening of Gerota's fascia, perinephric fat stranding, bulky psoas muscle, perinephric collection and reactive pleural effusion. Patchy/decreased enhancement in the adjacent organs such as the spleen, colon, and pancreas, suggest the invasive nature of the disease.[3]

Mucormycosis is known for angioinvasion which may result in bilateral renal artery thrombosis. Even though main renal artery/vein can be involved it's the segmental branches more commonly affected resulting in intra renal segmental infarcts.[4] In all these cases, the antifungal drug may not reach the targeted site compromising its efficacy.[5] MRI findings include T1 and T2 hypointense areas (unlike T2 hyperintense areas in other pyelonephritis) with diffusion restriction. The T2 hypointensity is due to fungal components which exhibit paramagnetic effect (due to iron) and the infarcted tissues show diffusion restriction.[4]

Even in a case of disseminated mucormycosis involvement of kidney is not a common finding. However, in the presence of suspicious radiologic findings, a biopsy is indicated to confirm the diagnosis as IRM can also clinically masquerade as RPGN—rapidly progressive glomerulonephritis, pyelonephritis, renal abscess and acute interstitial nephritis. Hence, even in immunocompetent patients, nonresolving pyelonephritis should prompt the possibility of a fungal infection. Hence, urine specimens and blood cultures for fungal hyphae should be strongly considered to make an early diagnosis.[2,5]

REFERENCES

1. Didehdar M, Chegini Z, Khoshbayan A, et al. Clinical presentations, diagnosis, management, and outcomes of renal mucormycosis: An overview of case reports. Front Med (Lausanne). 2022;9:983612.
2. Dharmendra Bhadauria, Praveen Etta, Anand Chelappan, et al. Isolated bilateral renal mucormycosis in apparently immunocompetent patients—a case series from India and review of the literature, Clinical Kidney Journal. 2018; 6: 769-76.
3. Devana SK, Gupta VG, Mavuduru RS, et al. Isolated Renal Mucormycosis in Immunocompetent Hosts: Clinical Spectrum and Management Approach. Am J Trop Med. 2019;100(4):791-7.
4. Madhumitha B, Ganesh R, Karunakaran N, et al. Post-Covid Renal Mucormycosis: A Case Report: J Gastrointestinal Abdominal Radiol ISGAR 2022;5:70-4.
5. Saneesh PS, Yelamanchi R, Pilllai S. Isolated renal mucormycosis presenting with bilateral renal artery thrombosis: a case report. Afr J Urol. 2021;27(1):86.

26 Bilateral Endometriotic Cysts with Possible Rupture on Right Side

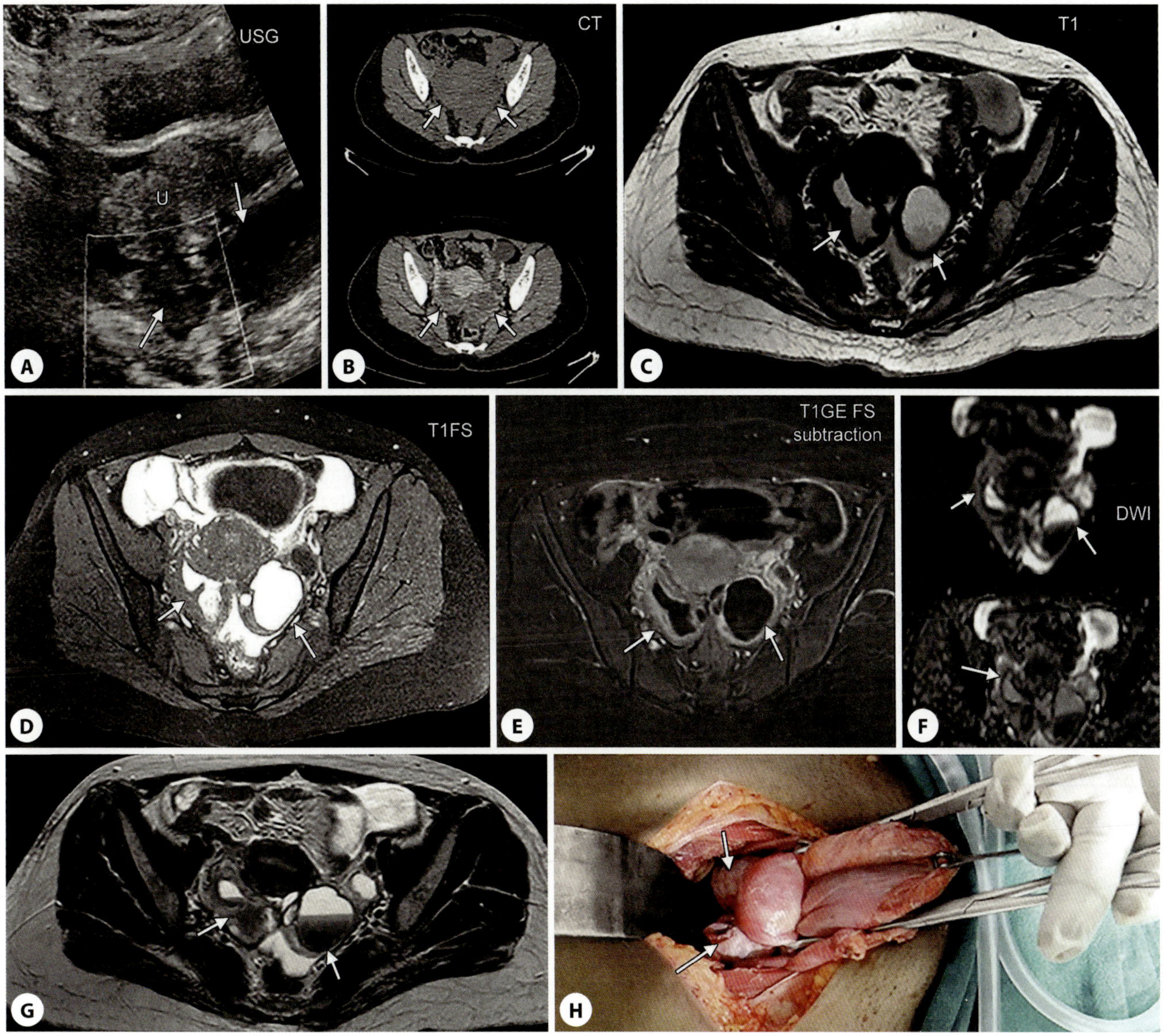

CLINICAL BACKGROUND

A 28-years-old-female patient with complaints of lower abdomen pain and irregular menstrual cycle and elevated CA 125.

IMAGING FINDINGS

Well defined thick walled cystic lesions with septations and low level internal echoes in bilateral adnexa. No demonstrable vascularity or mural nodule. The lesions show peripheral enhancement in CECT abdomen. No evidence of calcification or fat components. Mild free fluid in pelvis. Both ovaries are seen in close proximity to each other, posterior to uterus, ('Kissing ovaries') and show multiple T1/T2 hyperintense cysts. Low ADC without diffusion restriction seen. Internal T2 hypointense areas seen ('T2 shading') with fluid-fluid level. On T1 fat-sat, the cysts appear hyperintense (implying absent fat component). T1 Fat-sat post-contrast subtraction image shows peripheral enhancement of cysts without any enhancing mural nodule **(Figs. 1A to H)**.

DISCUSSION

Endometriosis is defined as the presence of ectopic endometrial tissue outside the uterine cavity. Rokitansky described endometriosis, for the first time, almost 150 years back. However, it was John A Sampson who provided an insight into the pathogenesis of this disease with his 'theory of retrograde menstruation'. It is a benign condition commonly observed in women of reproductive age group. Ovaries are the most common site. Endometrioma, also called as chocolate cyst or endometriotic cyst, is a localized form of the disease occurring in ovaries.[1]

MR plays an important role in the evaluation of complex indeterminate cystic ovary lesions. The characteristic T1 hyperintensity in cysts is seen in hemorrhagic cyst, endometriotic cyst, dermoid cyst and mucinous tumors. Fat saturation differentiates the dermoid and other fat containing cystic lesions from other T1 hyper-intense cysts, as they become hypointense on T1 fat-sat. "T2 shading sign" is a more specific sign for endometriosis. This T2 signal loss is due to high concentration of protein and iron within the endometrioma resulting from recurrent hemorrhage. Hemorrhagic cyst, although appear hyper-intense on T1, T2 shading is unlikely as there is no recurrent bleed within it. Endometriotic cyst can have low ADC values, due to 'T2 blackout' effects without diffusion restriction as seen in Tubo-ovarian abscess. 'Kissing ovaries' indicate pelvic adhesion associated with severe form of the disease.[2]

Of importance, endometriosis predisposes to clear cell and endometrioid sub-types of epithelial ovarian neoplasms. An estimated 2.5% of women with endometriosis develop ovarian cancer. Endometriosis, by itself, is one of the several benign causes of an elevated CA 125 levels (864 IU/mL). The role of imaging is not only to diagnose this condition but also to rule out extension and to exclude malignancy. Although wall thickness and thickness of septa are not very specific signs to exclude malignancy, absence of thick, irregular wall, thick septa; papillary projections; and large soft-tissue component with necrosis in combination can conclusively exclude malignancy in most cases with the help of contrast MRI.[3]

REFERENCES

1. Acién P, Velasco I. Endometriosis: a disease that remains enigmatic. ISRN Obstet Gynecol. 2013;17;2013.
2. Wasnik AP, Menias CO, Platt JF, Lalchandani UR, Bedi DG, Elsayes KM. Multimodality imaging of ovarian cystic lesions: Review with an imaging based algorithmic approach. World J Radiol. 2013;28;5(3):113-25.
3. Wei JJ, William J, Bulun S. Endometriosis and ovarian cancer: a review of clinical, pathologic, and molecular aspects. Int J Gynecol Pathol. 2011;30(6):553-68.

27 Giant Cell Tumor with Hemorrhage or Secondary Aneurysmal Bone Cyst Component

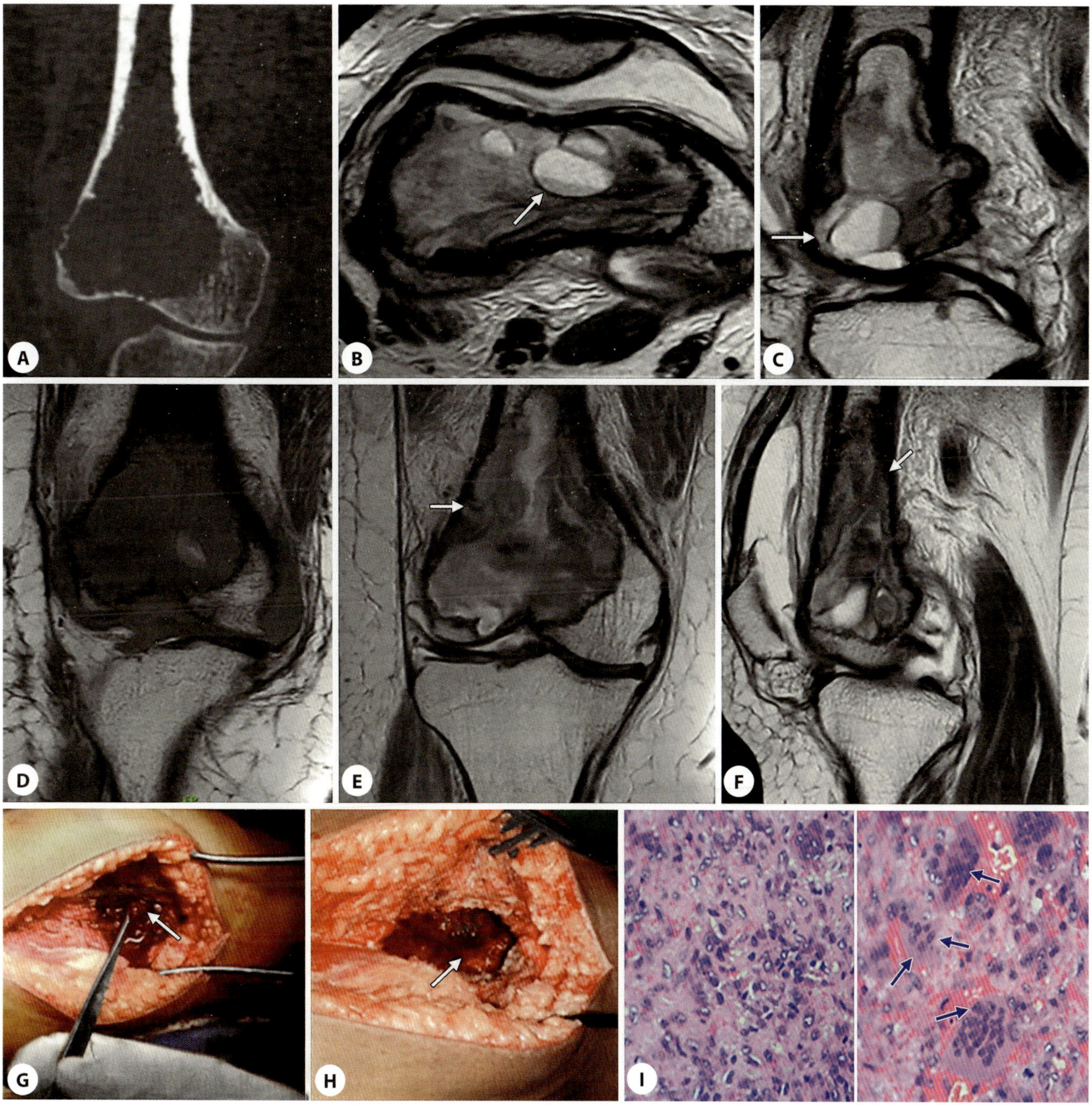

CLINICAL BACKGROUND

A 43-year-old female patient presented with acute knee pain. No history of trauma or fever.

IMAGING FINDINGS

Subarticular well defined eccentric lesion with narrow zone of transition and nonsclerotic margin. Note made of severe cortical thinning. T2 weighted MRI shows lesion showing heterogeneous hyperintense signals. Few fluid-fluid levels are noted in T2 weighted MRI corresponding with T1 hyperintense signals. Intraoperative images show highly vascular appearance of the lesion with clots. Histopathology confirmed GCT with possible ABC component **(Figs. 1A to I)**.

DISCUSSION

Giant cell tumor (GCT) of bone is generally a benign tumor composed of mononuclear stromal cells and characteristic multi nucleated giant cells that exhibit osteoclastic activity. It was first described by Cooper and Travers. Despite being categorized as a benign lesion, GCT may be locally aggressive and recur after surgical resection. GCT typically presents as a lytic lesion with well-defined and non-sclerotic margin, at eccentric location in patients with closed physes. It may also have aggressive features, such as a wide zone of transition, cortical thinning, expansile remodelling, or even cortical bone destruction and an associated soft-tissue mass.[1]

Campanacci et al. classified the GCT into three grades depending on their radiographic appearance:

- *Grade 1 lesion (latent):* Well-defined margin and an intact cortex;
- *Grade 2 lesion (active):* Relatively well-defined margin but no radiopaque rim, and the cortex is thinned and moderately expanded;
- *Grade 3 lesion (aggressive)* has indistinct borders and cortical destruction.

Enneking et al. proposed a clinico-radiological classification of three stages for benign bone tumors including GCT:

- Stage 1 (latent) refers to a confined totally by bone, asymptomatic, inactive on bone scan, histologically benign lesion;
- Stage 2 (active) refers to an expanded cortex with no breakthrough, symptomatic (often with a pathologic fracture), active on bone scan, histologically benign lesion;
- Stage 3 (aggressive) refers to a rapidly growing mass, cortical perforation with soft tissue mass, may metastasize, symptomatic, extensive activity on bone scan, histologically benign; stage 4 (malignant) refers to a sarcomatous lesion contiguous with a benign GCT.

The Campanacci grading system for GCT is similar to that proposed by Enneking for benign bone tumors overall.[2]

Uncommon manifestation in GCT include secondary ABC formation, benign lung metastases and rarely malignant transformation. Secondary aneurysmal bone cyst (ABC) formation (As in our case) is relatively more common among all three, that has been reported in up to 14% of cases presenting with fluid fluid levels. The differential diagnosis for GCT in children include chondroblastoma which is also an epiphyseal lesion. Fluid-fluid levels can be seen in both of these conditions, although presence of extensive surrounding soft-tissue and marrow edema at MR imaging may help to differentiate chondroblastoma from GCT. Chondroblastoma may also demonstrate a sclerotic margin and central calcification with a typical "rings-and-arcs" pattern.

Fluid-fluid levels can be seen in both primary ABC and GCT with secondary ABC. Presence of soft tissue component, which is seen in later, is used to differentiate above two conditions. Sometimes, hemorrhage within cystic spaces of a GCT can also lead to the fluid-fluid level within it and becomes difficult to differentiate. Telangiectasia osteosarcoma is one malignant lesion which demonstrates fluid-fluid levels at MRI.[1,2]

REFERENCES

1. Chakarun CJ, Forrester DM, Gottsegen CJ, et al. Giant Cell Tumor of Bone: Review, Mimics, and New Developments in Treatment. RadioGraphics 2013;33:1:197-211.
2. Mavrogenis AF, Igoumenou VG, Megaloikonomos PD, et al. Giant cell tumor of bone revisited. SICOT J. 2017;3:54.

28

Intraventricular Tuberculoma with Paradoxical Reaction

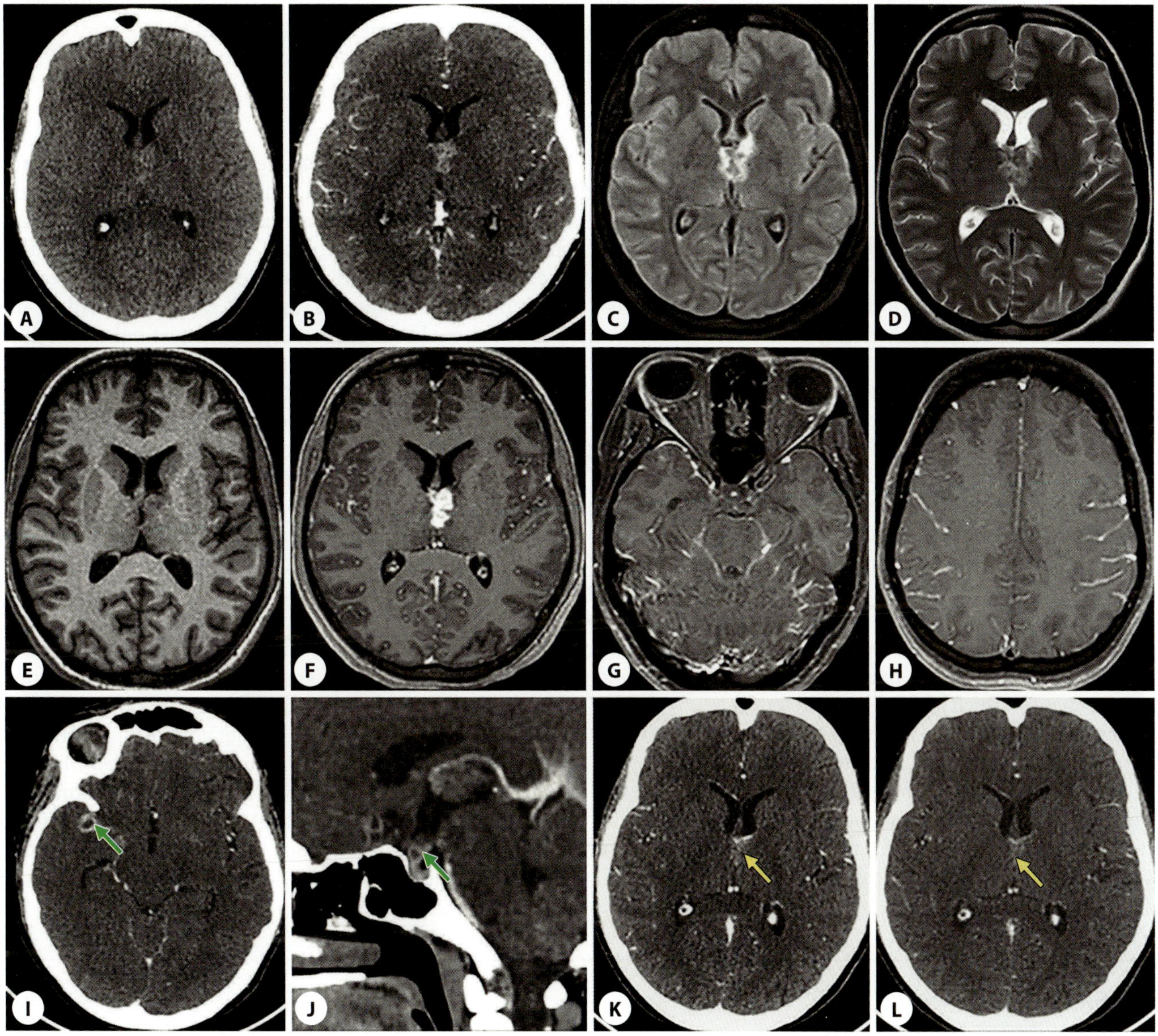

CLINICAL BACKGROUND

A 27-year-old female came with complaints of headache for past 10 days, history of fever for past 10 days, history of giddiness and vomiting for past 7 days.

IMAGING FINDINGS

Slightly hyperattenuating lesion in the region of inter ventricular foramen/roof of third ventricle showing enhancement on post CECT. No hydrocephalus. Well defined T2 hypo-intense and FLAIR hetero-intense lesion with mild surrounding edema noted. The lesion is iso to hypo-intense on T1 and conglomerate ring enhancement on post contrast T1 MRI. MRS shows lipid peak. Thickening and abnormal leptomeningeal enhancement along with basal cistern enhancement notedon postcontrast T1 MRI. Follow up CECT show regression in intensity of enhancement of the lesion following anti-TB drug treatment (yellow arrows). However, new enhancing lesion on right temporal region and in pituitary stalk (green arrows) paradoxical reaction likely **(Figs 1A to L)**.

DISCUSSION

CNS tuberculosis, though rare is not very uncommon. There are various manifestations of CNS TB which includes meningitis, tuberculoma, cerebritis, abscess etc. Tuberculoma can be staged into four groups based on stages of infection. This includes non caseating granuloma, caseating granuloma, caseating granuloma with central liquefaction and calcified granuloma.[1]

The intra-ventricular location of tuberculoma is rare and that in third ventricle is extremely rare, only one case reported in literature so far. The correct diagnosis is vital to avoid unnecessary surgical intervention especially when the size of the lesion is less than 2.5 cm and without hydrocephalus at the time of presentation. In our case, the case was referred as intraventricular hemorrhage as it was hyper-dense on plain CT. However, post contrast CT demonstrated significant enhancement of the lesion ruling out hemorrhage. The differential diagnoses include ependymoma, subependymoma, central neurocytoma, meningioma and granulomas for which MRI was considered.[2,3]

Ependymoma and subependymoma are relatively common in fourth ventricle, although they can occur at supra-tentorial location. They appear hyper-intense on T2 with areas of calcification and bleed giving heterogeneous appearance and areas of blooming on GRE. Central neurocytoma can typically mimic our case, as they are generally hyper-attenuating on CT. Punctuate calcifications are common. But they have multiple cystic areas on T2/FLAIR giving bubbly appearance. Choline and glycine peak are reported on MRS. Intraventricular meningioma though rare is also a possible differential diagnosis. These tumors appear hyper-attenuating on CT and show homogeneous post contrast enhancement. Alanine peak is noted on MRS at 1.4 ppm and a distinct peak at 3.8 ppm is also reported in literature.[2]

Among granulomatous lesions TB and NCC are the common differential diagnoses. Eccentric T2 hypo-intense scolex are characteristic for NCC. NCC is often distributed diffusely with milder perilesional edema whereas, edema is comparatively larger for TB. Cyst with dot sign is very specific for vesicular stage of NCC. TB caseating granuloma and caseating granuloma with central liquefaction are T2 hypo-intense, but the presence of T1 hyper-intense rim is specific for former and central T2 hypo-intense area is specific for the later. Presence of meningitis and basal exudates, as in our case, can give additional clues for TB infection as tuberculoma and meningitis often co-exist in 10–50% cases. Medical treatment with ATT can be considered in small lesions and in absence of hydrocephalus. ATT should be continued despite paradoxical reactions as these reactions do not warrant cessation of ATT.[3,4]

REFERENCES

1. Taheri MS, Karimi MA, Haghighatkhah H, et al. "Central Nervous System Tuberculosis: An Imaging-Focused Review of a Reemerging Disease", Radiology Research and Practice. 2015:1-8.
2. Varrassi M, Bellisari FC, De Donato MC, et al. Intracranial ependymomas: The role of advanced neuroimaging in diagnosis and management. Neuroradiol J. 2021;34(2):80-92.
3. Diker S, Ruso DÖ, Bayraktar N, Balyemez U. Intracranial tuberculomas or neurocysticercosis: differentiated by cervical lymph node pathology. Egypt J Neurol Psychiatr Neurosurg. 2022;58(1):117.
4. Zaki SA, Shenoy P. Paradoxical response to anti-tubercular treatment. Indian J Pharmacol. 2011;43(2):212-3.

29 Median Prostatic Cyst—Isolated Müllerian Duct Cyst

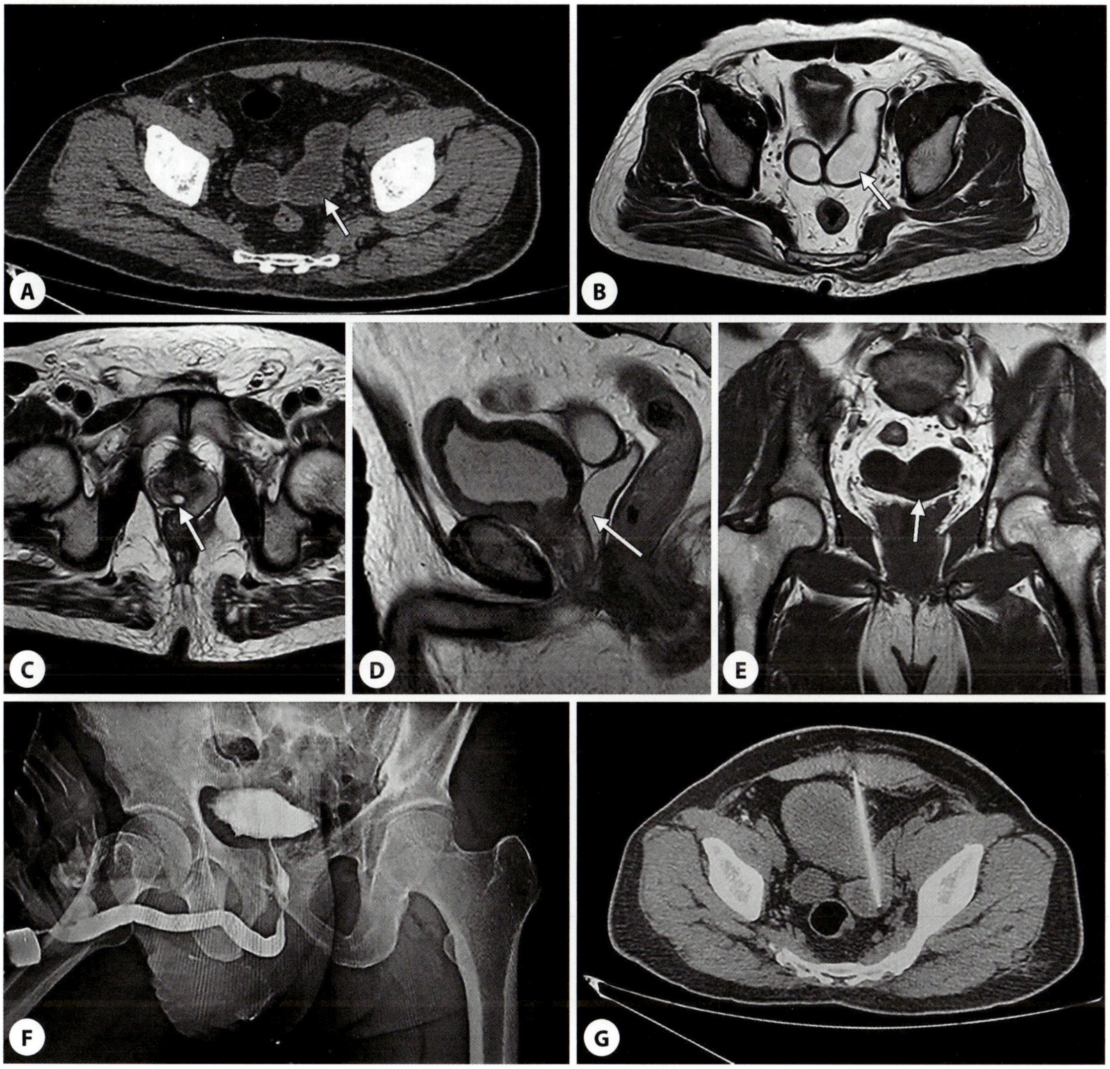

CLINICAL BACKGROUND

A 61-years-old male presented with dysuria and supra pubic tenderness.

IMAGING FINDINGS

CT shows moderate sized cystic lesion in midline pelvis possibly arising from prostrate and extending above prostatic base. Bilateral kidneys and ureters are normal. MR pelvis showing T1 hypo and T2 hyper intense lobulated cystic lesion arising from prostate at midline and extending above prostatic base. No demonstrable communication with urethra. AUG shows no communication of the cyst with urethra. CT guided aspiration performed and sent for cytology to look for spermatozoa in particular, which came as negative for spermatozoa **(Figs. 1A to G)**.

DISCUSSION

Cysts of the lower male genitourinary tract are not very common. Even though they are benign and often associated with a variety of genitourinary abnormalities. They can be classified into two main groups namely: intraprostatic cysts and extraprostatic cysts.[1]

Intraprostatic cysts can be further classified into median cysts (prostatic utricle cysts, müllerian duct cysts), paramedian cysts (ejaculatory duct cysts), and lateral cysts (prostatic retention cysts, cystic degeneration of benign prostatic hypertrophy, cysts associated with tumors, prostatic abscess). Extraprostatic cysts include cysts of the seminal vesicle, vas deferens, and Cowper duct.[1,2]

Müllerian duct cyst and prostatic utricle cysts are the two median cysts which can be sometimes difficult to differentiate on imaging. Utricle cysts are pear-shaped structures that are commonly seen under 20 years of age and communicate freely with the prostatic urethra. They are typically smaller than müllerian cyst (usually <1cm), however larger one are reported in literature known as giant utricle cysts.[3]

These prostatic utricle cysts are often associated with various GU abnormalities like hypospadias, intersex disorders, cryptorchidism, and ipsilateral renal agenesis. Müllerian duct cyst, on the other hand are associated with normal external genitalia and occasional renal agenesis. Müllerian duct cysts appear as teardrop-shaped midline cysts extending above the prostate base. Unlike utricle cyst, Müllerian duct cysts do not communicate with posterior urethra. These cysts do not contain spermatozoa, unlike the utricle cysts.[4]

To note, the importance of these two generally asymptomatic cysts is that they can get infected and result in abscess formation. Another important point to note is that incidence of malignancy is reported in both of these median cysts. Hence, prompt diagnosis based on the location and imaging findings will be key for early intervention.

REFERENCES

1. Shebel HM, Farg HM, Kolokythas O, et al. Cysts of the lower male genitourinary tract: embryologic and anatomic considerations and differential diagnosis. Radiographics. 2013;33(4):1125-43.
2. Feutry G, De Perrot T, Wirth GJ, at el. Prostatic Utricle Cyst as the Most Likely Cause in a Case of Recurrent Episodes of Hematospermia. Case Rep Urol. 2017;2017.
3. Trivedi, J, Sutherland T, Page M. Incidental findings in and around the prostate on prostate MRI: a pictorial review. Insights Imaging. 2021;12:37.
4. Priyadarshi V, Singh JP, Mishra S, et al. Prostatic utricle cyst: a clinical dilemma. APSP J Case Rep. 2013;4(2):16.

30 Meningioma En Plaque

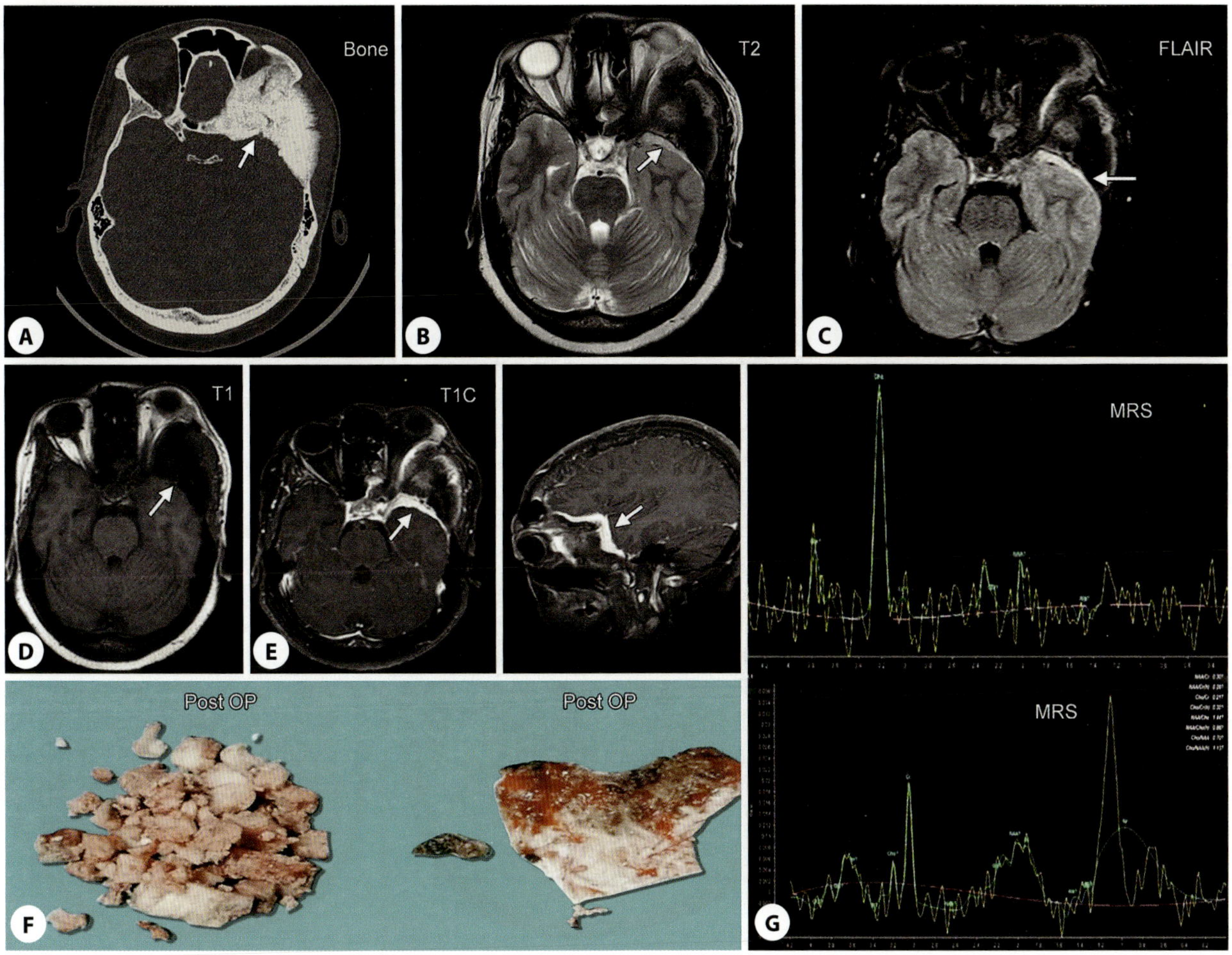

CLINICAL BACKGROUND

A 36-year-old female, history of left sided gradual onset proptosis with diplopia.

IMAGING FINDINGS

Marked hyperostosis seen in the left frontal and temporal bones, extending into sphenoid wing, superior/lateral walls of left orbit and lateral wall of posterior ethmoid and sphenoid sinus, on left side. Displacement of lateral rectus muscle and moderate degree of proptosis noted. Flat dural thickening, appearing iso-intense on T1-weighted images and iso-to-hyperintense on T2-weighted images, noted in left frontal-temporal convexity adjacent to the bone changes. Transgression across the sclerotic bone noted with extra-calvarial involvement. Indentation and compression of adjacent brain parenchyma seen. However, no demonstrable edema seen on T2/FLAIR images. The lesion shows intense and homogeneous post contrast enhancement. Elevated lipid peak (in short TE) + alanine doublet inversion at 1.4 ppm (long TE) + distinct peak at 3.8 ppm (long TE)—Noted in MRS. The intraoperative images are attached showing the dura with tumor and the excised bony components of the lesion **(Figs. 1A to G)**.

DISCUSSION

The term 'meningioma en plaque (MEP)' was coined by cushing and Eisenhardt in 1938 to differentiate these uncommon sheet-like meningiomas from the more common globular variety, 'meningioma en masse'. They constitute 2–4% of all intracranial meningiomas. Morphologically these are carpet or sheet-like lesions that grow in a radial fashion along the meninges. They tend to invade the adjacent bone resulting in bony hyperostosis which is disproportionately greater than the size of the intracranial mass itself. Hence, unlike in globular meningiomas, the bony hyperostosis in meningiomas en plaque is more likely to be secondary to tumor invasion. Although locally invasive, they usually correspond to a WHO grade I meningioma.[1]

Contrast enhanced MRI is the preferred imaging modality. En plaque meningiomas may have varied appearances, ranging from a smooth thin extra-axial mass to a highly irregular lobulated lesion. The lesion tends to grow radially or in a sheet-like manner along the dura, as described in our case above, with prominent calvarial thickening. CT is always superior to demonstrate the osseous changes. Hyperostosis of the skull associated with MEP is often confused with other hyperostosing conditions such as fibrous dysplasia (FD) and osteoma.[2]

Unlike FD, which is characterized by ground glass matrix, the hyperostosis in MEP is characterized by indolent growth and a sclerotic pattern. Periosteal hyperostosis pattern when seen in MEP can confidently differentiate this condition from FD, as periosteal new bone formation is not seen in later. Another clue is, the surface of the bony hyperostosis is irregular in MEP whereas, it is smooth in FD. In FD, the curvature of the inner table is usually preserved and the pressure effect on the adjacent brain is unusual. Osteoma usually arises from the outer table of the skull and rarely from the inner table, but as a rule, does not extend into the diploe. A biconvex appearance with inward and outward bulging has not been reported in osteoma and is characteristic of MEP. Another differential point is that osteomas do not extend across suture lines, whereas hyperostosis from MEP may do.[2–4]

Dural metastasis can appear as focal nodular dural thickening or as diffuse smooth dural thickening showing intense enhancement like meningioma on post contrast study. In such scenario MR spectroscopy could help as metastases have high choline, low NAA: creatinine ratios and high lipid: creatinine ratios without the alanine peak, which is characteristic of meningiomas, as shown in our case. Diffuse dural lymphoma cam mimic MEP, as these highly cellular neoplasms appear hyperdense on CT and show intense homogeneous post contrast enhancement. However, they show restricted diffusion more often than meningioma or metastases. MR perfusion will be also be helpful in these cases.[4]

To conclude, en plaque meningiomas are a rare flat variety of intracranial meningiomas which grow along the planes of the meninges. Their diagnosis remains difficult but should be considered when linear or lobulated enhancing dural-based mass lesion is seen with disproportionate underlying bone changes. Complete tumour excision is necessary to prevent recurrence. But most times, complete resection is impossible due to the close proximity of vital structures.

REFERENCES

1. Delgado R, Bahmad HF, Bhatia V, et al. Intraosseous meningioma mimicking osteosarcoma. Autops Case Rep. 2021;29:11.
2. Watts J, Box G, Galvin A, et al. Magnetic resonance imaging of meningiomas: a pictorial review. Insights Imaging. 201;5(1):113-22.
3. Kamaluddin NA, Samsudin AHZ, Wan Hitam WH, et al. Meningioma Mimicking Fibrous Dysplasia. Cureus. 2019;27:11(9):
4. Lyndon D, Lansley JA, Evanson J. et al. Dural masses: meningiomas and their mimics. Insights Imaging. 2019;10:11.

31 The Facet Joint Syndrome

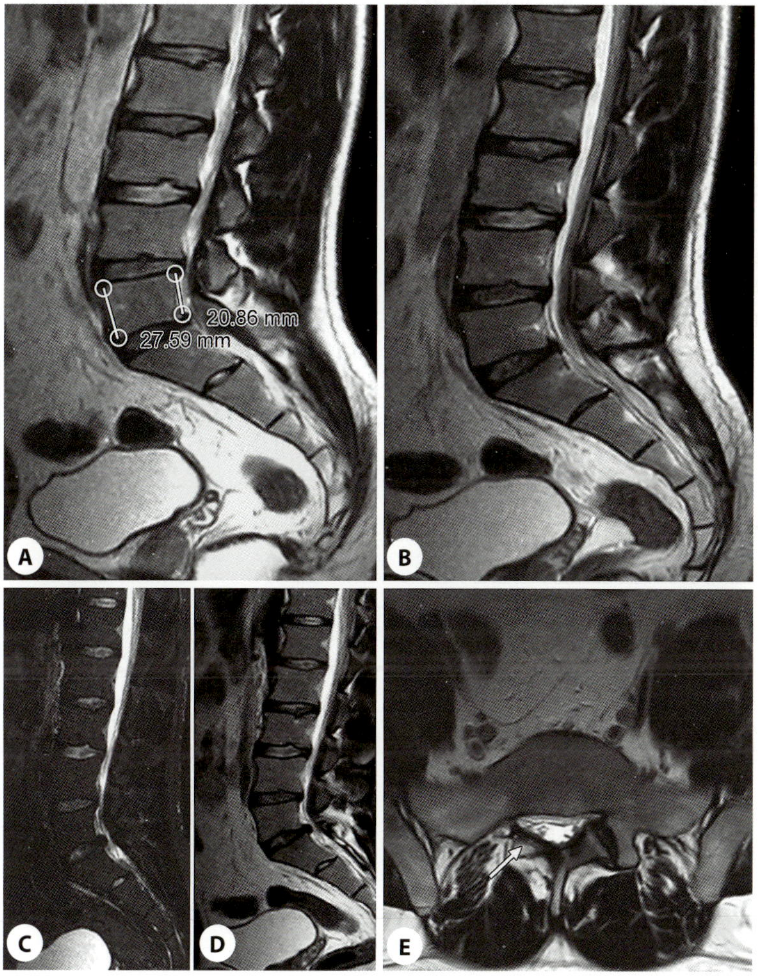

CLINICAL BACKGROUND

A 25-year-old male patient with complaints of right radicular pain.

IMAGING FINDINGS

Multi-level schmorl's nodes in lumbar spine. Characteristic hypoplasia of right inferior articulating process of L5 (white arrow) and facet joint hypoplasia. Associated disc protrusion at L5-S1 level. Also mild hypoplasia of L5 vertebra seen with posterior vertebral body height lower than the anterior vertebral body height **(Figs. 1A to E)**.

DISCUSSION

The facet joint is a true synovial joint, which has superior and inferior articulating processes arising vertically from the junction of pedicles and laminae, representing an important portion of posterior spine. Together with the intervertebral disk, they restrict vertebral movement while helping in load transmission and improving stability. CT is more accurate than MRI in the anatomic assessment of facet joints and to help distinguish bone pathologic conditions.[1]

Numerous anatomic variations and congenital anomalies in the neural arch and its process can affect the ossification process. Most of the patients are asymptomatic and these findings are incidentally noted on imaging for another cause. Some of the variations and anomalies can cause symptoms and the diagnosis is made on the imaging to rule out fracture, dislocation or degenerative changes.

Unilateral hypo-plastic facet joint is a rare cause of the chronic back pain also known as facet joint syndrome.[2]

In 1979, Frank and Miller were the first to describe hypoplasia of L5 vertebral body in patients with bilateral spondylolysis at L5, on conventional radiographs of the spine. They also noticed that not all patients with spondylolysis had anterior vertebral slippage. Therefore, they introduced the term pseudospondylolisthesis to designate the false impression of spondylolisthesis caused by the shortening of the anteroposterior diameter of L5. Another important finding was the abnormal posterior wedging of L5, which has been considered an important predictor of spondylolysis.[3]

The congenital hypoplastic facet joint and pedicle can be seen on conventional radiographs as an absent pedicle with associated abnormal enlargement of the neural foramen. Multidetector computed tomography and magnetic resonance imaging demonstrates additional findings such as small anteriorly displaced transverse process, hypoplastic pedicle and facet joint, tilt of the spinous process and contralateral facet joint or pedicle hypertrophy and sclerosis.[4] However, not all the cases will show the additional features and will present as isolated finding of unilateral hypoplastic facet joint and pedicle. If this is an isolated finding, conservative therapy is usually recommended. However, if there is associated disc herniation or canal stenosis, orthopaedic surgery should be sought if the condition is debilitating.

REFERENCES

1. Anaya JEC, Coelho SRN, Taneja AK, et al. Differential Diagnosis of Facet Joint Disorders; RadioGraphics. 2021;41:2:543-58.
2. Coskun H, Turan A, Kaplanoglu H. Frequency of Hypoplasia of the Vertebral Body at L5, and Its Relationship with Degeneration in Patients with Low Back Pain. Turk Neurosurg. 2022;32(4):641-8.
3. Wilms G, Maldague B, Parizel P, et al. Hypoplasia of L5 and wedging and pseudospondylolisthesis in patients with spondylolysis: study with MR imaging. Am J Neuroradiol. 2009;30:674-80.
4. Mellado JM, Larrosa R, Martín J, et al. Cozcolluela MR. MDCT of variations and anomalies of the neural arch and its processes: part 2—articular processes, transverse processes, and high cervical spine. AJR Am J Roentgenol. 2011;197(1):W114-21.

32 Hypervascular Liver Metastases with Possible Pancreatic or Renal Primary

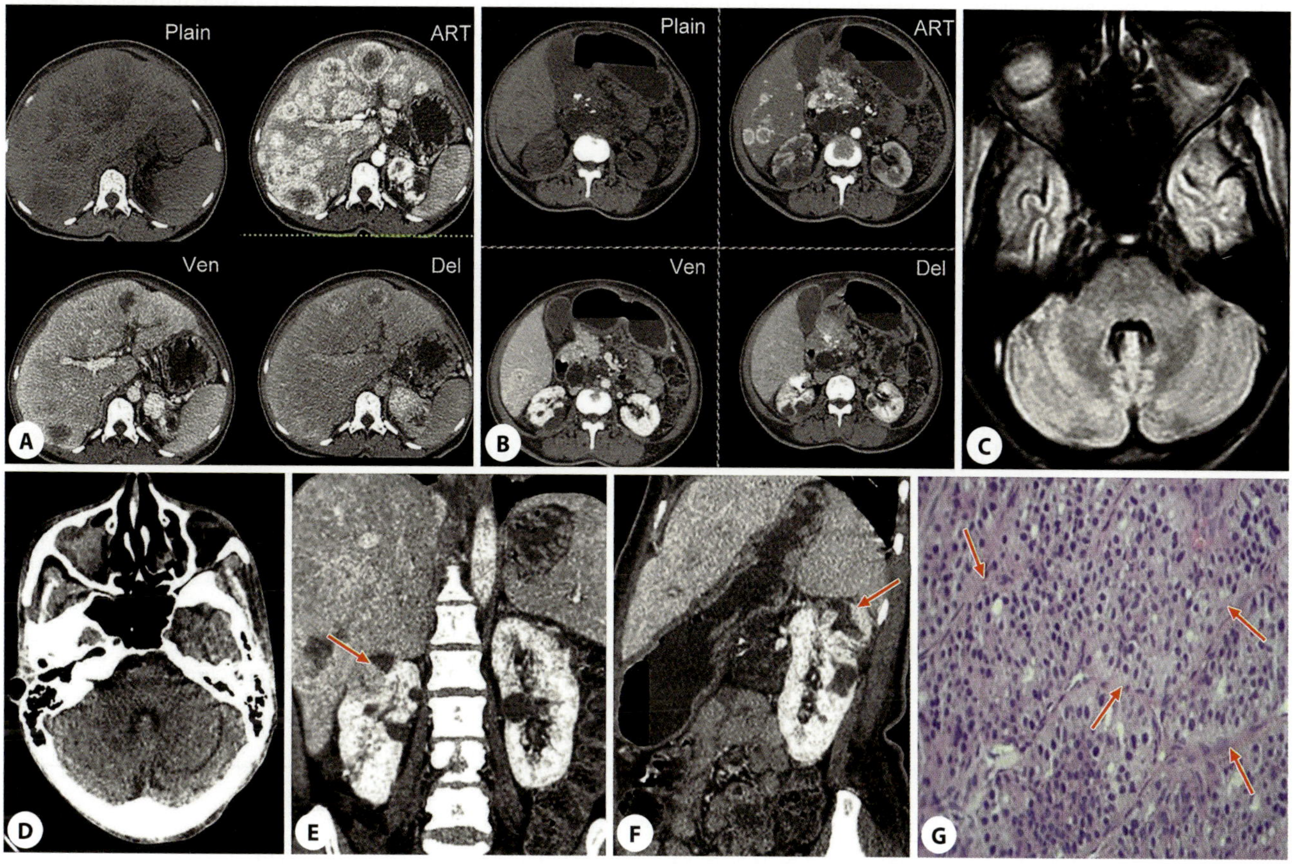

CLINICAL BACKGROUND

A 46-year-old female presented with complaints of weight loss and vague abdomen pain.

IMAGING FINDINGS

CECT shows an irregular lesion in the region of head of pancreas with calcifications and heterogeneous post contrast enhancement. CECT showing multiple arterial phase enhancing lesions without any scar or capsule on delayed images. The lesions show early washout pattern. CECT showing exophytic enhancing mass lesions in both kidneys. Plain CT brain and FLAIR show no demonstrable SOL (particularly in cerebellum). High power examination of the tumor showing back to back nodules/insular pattern of bland cells (× 400 H&E) and tumor cells without significant pleomorphism having round nucleus and moderate eosinophilic cytoplasm as indicated by red arrows. Necrosis or mitoses not seen (× 400 H&E). IHC + for CK, synaptophysin, CD56 and NSE **(Figs. 1A to G)**.

DISCUSSION

Triple phase CT used in the characterization of liver SOL is based on the principal of dual blood supply to liver. Liver gets its blood supply from both portal vein (80%) and hepatic artery (20%). The pathological lesions that derive its blood supply from the hepatic artery enhance early in the arterial phase (30–40 seconds), before the contrast reaches the portal venous system. All other hypo-vascular pathological lesions are better visualized in the portal venous phase (70–80 seconds) as hypo-dense lesions in background of enhancing liver. The third phase known as equilibrium (>180 seconds) is useful to assess the washout pattern of the lesion. The major differential diagnosis for the hypervascular lesions of liver include hemangioma, Focal nodular hyperplasia, adenoma, hepatocellular carcinoma and metastasis (especially from neuroendocrine tumor, sarcoma, renal cell carcinoma, breast malignancy and melanoma).[1,2]

Hemangioma is one of the most common liver SOL. It shows characteristic peripheral discontinuous nodular enhancement with progressive centripetal fill-in and matches blood pool in all phases. Of exception, is flash filling hemangioma which shows intense uniform enhancement in arterial phase and matches blood pool in all other phases. Focal nodular hyperplasia (FNH) is another benign hyper-vascular liver lesion. Typical FNH is characterized by its classical T2 hyper-intense central scar. Central scar can also be seen in fibrolamellar carcinoma (FLC), hemangioma, HCC and cholangio-carcinoma. However, the scar appears hypo-intense on both T1 and T2 in these lesions. Even though hyper-vascular lesions show enhancement in arterial phase, the scar tissue shows enhancement only on delayed phase.[2-4]

The other characteristic feature to look for is the capsule which is commonly seen in hepatic adenoma and HCC. Hepatic adenoma (common in patients on OCP or steroids) is characterized by thin capsule with subcapsular feeding vessels. Both HCC and adenoma can have fat and hemorrhagic components within it. Any enhancing lesion in the background of liver cirrhosis is considered as HCC unless proved otherwise.[4]

Hypervascular metastases are common with neuroendocrine tumor and other primary malignancies as stated above. These lesions show arterial phase enhancement with early washout pattern. The scar or capsule is not seen unlike in HCC. Ultrasound guided liver biopsy was performed from the lesion and histopathology confirmed the diagnosis of neuroendocrine metastases.[4]

Double malignancy (bilateral RCC and pancreatic neuroendocrine tumor) is not very common, as it highlights the rare occurrence, as it's in our case. Either a coincidence or syndromic association (like von Hippel-Lindau disease) is possible. CT brain however did not show hemangioblastoma in our case probably excluding the possibility of VHL. However, as the causative mutation can be detected by genetic tests in the most VHL cases and the surveillance outcome tends to be favourable, genetic examinations are advised in all suspected cases.

REFERENCES

1. Boas FE, Kamaya A, Do B, et al. Classification of hypervascular liver lesions based on hepatic artery and portal vein blood supply coefficients calculated from triphasic CT scans. J Digit Imaging. 2015;28(2):213-23.
2. Amico EC, Alves JR, Souza DLB, et al. Hypervascular Liver Lesions in Radiologically Normal Liver. Arq Bras Cir Dig. 2017;30(1):21-6.
3. Karahasanoglu R, Otcu H, Selcuk T, et al. Focal nodular hyperplasia vs. hemangioma: computed tomography and magnetic resonance imaging findings. Ann Hepatol. 2011;10(2):218-20.
4. Heiken JP. Distinguishing benign from malignant liver tumours. Cancer Imaging. 2007;1;7 Spec No A(Special issue A): S1-14.

33 Pott's Puffy Tumor

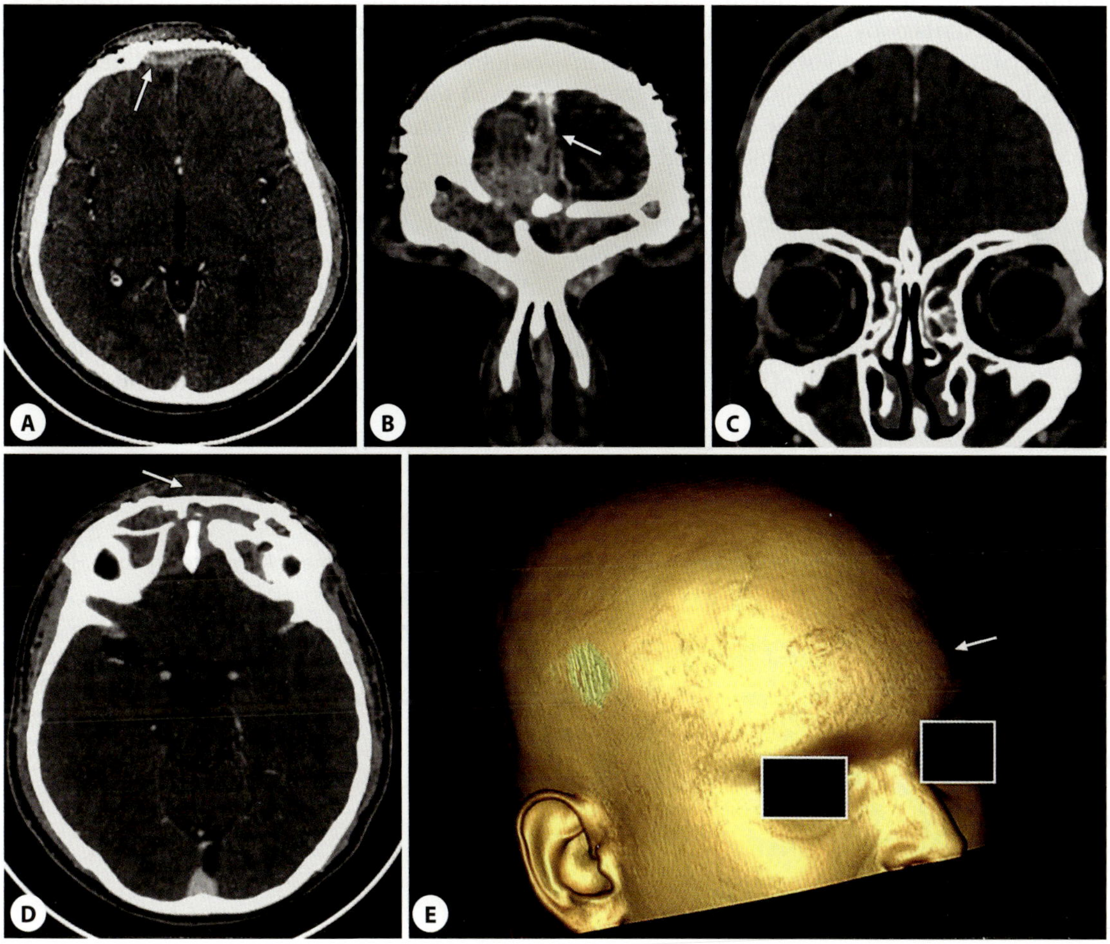

CLINICAL BACKGROUND

A 16-years-old male, post craniotomy with mesh repair. Now presented with recent onset forehead swelling and headache for 1 week.

IMAGING FINDINGS

Mild enhancing and extensive soft tissue density mucosal thickening in all paranasal sinuses. Peripherally enhancing extra axial collection of thickness 3 mm in frontal region. Associated subgaleal collection (thickness 3 mm) noted around the mesh. Filling defect seen in anterior portion of superior sagittal sinus thrombosis. No evidence of intra orbital extension or brain abscess **(Figs. 1A to E)**.

Pott's puffy tumor (likely secondary to pan-sinusitis) with associated superior sagittal sinus thrombosis and mesh infection.

DISCUSSION

Pott puffy tumor is a rare complication of sinusitis characterized by osteomyelitis of the frontal bone with subperiosteal abscess presenting as frontal swelling. This condition was first described by Sir Percival Pott in 1768 in relation to frontal head trauma. Later, it was found that this entity is more commonly related to frontal sinusitis. Initially the word "tumor" represented one of the four components of inflammation described by rubor (redness), tumor (swelling), color (warmth), and dolor (pain). The tumor in this case refers to the observable swelling of the forehead, rather than to any neoplasia. It can be found in all age groups, but occurs predominantly in adolescents.[1]

Clinical differential diagnosis for forehead swelling includes infected sebaceous cyst, benign tumors like dermoid cysts, lipomas, frontal sinus mucoceles and malignant tumors like metastases or aggressive frontal meningiomas. Clinical presentation in combination with imaging findings can easily differentiate this condition from others. Though the diagnosis of this condition is straightforward, we should be aware of this rare entity as the delay in diagnosis can lead to potential complications. Role of imaging is not only to diagnose this condition but also to exclude the complications associated with it.[2]

As venous drainage occurs through diploic veins that have communication with the dural venous sinuses, this condition can cause septic emboli and dural sinus thrombosis. Other important complications are brain abscess, subdural empyema, meningitis and orbital cellulitis. The commonly used modalities to diagnose are CT and MRI. MR is superior to CT in the demonstration of early brain parenchymal changes. However, CT can better demonstrate the bone changes and convincingly identify dural sinus thrombosis with greater sensitivity as in our case. Contrast CT can also identify the intracranial collection (as in our case) and can be a useful alternative modality in all such cases when MR is contraindicated.[3,4]

Early diagnosis and treatment of Pott puffy tumor is necessary. Broad-spectrum antibiotics for 4–6 weeks, along with surgical drainage, is the standard of care.

REFERENCES

1. Sandoval JI, De Jesus O. Pott Puffy Tumor. [Updated 2023 Aug 28]. In: StatPearls [Internet]. Treasure Island (FL): StatPearls Publishing; 2024.
2. Haider HR, Mayatepek E, Schaper J, et al. Pott's puffy tumor: a forgotten differential diagnosis of frontal swelling of the forehead. J Pediatr Surg. 2012;47(10):1919-21.
3. Germiller JA, Monin DL, Sparano AM, Tom LWC. Intracranial Complications of Sinusitis in Children and Adolescents and Their Outcomes. Arch Otolaryngol Head Neck Surg. 2006;132(9):969-76.
4. Bofares MK, Haqqar ZA, Ali IM. Pott's puffy tumor: as a very rare and unpredicted complication of ipsilateral pan sinusitis - case presentation and review of articles. Rhinology Online. 2021;4: 181-4.

34 Testicular Neoplasm—Seminoma

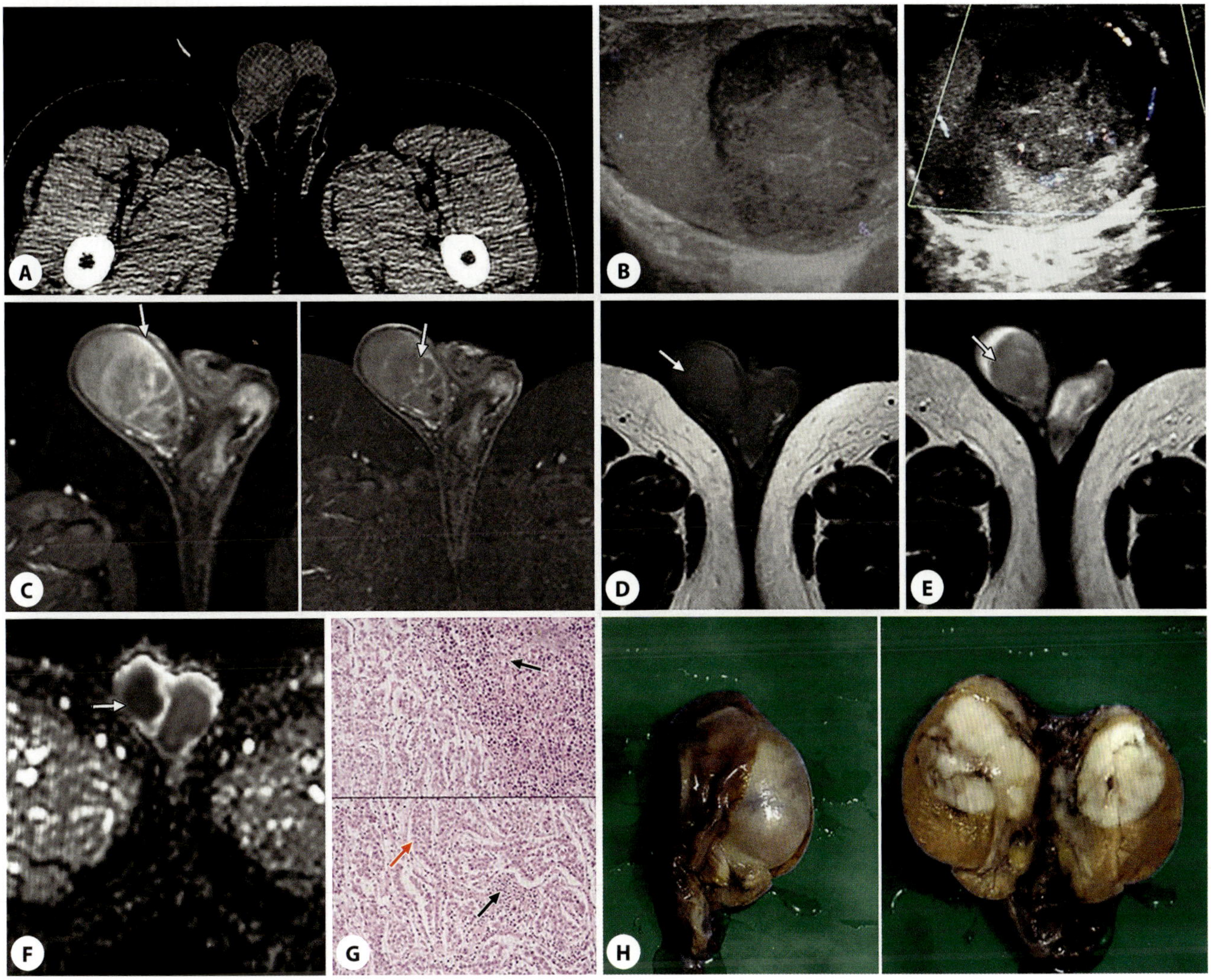

CLINICAL BACKGROUND

A 50-year-old male patient presented with palpable mass with dull aching pain in scrotum on right side. No history of trauma.

IMAGING FINDINGS

A well-defined, homogeneous, hypoechoic mass lesion with increased vascularity noted in right testis. No demonstrable calcifications or fatty components on CT. No retroperitoneal nodes. The lesion was T1 iso and T2 hyper-intense, showing significant enhancement (T1+C and subtraction images). Gross and histopathology images are shown. Histopathologic examination shows nests of tumor cells with necrosis (black arrows). Tumor cells (red arrows) with fibrous septae and mature lymphocytes (black arrows) **(Figs. 1A to H)**.

DISCUSSION

The testes are derived from three sources namely mesothelium, mesenchyme, and primordial germ cells. Mesothelial cells give rise to the tunica vaginalis, which is the serous covering of the testis. Mesenchymal cells give rise to the supporting stromal cells of the testicular interstitium, including endothelial cells and vascular smooth muscle cells. Primordial germ cells, pluripotent stem cells, is the source of most of testicular tumors. Cryptorchidism, family history, and infertility are the major risk factors for testicular cancer and seminoma is the most common testicular neoplasm. In general, intra testicular masses are generally malignant whereas, extra testicular masses are usually benign.[1]

Seminoma, the most common testicular neoplasm, is thought to arise from unipotential cell line and are usually hypo-echoic and homogeneous in US. Non-seminomatous germ cell tumors (NS-GCTs) on the other hand are heterogeneous with cystic areas and calcification more commonly seen than in former. Testicular lymphoma is difficult to differentiate from seminoma as they have similar imaging appearances but is more common in older age group (>60 years). Testicular infarction and hematoma are the common pseudomass that appear as focal hypo-echoic lesion in testes. However, absence of vascularity can differentiate these conditions from neoplasms. Adrenal rests also do appear hypo-echoic like seminoma, but they are usually bilateral and seen in patients with congenital adrenal hyperplasia.[1]

Granulomatous diseases and infections are the other common mimickers that needs to be excluded based on clinical history and presenting symptoms. Splenogonadal fusion, a rare condition—congenital fusion of the testis with ectopic splenic tissue (associated with cryptorchidism), like seminoma commonly presents as a painless mass. Central vascular pattern with vessels branching toward the periphery of lesion may be a helpful distinguishing feature. However, 99mTc sulfur colloid scans can only confirm the diagnosis as it can confirm activity in ectopic splenic tissue.[1,2]

Ultrasound (US) is the initial preferred imaging modality. US, performed with a high-frequency (7–10 MHz) transducer with pulsed and color Doppler modes, can not only differentiate the intratesticular mass from extra testicular mass but can also differentiate solid lesions (which are usually malignant) from cystic lesions (which are usually benign). Doppler is very useful to assess the vascularity of lesions and aid in diagnosis.[3]

MRI, although not first investigation of choice, is accurate for preoperative differentiation of benign from malignant testicular tumors, local staging of testicular malignant masses, and for guiding clinical decision making. Also, seminomas have enhancing fibrovascular septa which are not seen in NSGCT, and appreciated in contrast MR. NSGCT has mixed signal on T1WI and T2WI due to hemorrhagic or cystic degeneration unlike seminoma. MRI can be used as a problem solving modality and can distinguish seminoma from NSGCT based on the above imaging features.[3]

REFERENCES

1. Marko J, Wolfman DJ, Aubin AL, et al. Testicular Seminoma and Its Mimics: From the Radiologic Pathology Archives. Radiographics. 2017;37(4):1085-98.
2. Lopes RI, de Medeiros MT, Arap MA, et al. Splenogonadal fusion and testicular cancer: case report and review of the literature. Einstein (Sao Paulo). 2012;10(1):92-5.
3. Katabathina VS, Vargas-Zapata D, Monge RA, et al. Testicular Germ Cell Tumors: Classification, Pathologic Features, Imaging Findings, and Management. RadioGraphics. 2021;41:6:1698-716.

35

Focal Nodular Hyperplasia

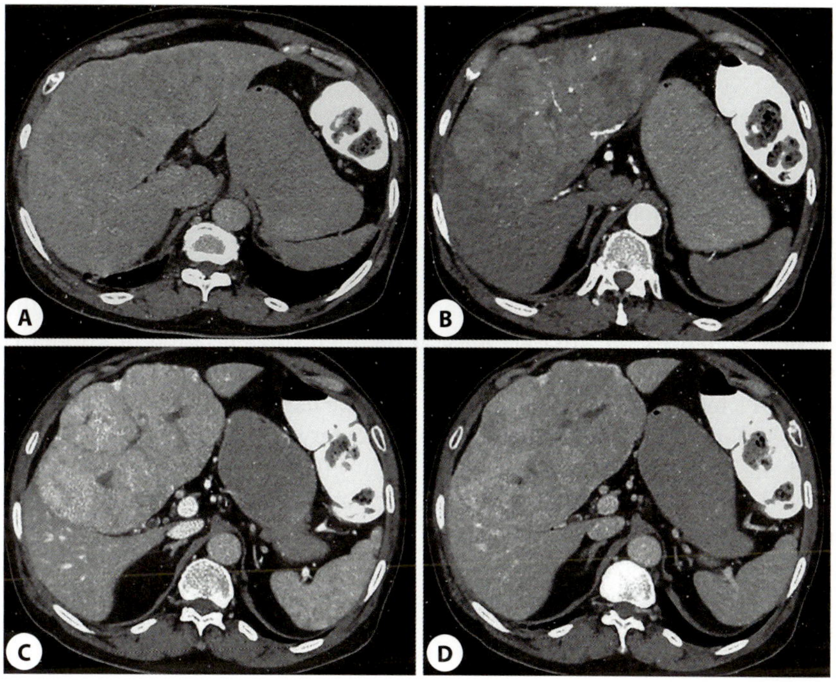

CLINICAL BACKGROUND

A 71-years-old male patient presented with no specific complaints.

IMAGING FINDINGS

Solitary well defined lobulated arterial phase enhancing lesion with non-enhancing scar noted in segment IV and V of liver, with dilated branches of hepatic arteries (Left > Right) supplying it. No demonstrable washout on portal venous phase. Lesion seen abutting the gallbladder **(Figs. 1A to D)**.

DISCUSSION

The term focal nodular hyperplasia (FNH) was coined by Edmondson in 1958 which refers to a relatively common benign hepatic tumor. Focal nodular hyperplasia is often an incidental finding that accounts for 8% of all primary liver tumors and 25% of benign ones (second most common benign tumor next to hepatic hemangioma). It is more common in females (8:1) in third/fourth decades, while FNH in males FNH are detected significantly later in life. Also to note that FNH in males display more severe morphological atypia and hence managed surgically.[1]

Multiple FNH is found to be associated with haemangiomas (23%), associated anomalies like congenital portal vein agenesis, inflammatory liver pseudotumors, hepatic vein thrombosis and intrahepatic AV shunting. FNH has also been found in association with extrahepatic pathology like cerebrovascular anomalies, sickle-cell anaemia, cystic dysplasia of kidney, Klippel–Trenaunay syndrome, cerebral meningiomas, astrocytomas, and hereditary hemorrhagic telangiectasia. Focal nodular hyperplasia has also been described in patients with glycogen-storage disease although the latter is much more frequently associated with hepatic adenomas. There have also been reports of FNH nodules adjacent to an adenoma and hydatid cyst in the same liver.[1]

On B-mode USG the FNH appearance is nonspecific and variable most of the lesion (80%) are isoechoic or mildly hypoechoic while hyperchoic nodules are less common. If the lesion is isoechoic, displacement of vascular structures may be the only sign of its presence. The central hyperchoic scar can be visualized in a limited percentage of cases (19–47%). In most cases, Doppler analysis will reveal color uptake in and around the lesion with a high peak systolic flow and low RI (0.50–0.55) differrentiating it metastatic lesion (RI > 0.70).[1]

MRI is the imaging method of choice to differentiate FNH from hepatic adenomas. FNH appears isointense to hypointense lesions on T1-weighted images and isointense to hyperintense on T2-weighted images. Similar to CT imaging, the lesion enhances on arterial phase images and is relatively obfuscated on venous and delayed phase images. The central T1 hypo and T2 hyperintense scar (due to the presence of blood vessels, bile ducts, and edema-inducing phenomena) can be identified in 50–70% of moderate-to-large- sized nodules and at a much lower percentage in small lesions (<3 cm). It also shows delayed enhancement. MRI with hepatobiliary scintigraphy is the most specific imaging modality to diagnose focal nodular hyperplasia with a sensitivity and specificity of 99% and 100%, respectively. FNH nodules, in MR contrast with superparamagnetics that are specific for Kupffer, appear isointense or mildly hyperintense in T1- weighted images whereas malignant hepatic lesions are hypointense because they lack structurally normal hepatocytes.[1,2]

Triphasic helical computed tomography with and without contrast, is a reliable imaging modality. Pre-contrast, focal nodular hyperplasia appears hypodense or isodense with a central scar evident in approximately one-third of cases. FNH appears hyperdense during the hepatic arterial phase and isodense during the portal venous phase rendering the lesion indistinguishable from the rest of the liver parenchyma.[2] The central scar remains hyperdense during the late phase due to slow wash-out of contrast medium from the myxomatous stroma that makes up the scar.

Scintigraphy with 99Tc reveals normal or increased uptake of the colloid at the level of the lesion, which reflects the high concentration of Kupffer cells in these nodules. Angiography (ideally with Lipiodol enhancement) can also be used for diagnosis of FNH. The latter study reveals a hypervascular formation with a central origin and centrifugal development. Fewer times, cytology may not be sufficient to distinguish FNH from well-differentiated HCC or Adenoma, especially in atypical variant that lack a central scar or other typical imaging findings and all those cases warrant USG guided biopsy.[1]

REFERENCES

1. Venturi A, Piscaglia F, Vidili G, et al. Diagnosis and management of hepatic focal nodular hyperplasia. J Ultrasound. 2007;10(3):116-27.
2. Hamad S, Willyard CE, Mukherjee S. Focal Nodular Hyperplasia. [Updated 2022 Sep 26]. In: StatPearls [Internet]. Treasure Island (FL): StatPearls Publishing; 2024.

36

Guillain–Barré Syndrome

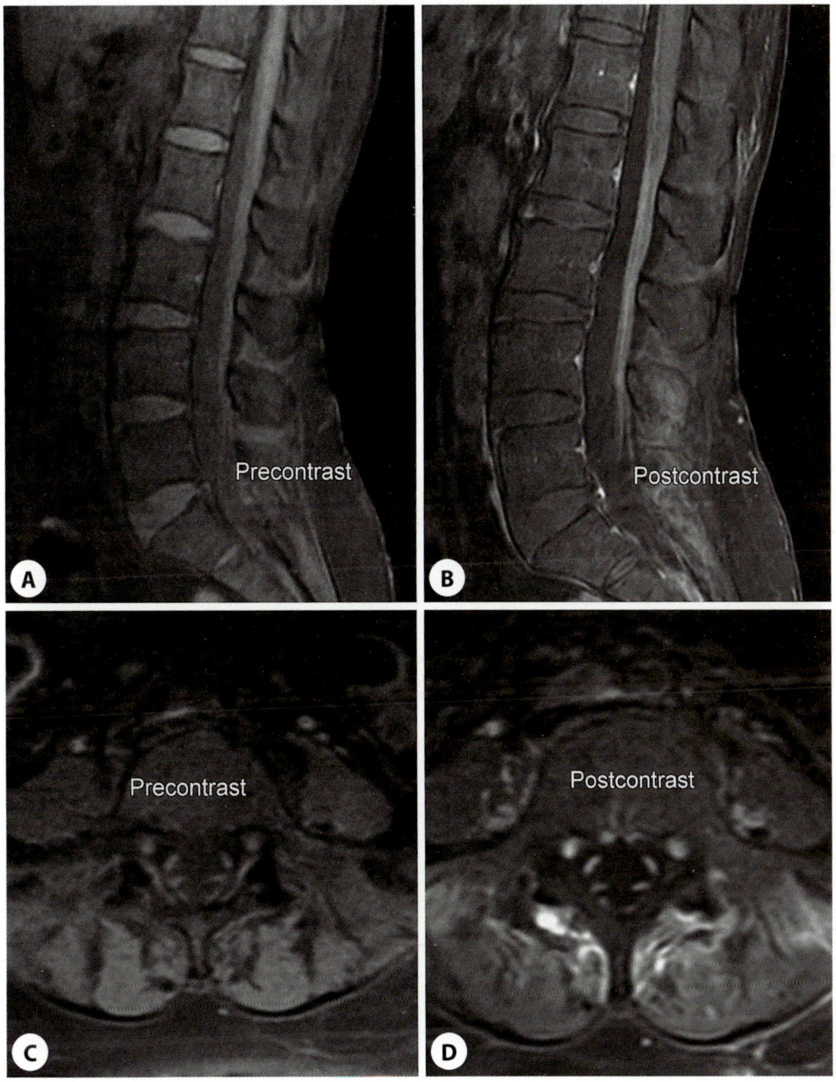

CLINICAL BACKGROUND

A 35-Year-old young female present with 1 week of fever followed by lower limb weakness.

IMAGING FINDINGS

Enhancing cauda equina nerve roots following postcontrast MRI. No disc or osseous pathology **(Figs. 1A to D)**.

DISCUSSION

Guillain–Barré syndrome (GBS) is marked by the sudden development of progressive, ascending, and symmetrical weakness in the limbs, accompanied by significantly reduced or absent reflexes. This condition is an inflammatory demyelinating polyneuropathy, characterized by its symmetrical progression, and is the most common cause of acute flaccid paralysis. Diagnosis is primarily based on clinical symptoms and physical examination, with confirmation from cerebrospinal fluid analysis (showing albuminocytologic dissociation) and electrophysiological studies. Radiological imaging is mainly used to exclude other spinal pathologies.[1]

GBS is often preceded by infections of the gastrointestinal or upper respiratory tracts, and in some cases, can be linked to vaccinations. Pathogens like *Campylobacter jejuni*, cytomegalovirus, Epstein–Barr virus, *Mycoplasma pneumoniae*, and HIV are known to trigger GBS. Recent reports also indicate a possible connection between COVID-19 infection and GBS. While the exact pathophysiology of GBS remains uncertain, immunologic responses and molecular mimicry are widely believed to play a role.[2]

In enhanced MRI, the spinal cord and nerve roots within the thecal sac usually show minimal gadolinium uptake due to the blood-nerve and blood–brain barriers. Significant enhancement of nerve roots, however, signals a breakdown in the blood-nerve barrier, which is thought to reflect the inflammatory process associated with GBS.[1,3]

Cranial nerves are involved in 30–40% of GBS cases, primarily affecting the facial and lower cranial nerves. The lower cranial nerves include CN IX, X, XI, and XII. Involvement of the abducens and trigeminal nerves is less common. It is important to note that in GBS, cranial nerve involvement can occur in addition to the more commonly affected cauda equina nerve roots in the spine.[2]

REFERENCES

1. Alkan O, Yildirim T, Tokmak N, et al. Spinal MRI findings of guillain-barré syndrome. J Radiol Case Rep. 2009;3(3):25-8.
2. Soh Y, Yoo EA, Kim ES, et al. MRI Features of Multiple Cranial Neuropathies in Guillain-Barré Syndrome Occurring after COVID-19 Vaccination: A Case Report. J Korean Soc Radiol. 2023;84(4):964-9.
3. Matsuki M, Okada N, Matsuo M. Case report: MR findings of Guillain-Barré syndrome. Radiat Med. 1998;16(2):133-5.

37

Pituitary Macroadenoma with Cavernous Sinus Invasion

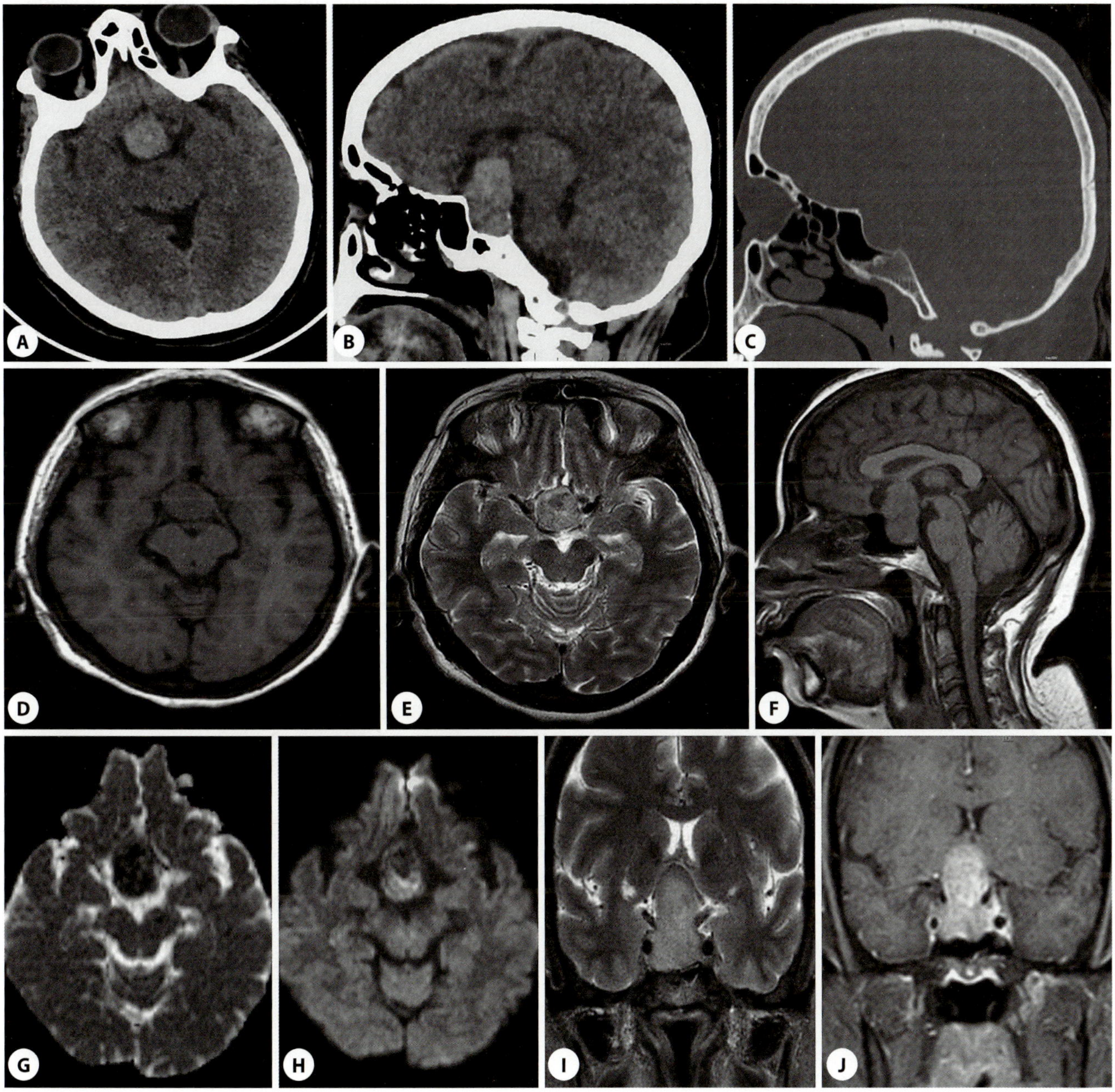

CLINICAL BACKGROUND

A 58-year-old female patient presented to the neurology OPD with complaints of headache and vomiting for past 1 month.

IMAGING FINDINGS

NCCT showed well defined iso-hyper dense lesion in sellar and suprasellar region. Bone window showed enlarged and remodeled sella turcica. No evidence of bony erosion or sphenoid sinus invasion. MRI findings-T1-isointense and T2–hyperintense well defined lesion in sellar/suprasellar region. Pituitary infundibulum not visualized separately. PPBS not seen. The lesion shows heterogeneous post contrast enhancement. The lesion causes mass effect and displacement of optic chiasm and bilateral ACA/ACOM. The lesion also causes mass effect over hypothalamus and mild abutment of third ventricle. No signs of hydrocephalus seen at present. Right grade 1 and left grade 0 cavernous sinus invasion noted **(Figs. 1A to J)**.

DISCUSSION

Pituitary tumors are the second most common type of primary central nervous system (CNS) tumors, making up a significant portion of cases across all age groups, and they are the most prevalent in adolescents and young adults. The majority of these tumors, particularly pituitary adenomas (PA), originate from the adenohypophysis, with two-thirds of them being functional (hormone-producing). Women generally present with symptoms of hyperprolactinemia earlier in life, whereas, men are typically diagnosed later, often with non-functional or non-secreting macroadenomas.[1]

Macroadenomas, which are larger than 10 mm, may also present with symptoms such as headaches and visual field impairments. When these tumors extend into the parasellar region or invade the cavernous sinus, they may cause cranial nerve palsies affecting cranial nerves III, IV, or VI. Compression of the pituitary gland or stalk can lead to hypopituitarism or even pituitary apoplexy. Factors that predispose individuals to pituitary apoplexy include hypertension, pregnancy, major surgeries, hypotension, dopamine agonist therapy, and anticoagulant use.[2]

Several classification systems are utilized to evaluate pituitary adenomas:

- Hardy's classification: Assesses the tumor in only one direction.
- Wilson's modification: A grading system useful for treatment planning with good prognostic significance.
- SIPAP classification: Based on post-contrast coronal and sagittal T1-weighted MRI images, combining elements of the Knosp, Hardy, and Wilson classifications, providing a comprehensive description of tumor growth, but not including size.

MRI is the preferred imaging modality for diagnosing pituitary macroadenomas. On MRI, these tumors typically appear isointense to gray matter on both T1-weighted and T2-weighted images. Most lesions demonstrate moderate, heterogeneous enhancement after contrast administration, although some may appear hypoenhancing. The characteristic 'snowman' appearance is due to constriction by the diaphragm sella. Cysts and necrosis are seen in approximately 15–20% of cases, while hemorrhage occurs in 10% and calcification is observed in 1–2% of cases.[3]

Post-contrast coronal MRI images are particularly useful for identifying lateral extension of pituitary macroadenomas and their relationship with adjacent parasellar structures, especially the internal carotid arteries, which are at risk during surgery. The Knosp-Steiner grading system, known for its practicality, is widely used to predict parasellar tumor growth into the cavernous sinus. Tumors with Knosp scores of 3–4 are classified as invasive pituitary adenomas. The revised Knosp classification subdivides grade 3 into two subtypes:

- Knosp 3A: Where the tumor extends above the intracavernous internal carotid artery (ICA) into the superior cavernous sinus.
- Knosp 3B: Where the tumor extends below the intracavernous ICA into the inferior cavernous sinus.[4]

In cases of ischemic pituitary apoplexy, characteristic MRI findings include an enlarged sellar or suprasellar mass with peripheral enhancement. Diffusion-weighted imaging is also helpful for identifying ischemic tissue. T1-weighted MRI often shows a lesion in the sellar/suprasellar area with high signal intensity, indicating the presence of blood. Gradient-echo sequences (T2-weighted MRI) are especially sensitive in detecting hemosiderin deposits.[5]

REFERENCES

1. Shih RY, Schroeder JW, Koeller KK. Primary Tumors of the Pituitary Gland: Radiologic-Pathologic Correlation. Radiographics 2021.
2. Anwar SSM, Hilal K, Khan A, et al. Magnetic resonance imaging grading of pituitary macroadenoma - SIPAP classification revisited. Eur J Radiol Open. 2023;10:100486.
3. Gupta K, Sahni S, Saggar K, et al. Evaluation of Clinical and Magnetic Resonance Imaging Profile of Pituitary Macroadenoma: A Prospective Study. J Nat Sci Biol Med. 2018;9(1):34-8.
4. Araujo-Castro M, Acitores Cancela A, Vior C, et al. Radiological Knosp, Revised-Knosp, and Hardy-Wilson Classifications for the Prediction of Surgical Outcomes in the Endoscopic Endonasal Surgery of Pituitary Adenomas: Study of 228 Cases. Front Oncol. 2022;11:807040.
5. Mayol Del Valle M, De Jesus O. Pituitary Apoplexy. [Updated 2023 Aug 23]. In: StatPearls [Internet]. Treasure Island (FL): StatPearls Publishing; 2024.

38 Primary Extradural (Intraosseous) Meningioma

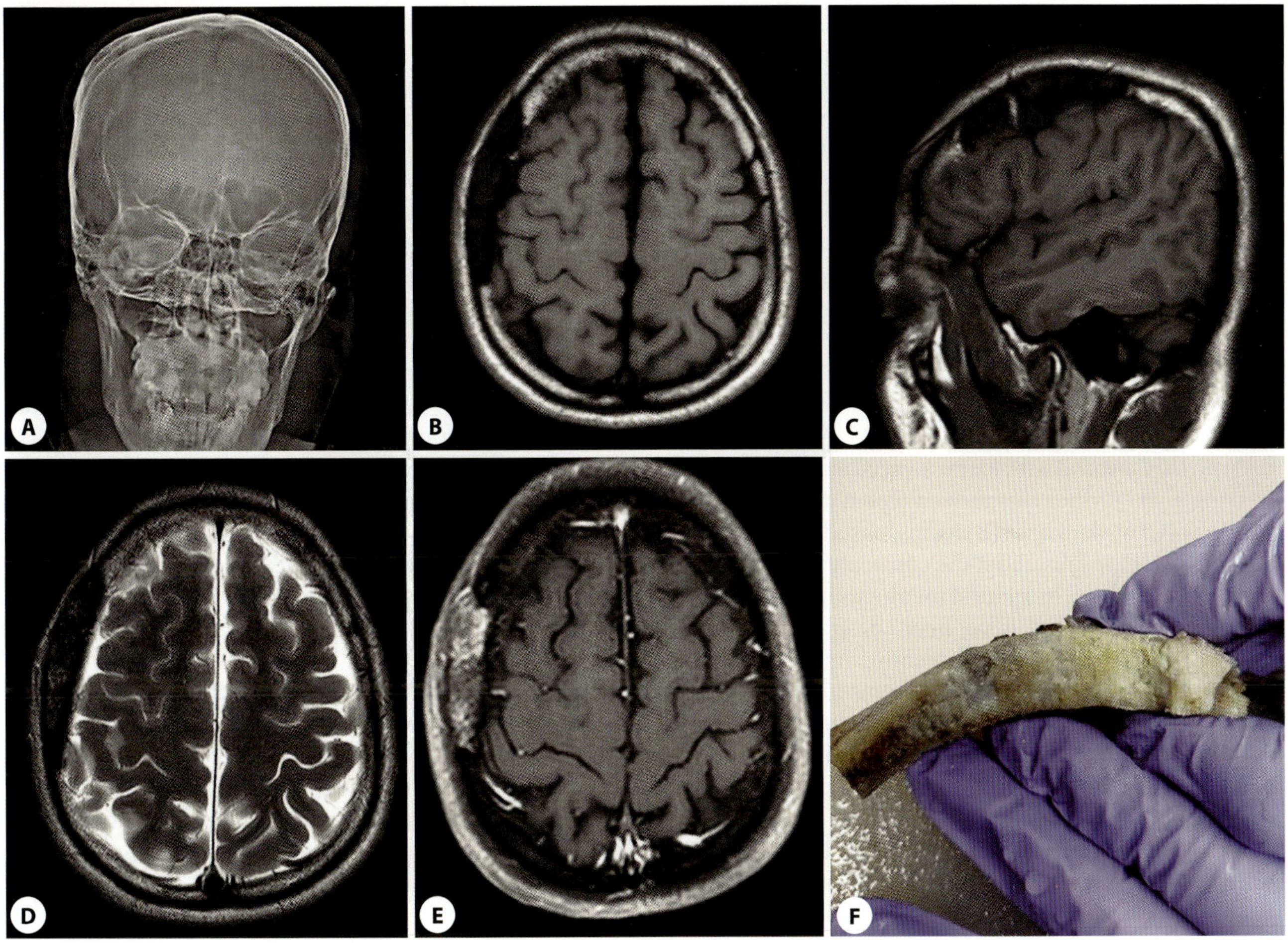

CLINICAL BACKGROUND

A 30-year-old male presented with nonspecific headache on and off for 2 weeks. Gives history of right side fronto-parietal swelling for last 10 years.

IMAGING FINDINGS

Patient taken X-ray PNS to rule out sinusitis. Incidentally detected sclerotic lesion in right side skull vault. MRI showed a T1 hypo and T2 hyperintense lesion in right fronto-partial skull vault adjacent to coronal suture with post contrast enhancement. No intracranial component. CT could not be obtained as patient denied consent and went for tumor excision. The postoperative image is shown **(Figs. 1A to F)**.

DISCUSSION

Extracranial Meningiomas: Incidence and Overview

The incidence of extracranial meningiomas is reported to be 1–2% of all meningiomas, making them rare. These meningiomas, originating outside the dura, have been labeled by various terms such as ectopic, extradural (epidural), calvarial, cutaneous, extracranial, extraneuraxial, or intraosseous meningiomas (1). Lang et al. (2) proposed the use of the term "primary extradural meningioma" to encompass all such tumors. This term emphasizes that the tumor originates outside the dural coverings of the brain or spinal cord, differentiating it from "primary intradural meningiomas," which may extend extracranially or metastasize. Tumors invading only the outer layer of the dura, with an extracranial epicenter, are classified as primary extradural meningiomas.[1,2]

Primary extradural meningiomas are classified into three types:

1. *Type I:* Purely extracalvarial
2. *Type II:* Purely calvarial
3. *Type III:* Calvarial with extracalvarial extension.

Lang et al.[3] further categorized type ii and type III into convexity (C) or skull base (B) forms, based on the tumor's location. Our case falls under the convexity type, identified as a purely calvarial, extradural meningioma.

Several hypotheses have been proposed regarding the origin of primary calvarial meningiomas. One theory suggests these tumors arise from ectopic meningocytes or arachnoid cap cells trapped in cranial sutures during birth molding, supported by their proximity to sutures. Another theory posits that meningothelial cells become trapped in sutures or fracture lines. However, only 8% of reported calvarial meningiomas were associated with cranial sutures, and only 5 out of 36 cases of primary intraosseous meningiomas had a history of head trauma in the region where the tumor later developed. In our case, no history of trauma was present.[1]

According to the literature, 68% of primary extradural meningiomas involve the calvaria. The most common locations for intraosseous meningiomas are the frontoparietal (as in this case) and orbital regions. These tumors often present as slow-growing scalp swellings, which may or may not be painful. Neurologic symptoms typically do not occur unless the lesion extends through the inner table and compresses intracranial structures. Many of these tumors are asymptomatic and found incidentally.

Although calvarial meningiomas are generally benign and slow-growing, they carry a higher risk of malignant transformation (11%) compared to intracranial meningiomas (2%).[1,2] The most common radiographic finding is hyperostosis, reported in 59% of cases, while osteolysis (35%) and a mixed presentation of hyperostosis and osteolysis (6%) have also been noted in the literature.[1] It is important to remember that osteolytic meningiomas with soft-tissue components should be considered "malignant until proven otherwise".[3,4]

Conventional radiographs are typically of limited value for diagnosing calvarial meningiomas due to overlapping bony structures. CT scans with bone windows are necessary to detect the tumor, identify cortical destruction, and assess intra- and extraosseous extension. MRI is more effective for evaluating the soft-tissue components and extradural extension of the lesion. The differential diagnosis for osteolytic intraosseous meningiomas includes metastatic cancer, plasmacytoma, giant cell tumor, hemangioma, epidermoid cyst, osteogenic sarcoma, eosinophilic granuloma, aneurysmal bone cyst, and fibrous dysplasia. In rare cases, malignant intraosseous meningioma must be ruled out when osteolytic skull lesions with soft-tissue components are observed.[1]

REFERENCES

1. Tokgoz N, Oner YA, Kaymaz M, et al. Primary intraosseous meningioma: CT and MRI appearance. AJNR Am J Neuroradiol. 2005;26(8):2053-6.
2. Lang FF, Macdonald OK, Fuller GN, et al. Primary extradural meningiomas: a report on nine cases and review of literature from the era of computerized tomography scanning. J Neurosurg. 2000;93:940-50.
3. Muthukumar N. Primary calvarial meningiomas. Br J Neurosurg. 1997;11:388-92.
4. Younis G, Sawaya R. Intracranial osteolytic malignant meningiomas appearing as soft-tissue masses. Neurosurgery. 1992;30:932.

39 Adnexal Torsion—Paraovarian Cyst

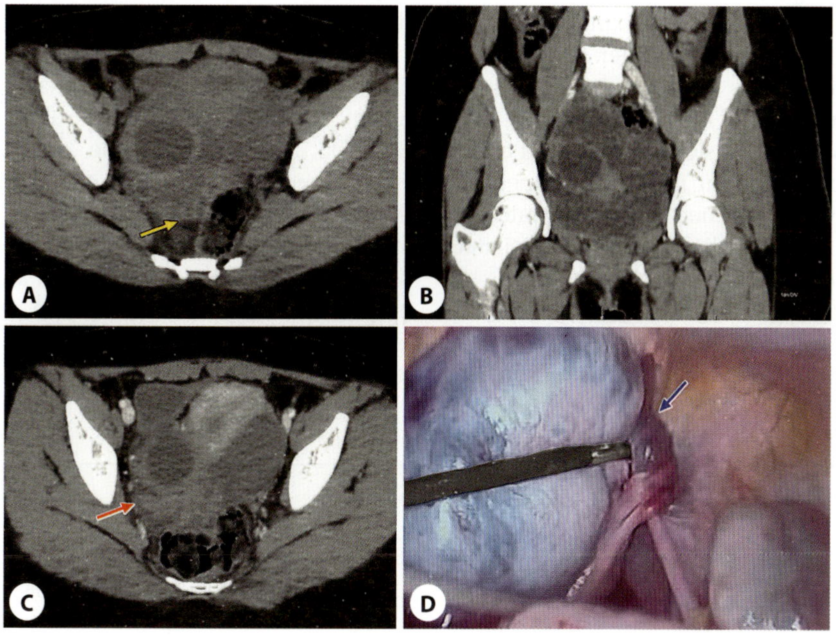

CLINICAL BACKGROUND

A 29-year-old young female with acute onset of lower abdomen pain. Previous history of left oophorectomy for ovary torsion.

IMAGING FINDINGS

Large heterodense complex cystic lesion in right adnexa, posterior to the uterus. Multiple peripherally arranged follicles seen (yellow arrow) **(Figs. 1A to D)**.

The lesion shows poor contrast enhancement on post contrast study (red arrow). Non enhancing simple cyst noted adjacent to lesion along left lateral wall. Surrounding inflammatory fat strandings. Minimal free fluid noted in pelvis. Intra-OP image is shown (blue arrow).

DISCUSSION

Adnexal Torsion: A Gynecologic Emergency

Adnexal torsion is a medical emergency in gynecology, affecting about 2–3% of females who report acute pelvic pain. This condition generally involves both the ovary and the fallopian tube, which is why "adnexal torsion" is the preferred term over "ovarian torsion." While isolated ovarian torsion, sparing the fallopian tube, can happen, it is rare due to the broad attachment of the ovary to the broad ligament. In rarer cases, torsion of the fallopian tube alone or extra-ovarian cysts such as paratubal or paraovarian cysts can occur. Early detection through imaging is crucial.[1]

Ultrasound (US) is the first imaging choice when adnexal torsion is suspected. A notably enlarged ovary with peripherally displaced follicles, known as the "string of pearls" appearance, is the primary and sometimes only finding. Central ovarian edema, which appears as a hypoechoic and heterogeneous central medulla, is seen in up to 79% of cases. Areas of increased echogenicity within the ovary may indicate hemorrhagic infarction (1). Another key US sign is the "follicular ring" sign, where a hyperechoic rim, 1-2 mm thick, surrounds the displaced antral follicles, which is best seen on transvaginal ultrasound.[2]

The twisted vascular pedicle often produces the classic "whirlpool" sign on US, showing twisting hypoechoic vessels, with or without a color Doppler signal, or the "target" sign, which consists of concentric rings that alternate between hypo- and hyperechoic areas when viewed perpendicular to the torsion axis. Isolated torsion of the fallopian tube is rare, but it typically appears on US as a dilated tube with thickened echogenic walls. This dilated tube, usually found medial to a normal ipsilateral ovary, tapers at both ends, creating the "beak" sign.[3]

CT scans, although not routinely recommended for diagnosing torsion, are often performed when women present with nonspecific abdominal pain and vomiting. The main finding on CT in adnexal torsion is a large pelvic mass, typically located superior to the uterus at the midline, present in most cases. A cyst acting as a lead mass may display smooth, concentric wall thickening, suggesting simple edema, while irregular or eccentric thickening may point to hemorrhagic infarction. Free fluid and inflammatory stranding of peritoneal fat may be seen, especially in chronic torsion, and should not be mistaken for peritoneal malignancy.[1]

MRI is mainly used for complex gynecologic cases, as it allows for better tissue differentiation. MRI is particularly useful for characterizing adnexal masses in torsion cases. Like US, MRI can show the "string of pearls" sign. The swollen, edematous ovary's central medulla often exhibits high signal intensity on T2-weighted images. Hemorrhage can appear as areas of high signal intensity on T1-weighted images with diffusion restriction, and this should not be misinterpreted as malignancy. A lack of enhancement strongly suggests ischemia, necrosis, and nonviability of the ovary.[1]

REFERENCES

1. Dawood MT, Naik M, Bharwani N et al., Adnexal torsion: Review of radiologic appearances; RadioGraphics. 2021;41(2):609-24.
2. Sibal M. Follicular ring sign: a simple sonographic sign for early diagnosis of ovarian torsion. J Ultrasound Med. 2012;31(11):1803-9.
3. Narayanan S, Bandarkar A, Bulas DI. Fallopian tube torsion in the pediatric age group: radiologic evaluation. J Ultrasound Med. 2014;33(9):1697-704.

40 Dysembryoplastic Neuroepithelial Tumor

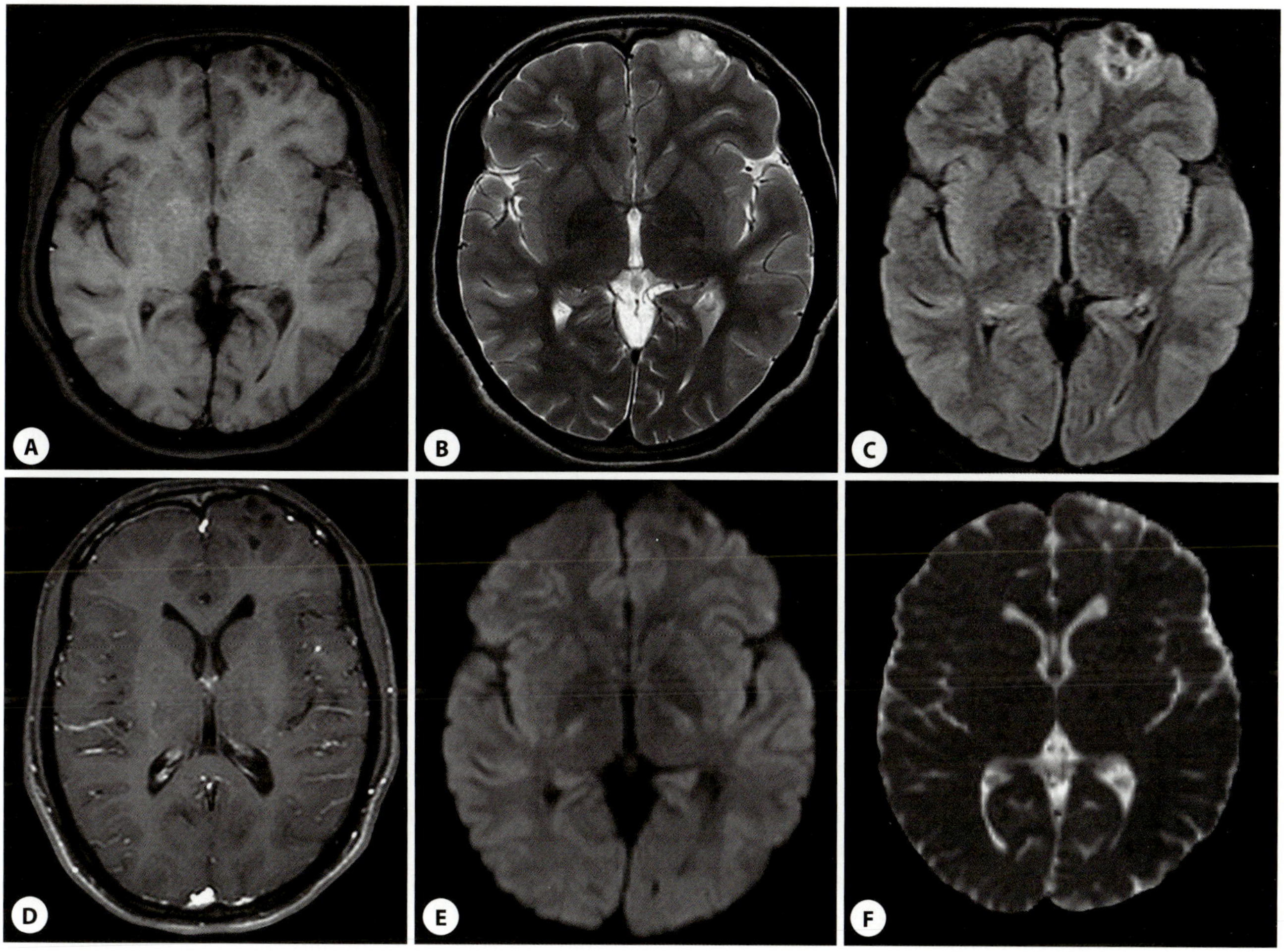

CLINICAL BACKGROUND

Young male presented with drug resistant seizure.

IMAGING FINDINGS

Cortical based T1 hypo and T2 hyperintense lesion with suppression on FLAIR noted in frontal lobe. The lesion shows bubbly appearance with surrounding oedema. No post contrast enhancement or diffusion restriction seen **(Figs. 1A to F)**.

DISCUSSION

Dysembryoplastic Neuroepithelial Tumor (DNET): Overview

Dysembryoplastic neuroepithelial tumor is a distinct low-grade glioneuronal tumor that primarily affects young children and adolescents. It is strongly associated with epilepsy that is resistant to medical treatment. First identified in 1988 by Daumas-Duport and colleagues, DNET is classified separately from more common glioneuronal tumors such as gangliogliomas.[1] The most frequent symptom of DNET is focal seizures, which may or may not impair awareness. These seizures rarely progress to more generalized forms, but over time, patients often develop chronic, drug-resistant epilepsy.[2]

DNETs typically originate in the cerebral cortex and may involve a complete gyrus or a segment of a cerebral lobe. The temporal lobe is the most commonly affected area, though the tumor can occur anywhere in the cortex. This cortical positioning, especially in the temporal lobe, makes DNETs highly prone to triggering epileptic seizures. Their dysplastic nature further adds to their epileptogenic potential. In more complex forms, DNETs consist of a tumor core surrounded by a dysplastic cortex, which is believed to be a significant cause of seizures. In simpler forms, the surrounding dysplastic cortex is absent, and the seizure activity is confined to the tumor area.[1,2]

In 2012, Chassoux and colleagues[3] classified DNETs into three types based on MRI appearance: Type 1 (polycystic), type 2 (nodular), and type 3 (diffuse or dysplastic). Type 1 was found to correlate with simple and complex histologies, while types 2 and 3 showed more nonspecific histologies. The MRI classification also proved useful in predicting the extent of the epileptogenic zone and outcomes following surgery, particularly concerning seizure control. However, this classification is not yet universally accepted, and further research is required to establish its clinical significance.

Imaging, particularly MRI, is essential for diagnosing DNETs. On MRI, DNETs often appear as a low-attenuation mass involving both the cortex and subcortical white matter, displaying a characteristic "bubble-like" or "popcorn-like" multinodular shape. These tumors exhibit low signal intensity on T1-weighted images and high signal intensity on T2-weighted and FLAIR images. They generally show minimal contrast enhancement after gadolinium administration, though patchy or partial enhancement may occur in some cases. Distinguishing DNETs from gangliogliomas can be challenging because both types of tumors commonly affect the temporal lobe and may have overlapping radiologic features. Gangliogliomas, however, often demonstrate stronger gadolinium enhancement and have a cystic or nodular structure. In cases where differentiation remains difficult, 11C-methionine positron emission tomography (PET) can be beneficial, as gangliogliomas tend to exhibit hypermetabolism, while DNETs typically show lower metabolic activity.[2]

Pros and Cons of DNET Diagnosis and Treatment

Advantages:

- *Surgical cure:* DNET is often surgically treatable, especially in cases where the tumor can be completely resected, leading to a potential cure for drug-resistant epilepsy.
- *Early diagnosis via MRI:* MRI provides excellent visualization, which helps in identifying the tumor and guiding treatment options.
- *Low malignancy:* DNETs are benign tumors with low malignant potential, making their management less aggressive than other tumors.

Disadvantages:

- *Chronic epilepsy risk:* Despite surgical intervention, some patients may continue to experience seizures, requiring long-term epilepsy management.
- *Challenging differentiation:* It can be difficult to differentiate DNETs from other glioneuronal tumors, especially in non-enhancing cases, which may complicate the diagnostic process.
- *Surgical complexity:* In complex cases, especially if the tumor is near critical brain structures, surgery can be risky, with potential side effects affecting neurological function.

REFERENCES

1. Daumas-Duport C, Scheithauer BW, Chodkiewicz JP, et al. Dysembryoplastic neuroepithelial tumor: a surgically curable tumor of young patients with intractable partial seizures. Report of thirty-nine cases. Neurosurgery. 1988;23:545–556.
2. Phi JH, Kim SH. Dysembryoplastic Neuroepithelial Tumor: A Benign but Complex Tumor of the Cerebral Cortex. Brain Tumor Res Treat. 2022;10(3):144-50.
3. Chassoux F, Rodrigo S, Mellerio C, et al. Dysembryoplastic neuroepithelial tumors: an MRI-based scheme for epilepsy surgery. Neurology. 2012;79:1699–707.

41 Idiopathic Thyroid Cartilage Purulent Chondritis

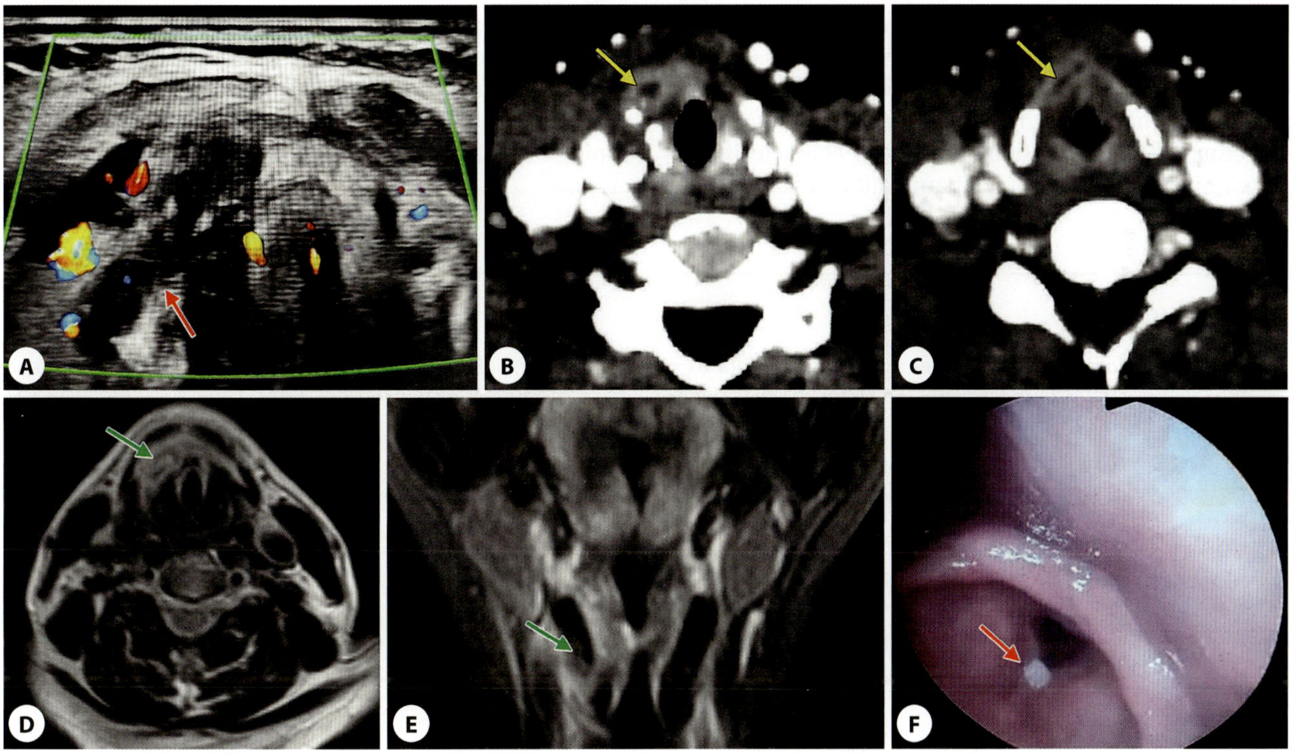

CLINICAL BACKGROUND

A 45-year-old female patient came with complaints of throat pain, neck swelling and pain for past 10 days.

IMAGING FINDINGS

Peripheral rim like enhancing hypodense area seen in perichondral space of thyroid cartilage on right side, extending up to anterior commissure with expansion of thyroid cartilage, there is tract seen extending from anterior commissure to anterior wall of hypopharynx. USG screening shows ill-defined hypoechoic area, anterior to right thyroid cartilage. Video laryngoscopy shows small whitish nodule in anterior commissure **(Figs. 1A to F)**.

DISCUSSION

Purulent chondritis of the laryngeal cartilage is an infection of the laryngeal framework cartilage that leads to abscess formation between the inner and outer layers of the perichondrium. On CT scans, this condition is identified by the expansion of laryngeal cartilage, rim enhancement, and fluid-filled areas, which are suggestive of an abscess.

Potential causes of this condition include extended intubation, autoimmune disorders such as relapsing polychondritis, prior radiation therapy, trauma, or unknown factors. Proper diagnosis before surgery is essential for effective treatment, which typically involves incision and drainage of the infected thyroid cartilage.[1]

Autoimmune diseases that can cause laryngeal symptoms in adults include relapsing polychondritis and granulomatosis with polyangiitis. Relapsing polychondritis is a condition marked by inflammation and destruction of cartilaginous structures in the body, including the ears, nose, larynx, trachea, bronchi, joints, and heart tissues. It is associated with other autoimmune conditions in about 30% of cases. Common CT features of this disease include subglottic stenosis, thickened tracheobronchial walls with calcifications, sparing of the posterior wall, and calcification or collapse of nasal cartilage.[2]

Granulomatosis with polyangiitis, a form of vasculitis affecting medium and small arteries, is characterized by necrotizing granulomatous inflammation. This condition usually involves the upper and lower respiratory tracts and often coexists with glomerulonephritis. It is generally diagnosed by detecting antineutrophil cytoplasmic antibodies.[2]

The differential diagnosis for purulent chondritis includes malignant conditions such as squamous cell carcinoma and chondrosarcoma. Chondrosarcoma, a rare cancer that makes up less than 1% of all laryngeal tumors, typically affects males in their sixth decade of life and arises more commonly from the cricoid cartilage than the thyroid cartilage. Imaging often shows a large, low-density mass with calcifications. Ultrasound-guided fine-needle aspiration (FNA) is useful for obtaining a biopsy and culture.[3]

REFERENCES

1. Eliashar R, Gross M, Goldfarb A, et al. Purulent chondritis of the laryngeal framework cartilages. Ann Otol Rhinol Laryngol. 2005;114:219-22.
2. Learned KO, Vu TH, Choi JM, et al. Purulent chondritis of thyroid cartilage. BJR Case Rep. 2020;6(3):20200013.
3. Chin OY, Dubal PM, Sheikh AB, et al. Laryngeal chondrosarcoma: a systematic review of 592 cases. Laryngoscope. 2017;127:430-9.

42 Rectal Malignancy: Role of MRI

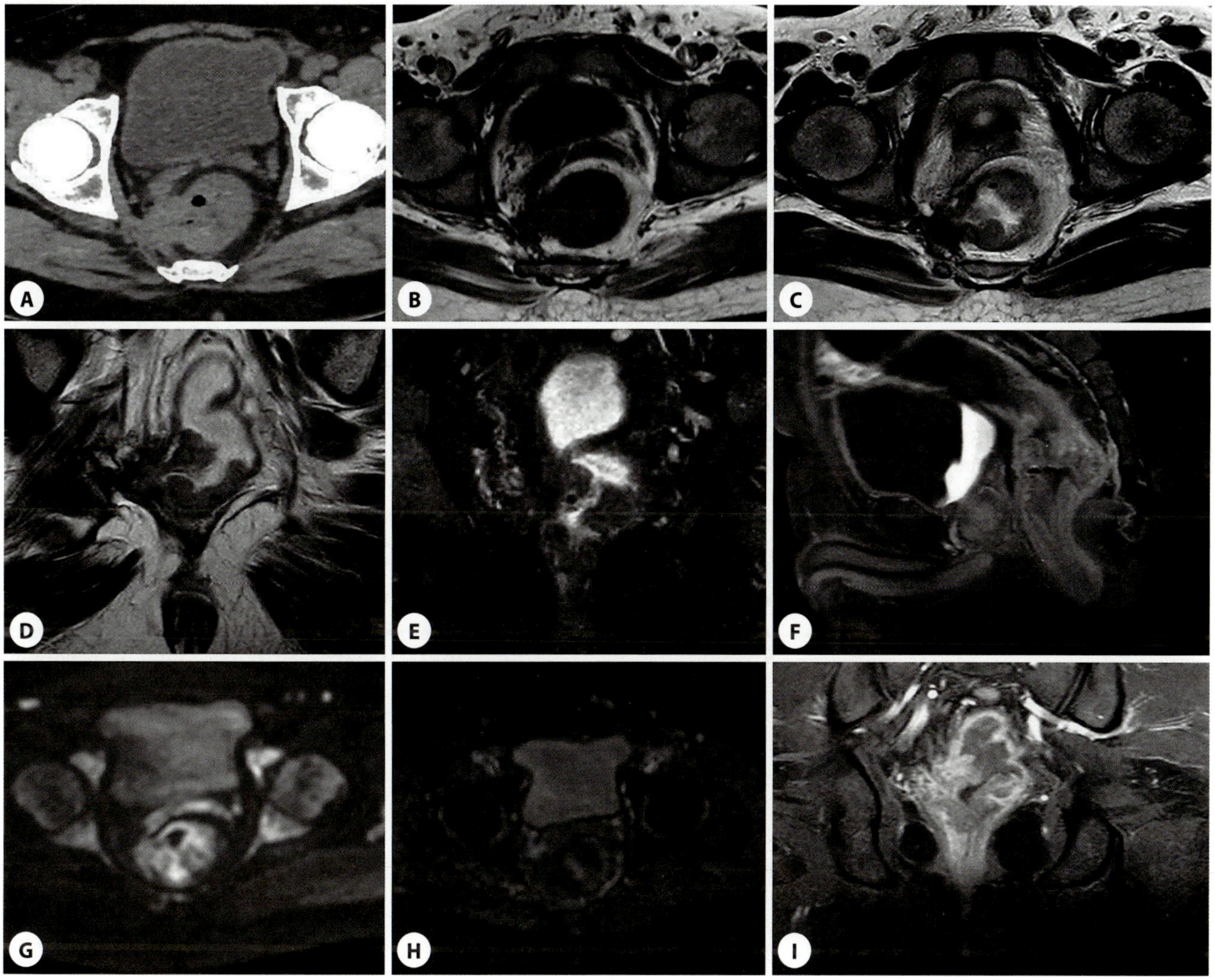

CLINICAL BACKGROUND

A 49-year-old male patient came with complaints of altered bowel habits.

IMAGING FINDINGS

Circumferential growth involving mid and lower rectum, below the peritoneal reflection. The lesion seen extending till anorectal junction **(Figs. 1A to I)**.

- Serosal breach in right lateral wall with involvement of adjacent mesorectal fat and mesorectal fascia with mesorectal deposits noted. Infiltration of levator ani muscle sphincter complex noted on right side. Subtle loss of fat plane with posterior wall of right lobe of prostate. Infiltration of right seminal vesicle with loss of T2 hyperintense signals.

- Poor flow related signals in right internal iliac artery branches adjacent to the lesion, likely extramural vascular invasion. Lesion shows diffusion restriction with intense enhancement, on post-contrast study. Few enlarged internal iliac and mesorectal lymph nodes noted.

DISCUSSION

Magnetic resonance imaging (MRI) is the preferred imaging method for rectal cancer staging due to its superior soft-tissue contrast resolution. It accurately assesses tumor spread beyond the rectal wall and its relationship to the mesorectal fascia (MRF) and sphincter complex. MRI staging of rectal cancer includes evaluating the tumor's location and its relation to the MRF and sphincters, tumor size, depth of extramural spread (T stage), involvement of the peritoneal reflection, presence of extramural vascular invasion (EMVI), lymph nodes, and bony metastasis.[1]

- Tumor localization: The distance from the lowest part of the tumor to the anal verge is measured:
  - Low rectal tumor: <5 cm from the anal verge
  - Middle rectal tumor: 5–10 cm from the anal verge
  - High rectal tumor: >10 cm from the anal verge

  In the lower rectum, the mesorectal fat is circumferentially bound by the MRF, whereas in higher sections, the peritoneum covers the anterior portion of the mesorectal fat up to the "anterior peritoneal reflection".[1]
- Tumor signal characteristics: On T2-weighted images, rectal tumors typically show signal intensity intermediate between the muscularis propria and mucosa. Differentiating between T1 and T2 tumors is challenging without using an endorectal coil, and these tumors are often collectively staged as "T1/T2."
- T3 tumor staging: A tumor is staged as T3 when it extends into the mesorectal fat. For T3 tumors, measuring the shortest distance between the tumor and the MRF is critical. A tumor-MRF distance greater than 1 mm is a good predictor of negative surgical margins after total mesorectal excision.[1]
- Sphincter involvement: For low rectal tumors, measuring the distance from the inferior tumor border to the top of the anal sphincters is crucial for planning sphincter-preserving surgery. Advanced T2, T3, and high rectal tumors involving the levator muscles often require abdominoperineal resection (APR). In cases with invasion of adjacent organs, pelvic exenteration may be needed.
- Nodal and EMVI evaluation: Regional lymph nodes, including mesorectal and internal iliac nodes, contribute to the N stage, while involvement of other lymph nodes is classified as metastasis. EMVI, although not part of the TNM staging system, is a recognized independent prognostic factor linked to higher rates of metastasis, local recurrence, poorer treatment response, and reduced survival.[1]

REFERENCE

1. Jhaveri KS Hosseini-Nik H. MRI of rectal cancer: An overview and update on recent advances. Am J Roentgenol. 2015;205(1):W42-55.

43 Ortner's Syndrome (Cardiovocal Syndrome)

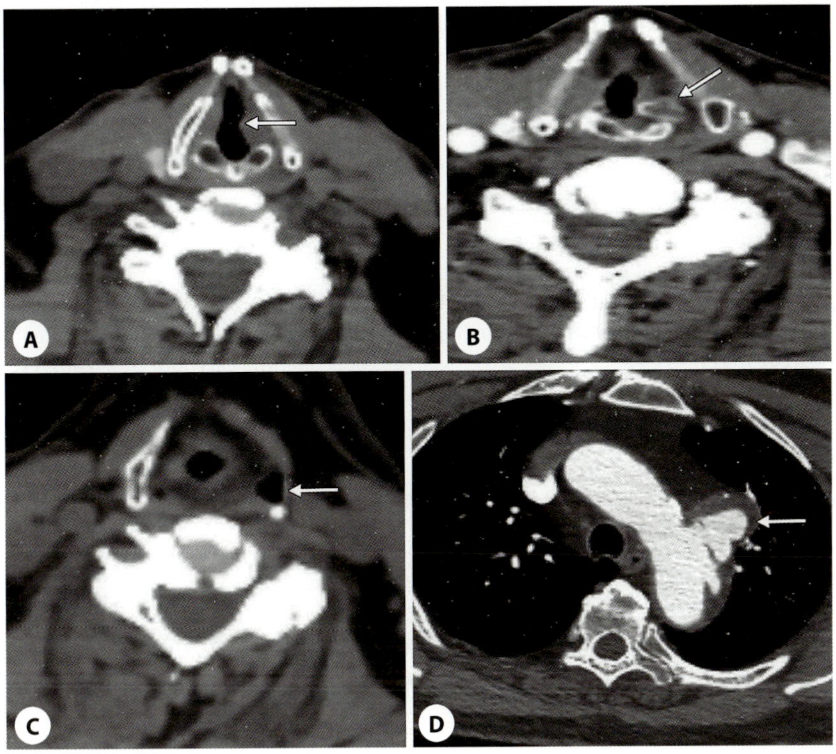

CLINICAL BACKGROUND

A 50-year-old male patient with dyspnea and hoarseness of voice.

IMAGING FINDINGS

Imaging findings of left vocal cord palsy, medial deviation of the aryepiglottic fold and abnormal dilatation of the ipsilateral pyriform sinus with saccular thoracic aortic aneurysm **(Figs. 1A to D)**.

DISCUSSION

Ortner's syndrome (OS), also referred to as cardiovocal syndrome, is a rare disorder in which the left recurrent laryngeal nerve is paralyzed due to an underlying heart or lung condition. The main symptoms include hoarseness, shortness of breath, cough, and difficulty swallowing. First described by Norbert Ortner in 1897 when he reported three cases involving severe mitral stenosis, the condition is most commonly linked to aortic aneurysms (41%), followed by pulmonary hypertension (35%), mitral stenosis (17%), and hypertension (12%).[1] OS is responsible for approximately 1.5%–6.3% of unilateral vocal cord palsy cases.[2]

The cause of OS can be traced to the anatomical path of the recurrent laryngeal nerve (RLN). As a branch of the vagus nerve (cranial nerve X), the RLN controls most of the larynx's intrinsic muscles except the cricothyroid muscle and also provides sensory feedback from below the vocal cords and the upper trachea. The right RLN loops around the right subclavian artery, while the left RLN loops around the ligamentum arteriosum, traveling between the trachea and esophagus. The left RLN is more prone to injury than the right due to its proximity to the aortopulmonary window and nearby structures.[3]

Diagnostic imaging for vocal cord palsy often reveals dilation of the pyriform sinus on the affected side, medial displacement of the aryepiglottic fold, and dilation of the ipsilateral laryngeal ventricle, forming the "sail sign".[2] Additional imaging signs include inward deviation of the arytenoid cartilage, fatty atrophy of the paralyzed vocal cord, flattening of the subglottic arch, thinning at the medial edge of the affected vocal cord (best seen on coronal reformatted images), and dilation of the vallecula on the same side.

A meta-analysis involving 256 OS cases identified that aortic abnormalities accounted for more than half of the cases. While aortic aneurysms are the primary cause, conditions like large vessel vasculitis and aortic fistulas are less frequently seen. Prompt treatment of OS can improve the prognosis, often resulting in recovery from hoarseness and swallowing difficulties. Vocal cord function may return after appropriate medical or surgical intervention.[2]

REFERENCES

1. Verma S, Talwar A, Talwar A, et al. Ortner's syndrome: A systematic review of presentation, diagnosis and management. Intractable Rare Dis Res. 2023;12(3):141-7.
2. SW Kheok, PR Salkade, A Bangaragiri, et al. Cardiovascular Hoarseness (Ortner's Syndrome): A Pictorial Review; Curr Probl Diagn Radiol. 2021;50(5):749-754.
3. Loughran S, Alves C, MacGregor FB. Current aetiology of unilateral vocal fold paralysis in a teaching hospital in the West of Scotland. J Laryngol Otol. 2002;116:907-10.

44 Mycotic Aneurysm

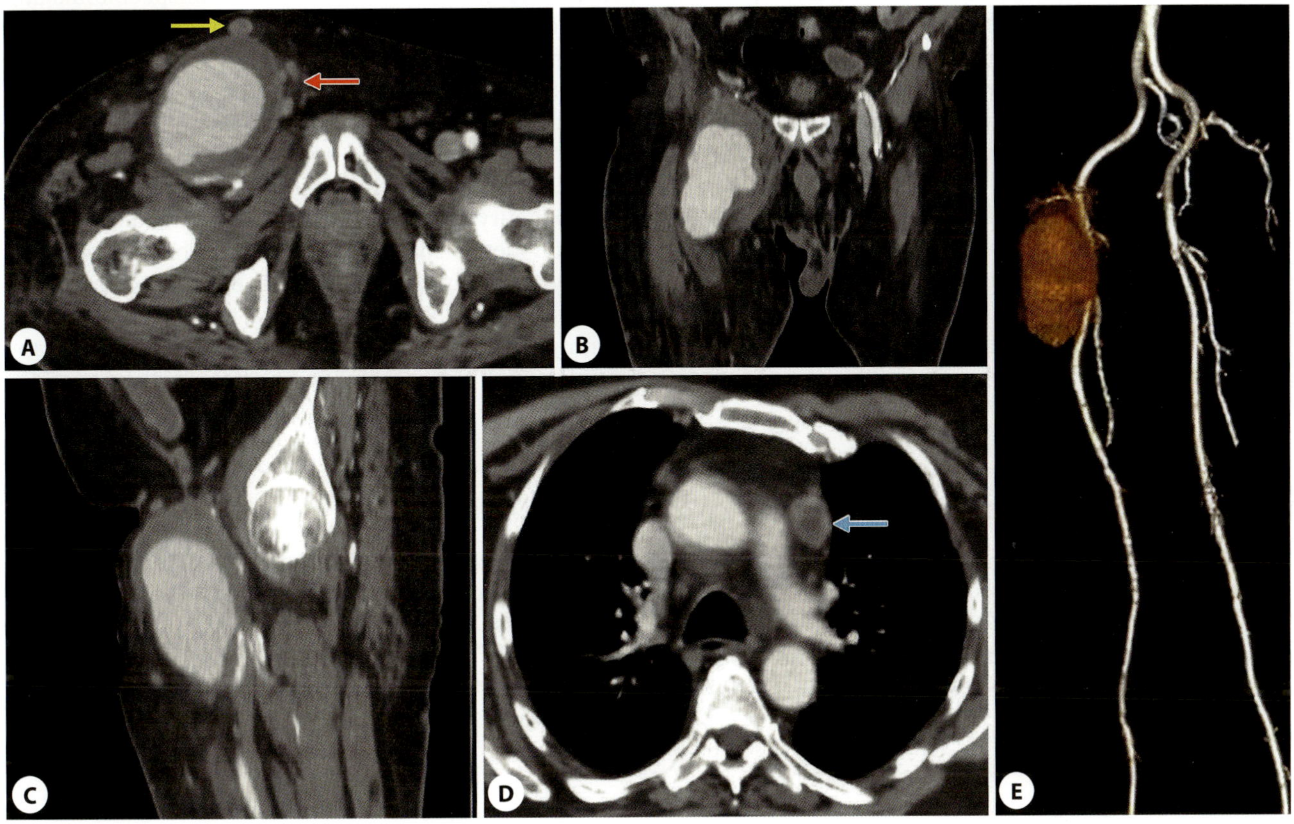

CLINICAL BACKGROUND

Known CKD with complaints of pain and swelling in right inguinal region for 3 months. History of catheter angiogram (2 years back) via right femoral approach. History of PTB completed ATT.

IMAGING FINDINGS

A saccular aneurysm outpouching from right common femoral artery with adjacent soft tissue inflammation (red arrow) and reactive nodes (yellow arrow). Multiple mediastinal lymph nodes present (blue arrow). No other aneurysm or thickening in visualized portions of thoracic and abdominal aorta **(Figs. 1A to E)**.

DISCUSSION

In 1885, the first description of mycotic aneurysms was provided by Osler. These aneurysms comprise about 2.5–3% of all aneurysms, with those affecting the femoral arteries being particularly rare, representing only 0.8% of cases. The term "mycotic" originates from the mushroom-like appearance of these aneurysms and does not indicate the infection's cause. There are four primary mechanisms through which arteries can become infected:

- Septic emboli originating from the heart, as described by Osler;

- Infection of an existing aneurysm due to either bacteremia or contiguous spread;
- Infected pseudoaneurysms resulting from trauma, especially in intravenous drug users; and
- Microbial arteritis stemming from bacteremia or local spread.[1]

Peripheral mycotic pseudoaneurysms are uncommon and can arise from either localized infections or systemic sepsis. The use of antibiotics has led to a decline in pseudoaneurysms resulting from infective endocarditis, while those from direct arterial trauma have become more frequent. The primary symptom reported by patients is pain (83.3%), followed by swelling (80%) and redness (78.5%), with only 30% of individuals presenting with fever.[2]

Doppler ultrasonography is a useful noninvasive technique for assessing infected aneurysms in peripheral arteries. However, multidetector computed tomography (MDCT) is the preferred imaging modality, crucial for establishing the diagnosis, localizing the aneurysm, characterizing its features, assessing complications, performing vascular mapping, and planning treatment. Typical imaging characteristics of infected aneurysms include a lobulated vascular mass, irregular arterial walls, perianeurysmal edema, and surrounding soft-tissue masses. Uncommon findings may include gas formation around the aneurysm, thrombosis within the aneurysm, calcification of the aneurysm wall, and disrupted arterial calcification at the infection site. Other nonspecific imaging indicators of infection include soft tissue stranding, adjacent lymphadenopathy, and fluid collections.[3]

While any vessel can be affected, it is important to note that "extra-organic visceral" pseudoaneurysms have a very high risk of spontaneous rupture, with a mortality rate of nearly 100%. The management of mycotic pseudoaneurysms should be tailored to individual patients based on factors such as location, morphology, bleeding severity, and available medical expertise. Treatment options may include open surgical repair, endovascular stenting, endovascular embolization, antibiotic therapy (intravenous), or a combination of these methods.[4]

REFERENCES

1. Fuente R, Medina FJ, Moradillo N, et al. Persistent mycotic superficial femoral artery pseudoaneurysm after endovascular treatment: A case report. J Vasc Bras. 2021;20:e20200095.
2. Vijay kumar K, Tay JS, Tang TY, et al. Spontaneous Superficial Femoral Artery Mycotic Aneurysm. Case Rep Surg. 2021;2021:6613914.
3. D'Souza D, Bell D, Vadera S, et al. Mycotic aneurysm. Reference article, Radiopaedia.org. (Accessed on 13 Mar 2024) https://doi.org/10.53347/rID-1706
4. Sharma PK, Garisa SS, Kumaran SV, et al. Mycotic (Infected) Pseudoaneurysm, a Diagnostic Challenge - Case Series. J Clin Imaging Sci. 2020;10:86.

45 Giant Pseudomeningocele

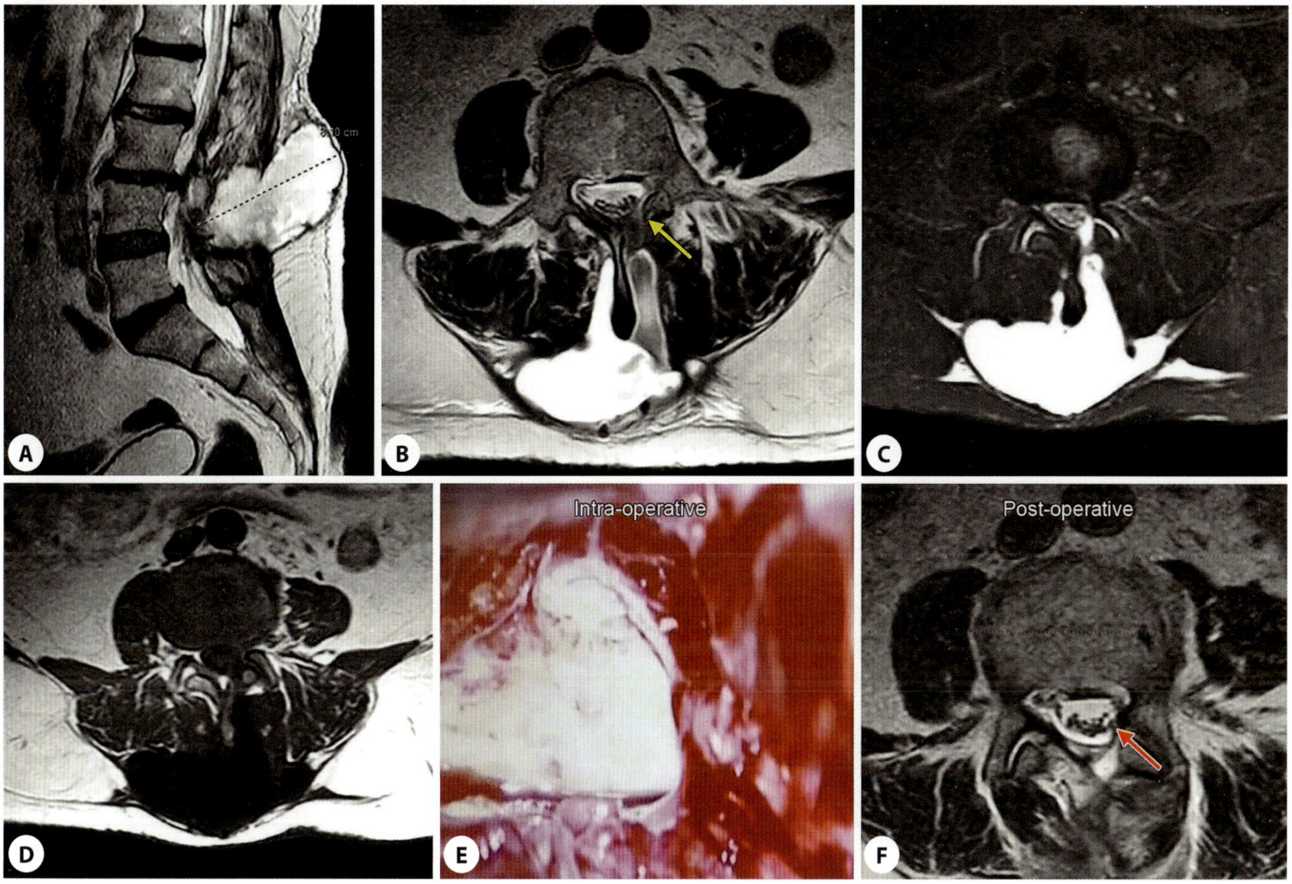

CLINICAL BACKGROUND

Postlumbar microdiscectomy (2 months) with complaints of swelling at postoperative site. Intermittent low-grade fever for 1 week.

IMAGING FINDINGS

Large CSF intense collection (> 8 cm) extending from a dural defect (yellow arrow) into the posterior para spinal muscles and subcutaneous plane. Intra-operative and Post-operative images are shown with closure of the dural defect (red arrow) **(Figs. 1A to F)**.

DISCUSSION

Pseudomeningocele is a relatively uncommon complication that can develop after spinal surgery. It is characterized by the extradural accumulation of cerebrospinal fluid (CSF) within the soft tissues of the back, resulting from fluid leakage through a tear in the dura mater. This condition is also known by various terms, including "spurious meningocele," "pseudocyst," and "false cyst." Pseudomeningoceles can be classified into three categories: Congenital, postoperative, and traumatic. Among these, postoperative pseudomeningoceles frequently arise following lumbar spinal surgeries. The phenomenon of "postlaminectomy pseudomeningocele" was first introduced in 1946 by Hyndman and Gerber, who studied extradural cysts. While the precise incidence of postoperative pseudomeningocele remains unclear, as many affected individuals do not exhibit symptoms, it can sometimes lead to nerve root entrapment, resulting in radicular pain.[1]

Giant pseudomeningoceles, which are defined as those exceeding 8 cm, are infrequently reported and not thoroughly addressed in the literature. The management of these large cysts typically requires a combined approach, which may include excision of the pseudomeningocele, repair of any dural tears, and placement of a subarachnoid catheter for drainage. Symptoms commonly associated with postoperative pseudomeningoceles include positional headaches, localized back pain, and radiculopathy. Herniation of nerve roots through tears in the dura and arachnoid membranes can occur, leading to potential strangulation of the nerve roots within the cyst, which may cause radicular pain and motor deficits. Headaches linked to larger pseudomeningoceles are often attributed to decreased CSF volume and lowered intracranial pressure.[1]

Magnetic resonance imaging (MRI) is the preferred imaging modality for evaluating suspected pseudomeningoceles in postoperative patients, particularly when no fusion hardware is present. MRI typically shows a fluid collection of varying sizes that has a CSF intensity signal along the surgical pathway, which may or may not be enclosed by deep muscular fascia. The fluid generally demonstrates a consistent CSF signal across all pulse sequences, including diffusion-weighted imaging. In postoperative lumbar cases, the fluid collection most commonly extends posteriorly from the lateral recess at the nerve root sleeve through the laminotomy. The presence of CSF pulsations or metallic implants can affect the fluid's appearance. Usually, there is no enhancing margin or muscle edema, except for what might be expected after recent surgical intervention. A CSF leak can lead to the engorgement or enlargement of the anterior epidural venous plexus. Dural thickening and enhancement may be observed in patients with symptomatic intracranial hypotension. The literature also reports instances of delayed infections in pseudomeningoceles. When examined via MRI, hematomas and abscesses typically display more complex signal characteristics, appearing inhomogeneous with thicker enhancing margins or capsules. Abscesses may also be associated with conditions like discitis or osteomyelitis. Hematomas are known to exhibit a "blooming" effect on T2-weighted (GRE) sequences. Importantly, patients with pseudomeningoceles generally do not show fever or other infection indicators unless the pseudocyst becomes secondarily infected.[2]

REFERENCES

1. Weng YJ, Cheng CC, Li YY, et al. Management of giant pseudomeningoceles after spinal surgery. BMC Musculoskelet Disord. 2010;11:53.
2. Jain NK, Dao K, Ortiz AO. Radiologic Evaluation and Management of Postoperative Spine Paraspinal Fluid Collections. Neuroimaging Clinics of North America. 2014;24:2:375-89.

46 Vestibular Schwannoma

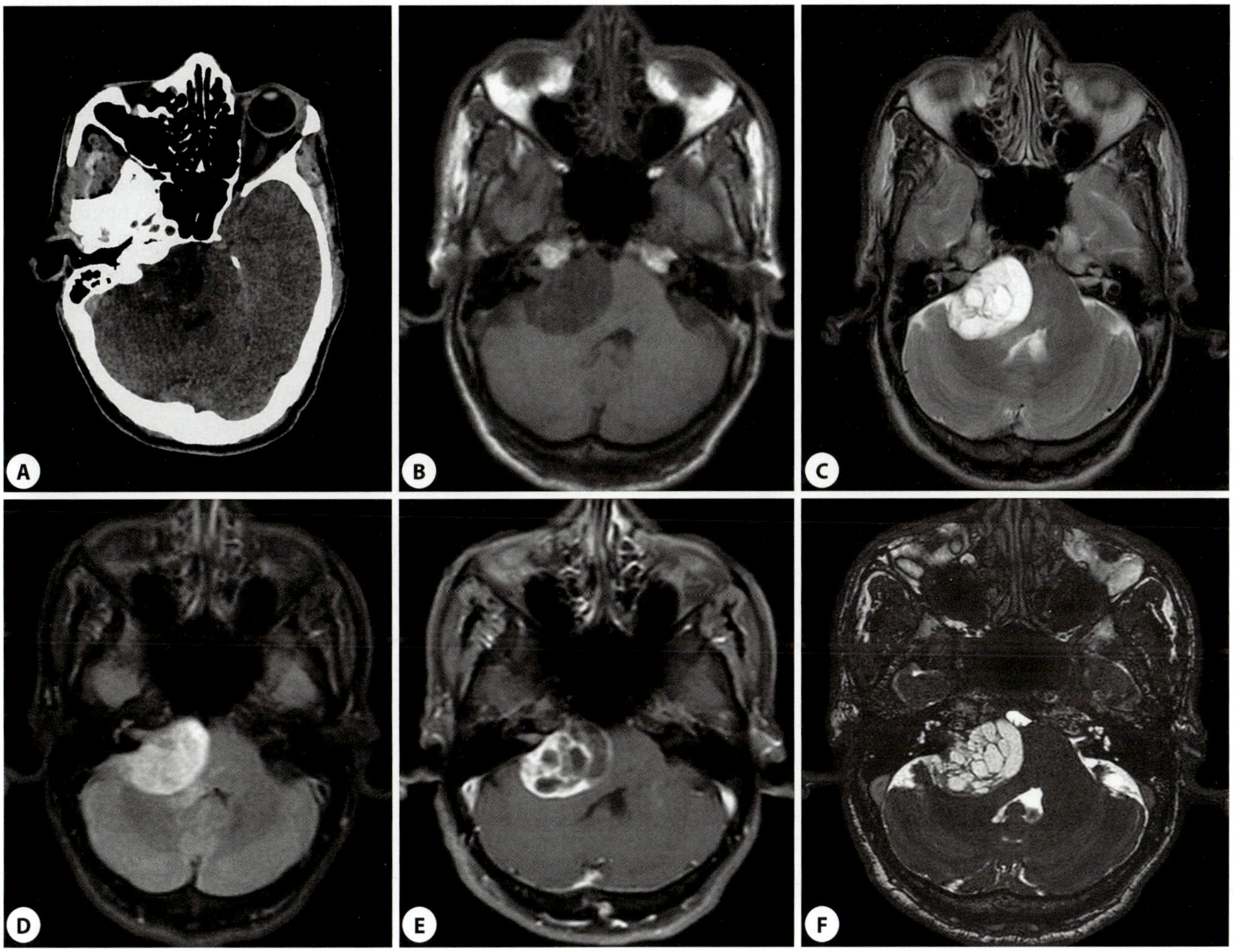

CLINICAL BACKGROUND

A 53-year-old male patient with complaints of hearing loss and headache.

IMAGING FINDINGS

Well defined T1 hypointense and T2/FLAIR heterointense, predominantly hyperintense lesion in right cerebello-pontine angle with internal auditory meatus extension **(Figs. 1A to F)**.

The lesion shows heterogeneous enhancement on postcontrast study with few nonenhancing areas within. Few foci of blooming in SWI seen within the lesion. The lesion shows no diffusion restriction. The lesion shows mass effect and compression of adjacent cerebellum, brainstem and fourth ventricle.

DISCUSSION

Vestibular schwannomas (VS), also known as acoustic neuromas, most often arise from the vestibular portion of the vestibulocochlear nerve sheath, typically at the junction between central and peripheral myelin near the vestibular ganglion in the internal auditory canal (IAC). These are benign tumors that account for 6–8% of all brain tumors and approximately 80% of cerebellopontine angle (CPA) tumors. They may remain within the IAC or grow into the CPA, leading to symptoms that result from pressure on nearby cranial nerves, the brainstem, or structures in the posterior fossa.[1]

Vestibular schwannomas is primarily associated with cranial nerve-related symptoms, with most patients experiencing long-term, asymmetric hearing loss, which is sensorineural in nature. Less common symptoms include tinnitus or balance issues, while more severe signs such as vertigo, sudden hearing loss, or facial numbness and weakness are rare due to the slow growth of the tumor. Audiometric testing and brainstem-evoked response audiometry can confirm hearing loss, with over 90% of patients showing abnormal results.[2]

Vestibular schwannomas represents the most common mass found in the CPA, accounting for 70–80% of these cases, followed by meningiomas (10–15%) and epidermoid cysts (5%). Other potential CPA and IAC masses include malignant tumors like leptomeningeal metastases, lymphoma, meningeal melanocytoma, or melanoma, along with inflammatory conditions like Bell's palsy and neurosarcoidosis, and aneurysms. Facial nerve involvement can help differentiate between a VS and other pathologies. Expansion of the IAC is often associated with poorer hearing before and after surgery. CPA meningiomas are dural-based tumors that grow along the petrous ridge and can invade the IAC. These tumors may contain calcifications, cause changes in bone structure, and show peritumoral edema if there is significant mass effect. Unlike meningiomas, VSs typically lack calcifications.

MRI typically shows VS as isointense to the cerebellum on T1-weighted images, with strong enhancement following contrast administration. Intralesional hemorrhage may appear as a hyperintense signal on T1 and cause susceptibility artifacts on T2* gradient-echo images. Larger tumors may show uneven enhancement due to hemorrhage or cyst formation. Indicators of concern include larger tumor size, compression of the brainstem or cerebellum, edema surrounding the tumor, hydrocephalus, and tonsillar herniation. CT scans can provide detailed information on bone involvement and may show bony destruction, helping to assess the surrounding anatomy.[3]

Cystic variants of VS can be mistaken for other cystic CPA lesions, such as epidermoid or arachnoid cysts. Cystic VSs account for around 10% of all cases and are linked to more significant hearing loss. These cysts likely result from recurrent minor hemorrhages or fluid expansion in trapped arachnoid tissue, which shows up as a hyperintense T2 signal with variable T1 signal. Enhancement of the cyst wall can help differentiate VS from other cystic lesions.[3]

REFERENCES

1. Mahaley MS Jr, Mettlin C, Natarajan N, et al. Analysis of patterns of care of brain tumor patients in the United States: a study of the Brain Tumor Section of the AANS and the CNS and the Commission on Cancer of the ACS. Clin Neurosurg. 1990;36:347-52.
2. Doyle KJ. Is there still a role for auditory brainstem response audiometry in the diagnosis of acoustic neuroma? Arch Otolaryngol Head Neck Surg. 1999;125:232.
3. Lin EP, Crane BT. The Management and Imaging of Vestibular Schwannomas. AJNR Am J Neuroradiol. 2017;38(11):2034-43.

47 SMA and Nutcracker Syndromes

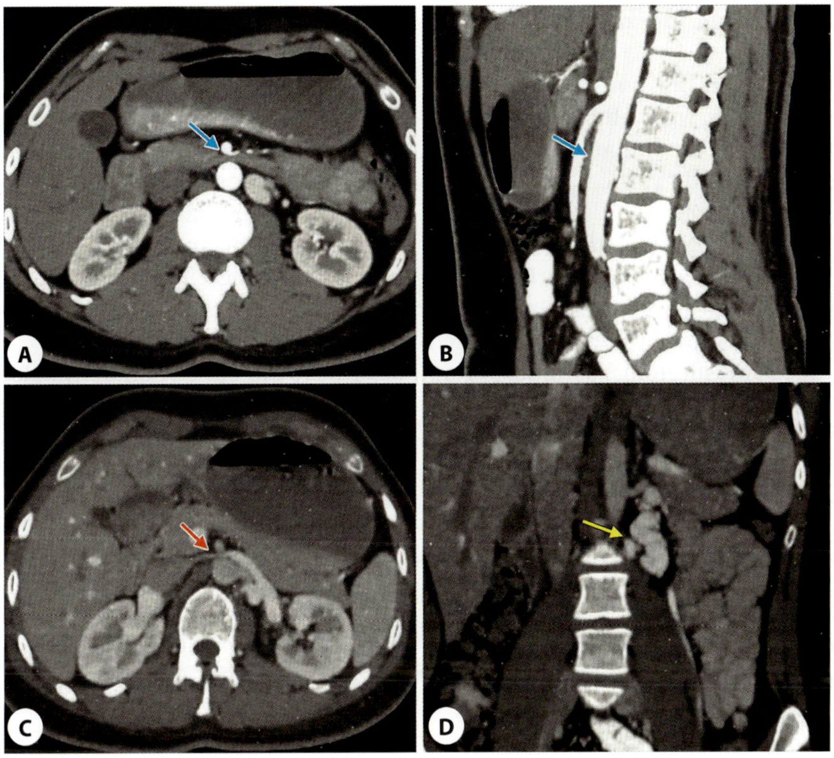

CLINICAL BACKGROUND

Young boy with complaints of abdomen pain (on and off - increased postprandial) and weight loss.

IMAGING FINDINGS

Aorto-mesenteric distance is reduced with loss of aorto-mesenteric fat planes, resulting in markedly upstream dilated stomach, I, II and III part of duodenum with abrupt narrowing at aorto-mesentric junction (blue arrows). Aorto-mesenteric angle is also reduced. Distally small and large bowel loops appear normal. Left renal vein is abruptly narrowed (red arrow) with dilated left distal gonadal vein (yellow arrow) **(Figs. 1A to D)**.

DISCUSSION

Superior mesenteric artery (SMA) syndrome, also known as Wilkie syndrome, was first described in detail by Wilkie in 1927. This rare condition results from the compression of the third part of the duodenum between the aorta and the SMA. Under normal circumstances, the duodenum is cushioned by mesenteric fat as it passes through the aorto-mesenteric angle, which prevents external pressure. However, significant weight loss (due to chronic illness, an acute catabolic state, or a low body mass index), as well as spine lengthening following scoliosis surgery, can reduce this fat layer and increase the risk of compression.[1]

Superior mesenteric artery syndrome affects females slightly more often and is estimated to occur in 0.013–0.3%

of the population. Typical symptoms include post-meal or intermittent abdominal pain, as well as signs of bowel obstruction like nausea, vomiting, and anorexia. CT imaging can reveal key diagnostic signs, including an aorto-mesenteric angle less than 22° (normal is around 90°) and an aorto-mesenteric distance of less than 8 mm (normal range is 10–28 mm). Additional signs include a dilated stomach and duodenum up to the point of compression, with a sudden narrowing where the duodenum passes under the SMA.[1]

On fluoroscopy, a common but nonspecific finding is dilation of the duodenum with abrupt narrowing at the third section, possibly accompanied by gastric distension. Other features include vertical compression of the mucosal folds at the same point, antiperistaltic movement of contrast material before the obstruction (causing a back-and-forth "rocking" flow of barium), and relief of the obstruction when the patient lies in a prone or left lateral decubitus position. However, recent research using CT as the main diagnostic tool has reported an 18.6% false-negative rate for barium studies.[1,2]

"Nutcracker syndrome," a term coined by Schepper, describes the compression of the left renal vein (LRV) between the aorta and SMA, also known as "anterior nutcracker syndrome." In some cases, the LRV may be compressed between the aorta and the vertebral body in a circumaortic (up to 17%) or retro-aortic (3%) position, referred to as "posterior nutcracker syndrome." This compression can lead to venous hypertension and the formation of periureteric varices.[2]

Patients with nutcracker syndrome may present with a range of symptoms, from being entirely asymptomatic to suffering from severe pelvic congestion. The most frequent symptom, however, is micro- or macroscopic hematuria. On CT scans, the "beak sign" – the abrupt narrowing of the LRV between the aorta and SMA with proximal dilatation – is characteristic of this condition. Other diagnostic features include an LRV diameter ratio (hilar to aortomesenteric) greater than 4.9, an aorto-mesenteric angle less than 41°, and a beak angle (measured between the anterior and posterior walls of the LRV as it passes under the SMA) greater than 32°.[1]

Due to the shared pathophysiology, radiologists should consider the possibility that both SMA and nutcracker syndromes may coexist in certain patients, as was the case here.

REFERENCES

1. Fong JKK, Poh ACC, Seng AG, et al. Imaging Findings and Clinical Features of Abdominal Vascular Compression Syndromes. Am J Roentgenol. 2014;203:29-36.
2. Lee TH, Lee JS, Jo Y, et al. Superior mesenteric artery syndrome: where do we stand today? J Gastrointest Surg. 2012;16:2203-11.

48 Psammomacarcinoma of Ovary

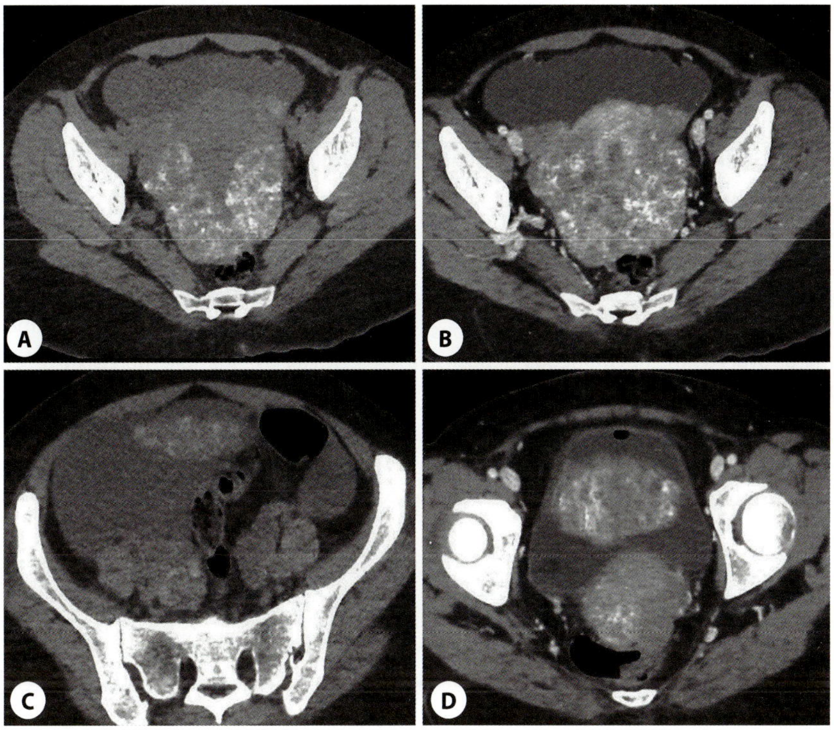

CLINICAL BACKGROUND

A 25-year-old young female presented with abdomen distension and pain.

IMAGING FINDINGS

Evidence of calcified lesion with post-contrast enhancement in both adnexa. Diffuse peritoneal thickening with calcific foci. Moderate ascites noted **(Figs. A to D)**.

DISCUSSION

Serous psammomacarcinoma, first reported by Grimaldi et al. in 1916, is a rare form of serous carcinoma that may develop in the ovary or peritoneum. It is characterized by a widespread presence of psammoma bodies, invasion into the ovarian stroma, peritoneum, or intraperitoneal organs, and moderate atypia in the cells. This tumor typically has a better prognosis compared to conventional serous carcinoma.[1] While it often originates from the ovary, it may also arise from the peritoneum. When confined to the pelvic region, it can resemble a calcified fibroma. The biomarker CA-125, frequently elevated in ovarian cancer cases, is typically raised in these instances.[2]

From an imaging perspective, serous psammomacarcinoma presents with distinct features. Calcifications are usually observed in one or both ovaries, and metastatic spread to the peritoneum or distant areas also shows calcification. Differential diagnoses for multiple calcified lesions in the abdomen include conditions like pseudomyxoma peritonei, undifferentiated malignancies in the abdomen, tuberculous peritonitis, meconium peritonitis, and mucinous stomach adenocarcinoma.[2]

A related condition is primary peritoneal serous carcinoma (PPSC), also known as primary peritoneal papillary serous carcinoma. This epithelial tumor primarily affects women in their fifth and sixth decades of life. PPSC extensively affects the peritoneal surface but usually spares or minimally involves the ovaries. The imaging features of PPSC resemble those of peritoneal carcinomatosis from ovarian cancer, with signs like ascites, omental nodules, fat stranding, and peritoneal thickening, though there is no visible adnexal mass. Elevated CA-125 levels are also common in PPSC.[3]

Psammomacarcinoma of the ovary is a rare type of tumor, typically showing radiological findings of multiple calcified lesions in both the abdomen and pelvis. When these calcified lesions are observed, this type of carcinoma should be considered as part of the differential diagnosis. These tumors generally respond well to chemotherapy, and the likelihood of recurrence after surgery is low.[4]

REFERENCES

1. Jena SK, Mishra P, Mohapatra V, et al. Bilateral Serous Psammocarcinoma of Ovary: Rare Variant Low Grade Serous Carcinoma. Case Rep Obstet Gynecol. 2015;2015:531242.
2. Diwakar N, Kamble RB, Dixit J, et al. Imaging of serous psammomacarcinoma of ovary with subcutaneous deposits: A case report. Indian J Radiol Imaging. 2011;21(2):150-2.
3. Míguez González J, Calaf Forn F, Pelegrí Martínez L, et al. Primary and secondary tumors of the peritoneum: key imaging features and differential diagnosis with surgical and pathological correlation. Insights Imaging. 2023;14:115.
4. Diwakar N, Kamble RB, Dixit J, et al. Imaging of serous psammomacarcinoma of ovary with subcutaneous deposits: A case report. Indian J Radiol Imaging. 2011;21:150-2.

49

Lipoma Arborescens

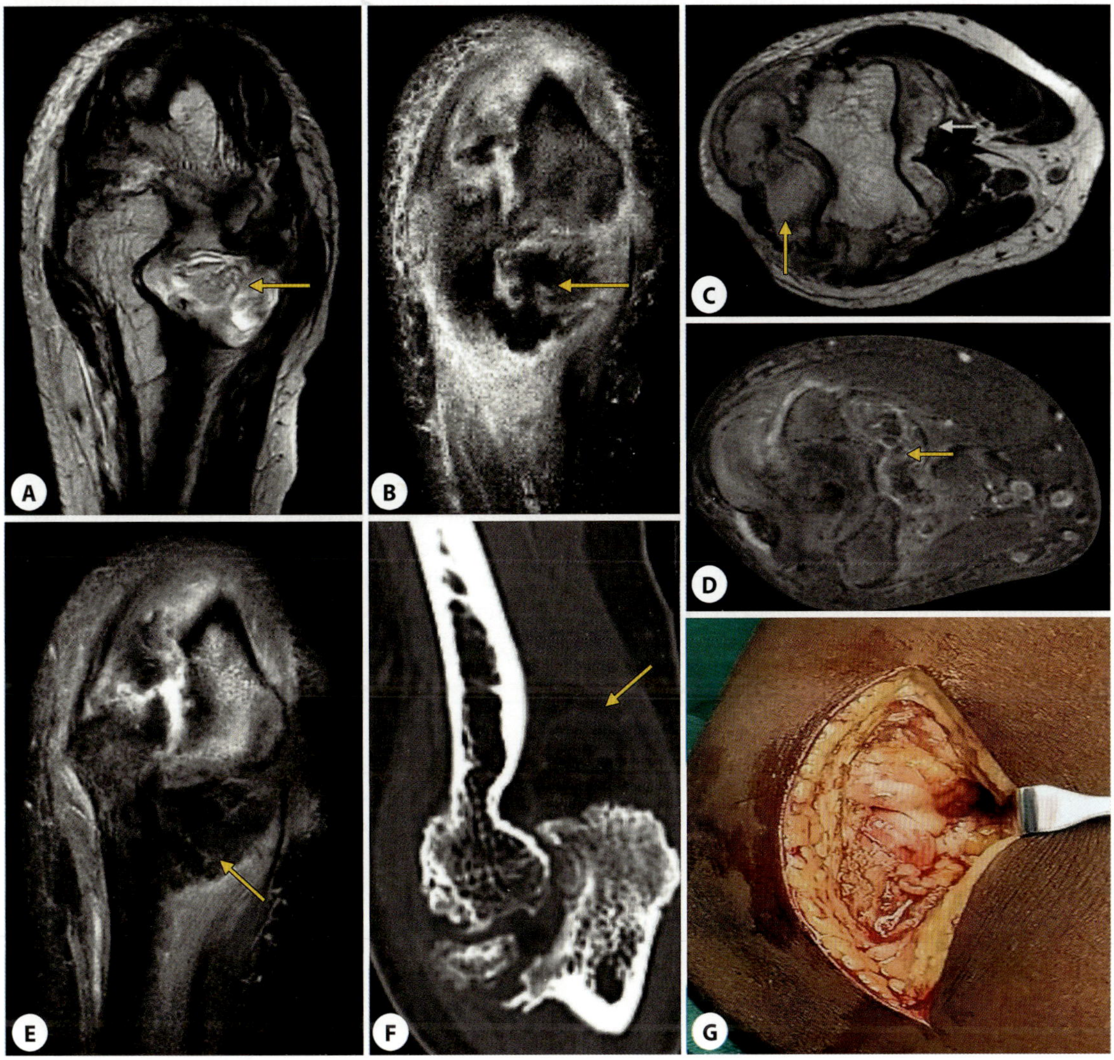

CLINICAL BACKGROUND

Young male patient with chronic left elbow joint pain.

IMAGING FINDINGS

Profound synovial thickening and enhancement seen, involving the elbow joint with minimal elbow joint effusion. Evidence of T1 hyperintense signals with fat saturation. Heterogeneous postcontrast enhancement of proliferated synovium. Articular surface erosions and irregularities involving head of radius, olecranon process of ulnar/distal humerus with subarticular edema in ulna. Surrounding soft tissue edema. Intra-operative image is shown **(Figs. 1A to G)**.

DISCUSSION

Lipoma arborescens is a benign condition resembling a "lipoma," where the synovium exhibits villous growth and the subsynovial connective tissue is replaced by mature fat cells. It is generally considered not a neoplasm, but rather a reactive response to chronic irritation of the synovium, whether caused by mechanical factors or inflammation. Various terms have been used to describe this condition, including diffuse lipoma of the joint, diffuse synovial lipoma, diffuse articular lipomatosis, fatty infiltration of the synovial membrane, and villous lipomatous proliferation of the synovium. These labels emphasize its non-neoplastic nature.[1]

Lipoma arborescens is typically seen in association with degenerative joint diseases, chronic rheumatoid arthritis, or previous trauma. Joint effusion is common and can be caused by the lesion itself or by the underlying arthritis. Though rare, some cases have been reported in the absence of any pre-existing chronic joint disease. Researchers have proposed two categories: An idiopathic "primary" type in younger patients and a more common "secondary" type in older individuals. The condition is usually unilateral, but in some cases with bilateral joint disease, both sides may be affected.[1]

MRI scans reveal characteristic frond-like projections originating from the synovium with a signal pattern identical to fat on all imaging sequences. If contrast is administered, the synovium, when inflamed, may enhance, but the fat content within the lesion does not. In some cases, the fatty tissue can form a visible mass, although mild cases typically exhibit diffuse villous growth. Villi can range from small and delicate to bulkier fatty lobules. Osseous erosions are infrequent but can occur as a secondary effect, although they are more commonly attributed to the underlying arthritis.[2]

Other fat-containing intra-articular lesions include true intra-articular lipomas and liposarcomas. A true intra-articular lipoma, though rare, is a localized mass of adipose tissue that lacks villous proliferation, and is surrounded by a thin fibrous capsule. These lipomas may either be sessile or pedunculated. In contrast, intra-articular liposarcoma, though even rarer and not observed in our practice, is a malignant condition. Liposarcomas typically appear in two forms: Low-grade myxoid liposarcoma, which is more common in younger adults, and high-grade pleomorphic liposarcoma, which is seen in older patients. These tumors are typically found near large joints like the knee or elbow, with the more aggressive forms more likely to appear in areas such as the buttocks, abdomen, or groin. Low-grade liposarcomas are well-differentiated and have a high fat content. Khan AM and colleagues recommend investigating lipomas in unusual locations to rule out malignancy.[3]

REFERENCES

1. Coll JP, Ragsdale BD, Chow B, et al. Best Cases from the AFIP: Lipoma Arborescens of the Knees in a Patient with Rheumatoid Arthritis. Radiographics. 2011;31(2):333-7.
2. Ryu KN, Jaovisidha S, Schweitzer M, et al. MR imaging of lipoma arborescens of the knee joint. AJR Am J Roentgenol. 1996;167(5):1229-32.
3. Khan AM, Cannon S, Levack B. Primary Intra-Articular Liposarcoma of the Knee. J Knee Surg. 2003;16(2):107-9.

50 Pigmented Villonodular Synovitis

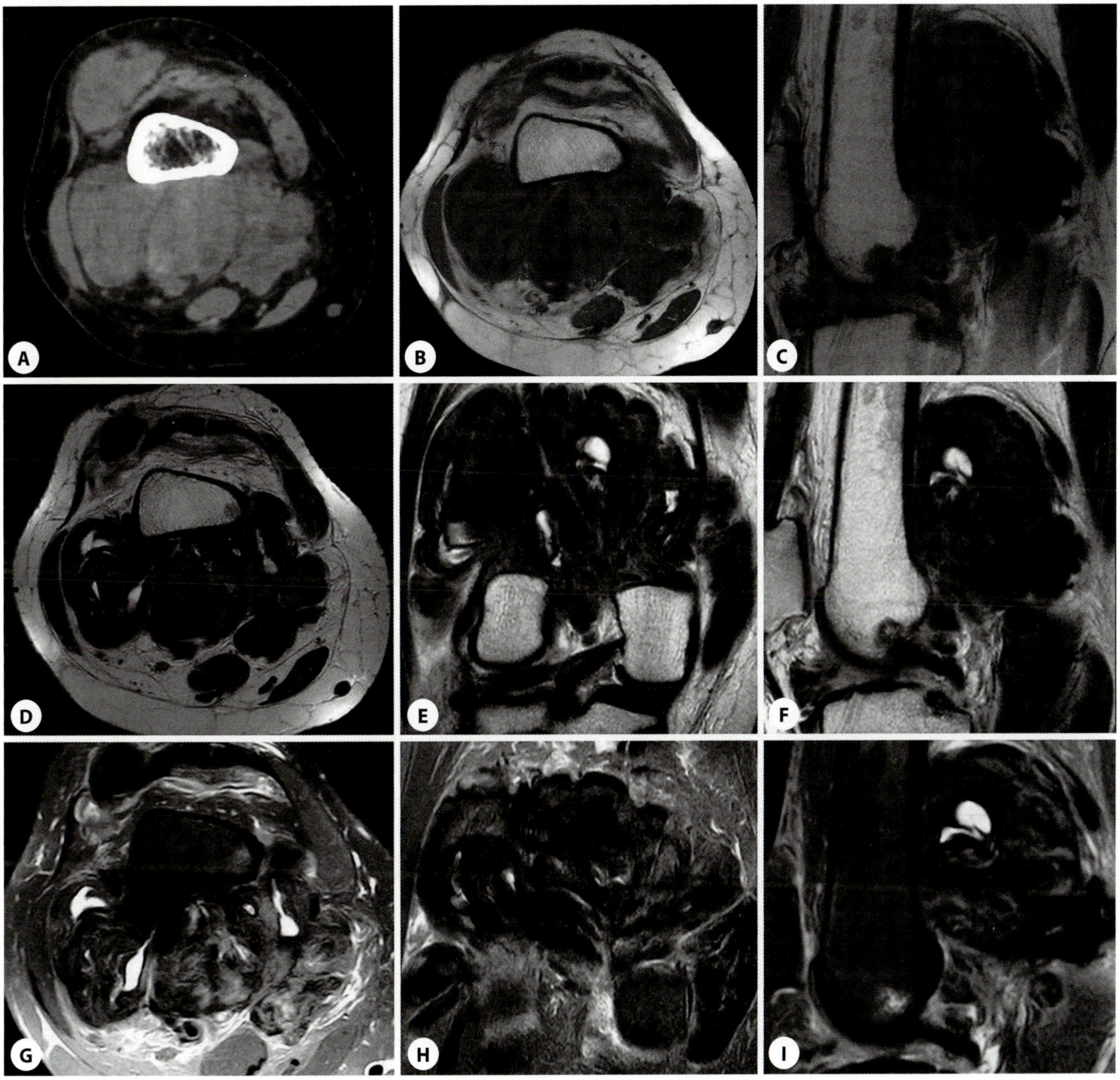

CLINICAL BACKGROUND

A 45-year-old female with complaints of knee pain and swelling.

IMAGING FINDINGS

Lobulated T1/T2 predominantly hypointense lesion with areas of T2 hyperintense foci noted in the intra-articular portion of the right knee joint/the lesion appears heterogeneously hyperintense on STIR/another similar lesion noted in the extra-articular location adjacent to lateral patellar retinaculum/Minimal joint effusion and subcutaneous edema noted/mild marrow edema noted in the distal aspect of femur/minimal degenerative cyst noted in intercondylar region of femur. Otherwise knee joint ligaments and menisci appear normal. CT screening shows no evidence of calcification, and the lesion appears slightly hyperdense to the adjacent muscles/mild cortical irregularity of femur noted **(Figs. 1A to I)**.

DISCUSSION

Pigmented villonodular synovitis (PVNS) is a condition involving the abnormal proliferation of synovial tissue, often accompanied by hemosiderin deposition in varying amounts. PVNS may affect a joint, bursa, or tendon sheath. When it involves the tendon sheath, it is commonly referred to as a giant cell tumor of the tendon sheath (GCTTS) or occasionally as nodular tenosynovitis. Typically, PVNS occurs in a single joint (monoarticular), regardless of whether it presents in the localized or diffuse form, and is most commonly seen in the knee. It predominantly affects individuals in their twenties to forties.[1]

On radiographs, PVNS typically lacks distinctive features. Bone demineralization is not a characteristic of PVNS, and joint spaces generally remain intact, although diffuse forms of PVNS may cause cartilage damage over time, leading to narrowing of the joint space. Unlike primary osteoarthritis, osteophytes are uncommon. In the diffuse form, subchondral cysts or marginal erosions with thin marginal sclerosis may appear. On CT scans, PVNS presents as isodense or slightly hyperdense in comparison to muscle, with visible synovial thickening. Subchondral cysts or erosions, when present, are better visualized using CT.[2]

MRI is often key to diagnosing PVNS, as it frequently shows heterogeneous signal intensity, typically a mix of intermediate and low signals on T1- and T2-weighted sequences. The low signal intensity correlates with hemosiderin accumulation. Gradient echo (GRE) sequences can further highlight the paramagnetic effects of hemosiderin, leading to pronounced low signal blooming. In rare cases, high T1 signal foci may be seen, likely due to the presence of trapped perisynovial fat. Though nonspecific, PVNS often shows heterogeneous enhancement on MRI.[2]

The diffuse form of PVNS manifests with significant synovial thickening and irregular, mass-like formations of various sizes scattered throughout the joint, accompanied by varying degrees of joint effusion. This form can also extend into the surrounding soft tissues, including pericapsular ganglia and bursae. Subchondral cysts and marginal erosions are often seen, with intraosseous PVNS extension sometimes present. When there is extracapsular extension, especially near neurovascular structures, surgical intervention may require a more extensive, open approach for resection.

The localized form of PVNS, primarily affecting the knee, especially the anterior compartment, presents as a well-circumscribed or irregularly shaped mass. It is generally less heterogeneous and more hyperintense on fluid-sensitive sequences than the diffuse form. Effusions are generally not observed in this form.[3]

REFERENCES

1. Murphey MD, Rhee JH, Lewis RB, et al. Pigmented villonodular synovitis: radiologic-pathologic correlation. RadioGraphics. 2008;28:1493-518.
2. Soubai RB, Tahiri L, Ibrahimi A. Bilateral pigmented villonodular synovitis of the knee. Joint Bone Spine. 2011;78(2):219-21.
3. Kim HS, Kwon JW, Ahn JH, et al. Localized tenosynovial giant cell tumor in both knee joints. Skeletal Radiol. 2010;39(9):923-6.

51 Disseminated Tuberculosis

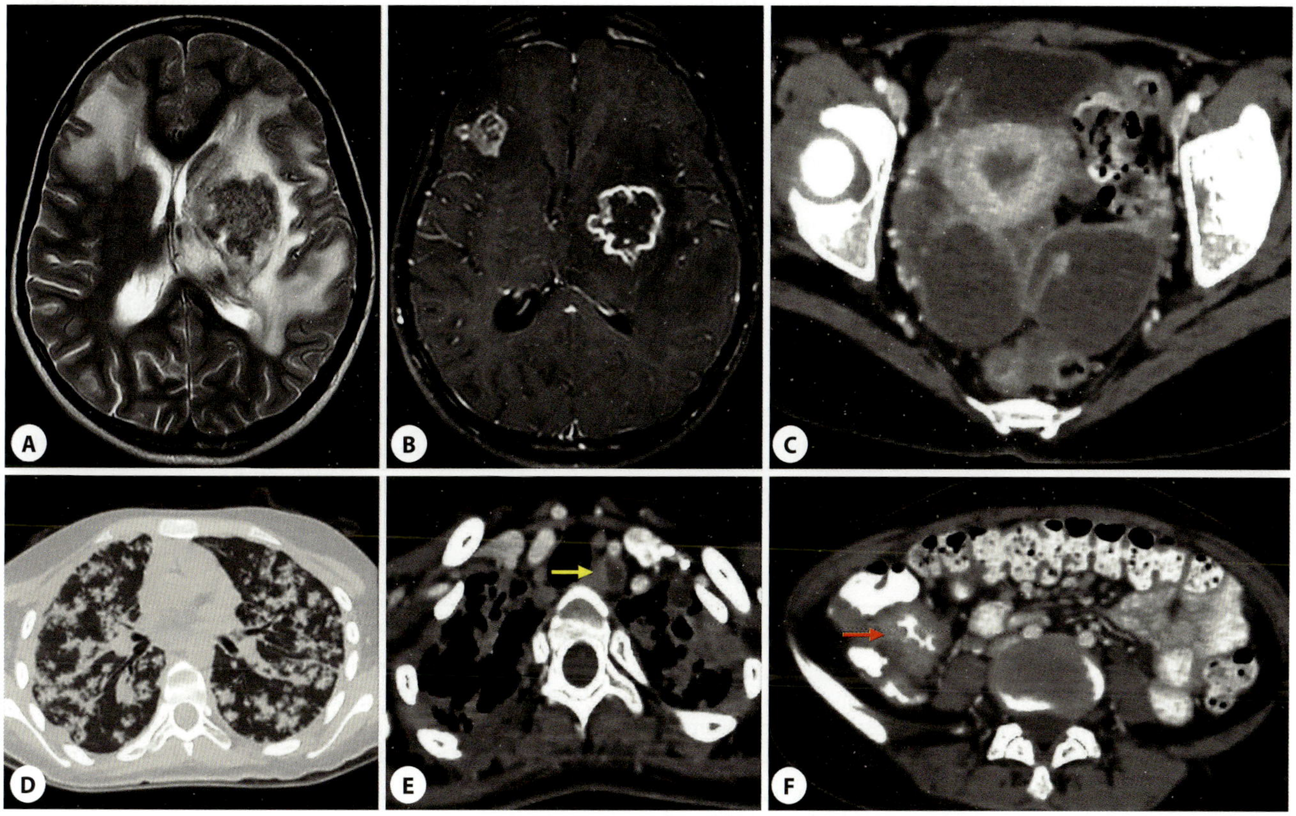

CLINICAL BACKGROUND

Young female patient with significant weight loss.

IMAGING FINDINGS

Ring enhancing conglomerated, T2 hetero predominantly hypointense lesions in left capsulo ganglionic region and right frontal lobe with severe surrounding parenchymal edema involving bilateral frontal and left parieto-temporal lobes **(Figs. 1A to F)**.

Bilateral adnexal peripherally enhancing cystic lesion.

Diffuse peribronchovascular consolidation/ground-glass opacities with centrilobular nodules in "tree in bud" appearance noted in bilateral lung parenchyma. Multiple enlarged bilateral paratracheal and pretracheal mediastinal lymph-nodes with central necrotic areas (yellow arrow).

Circumferential wall thickening with surrounding fat inflammation noted in distal ileum and ileocecal junction (red arrow).

DISCUSSION

Disseminated tuberculosis (TB) is a serious and potentially fatal condition caused by the spread of "*Mycobacterium tuberculosis*" through the bloodstream. Although the exact global prevalence remains uncertain, it is estimated to account for less than 2% of TB cases in immunocompetent adults and up to 20% of all extrapulmonary TB cases. This form of TB is a significant cause of illness and death in developing countries, particularly among children. The symptoms of disseminated TB vary widely, often presenting with subacute or chronic general symptoms like fever, weight loss, and night sweats. In some cases, patients may experience more severe clinical issues, such as anorexia, fever of unknown origin, or multiorgan failure, depending on the affected organs.[1]

Miliary TB, a specific form of disseminated TB, is caused by widespread dissemination of the bacteria via the bloodstream. It appears in 2–6% of primary TB cases and is more common in reactivation TB. Radiographic and high-resolution CT scans typically reveal numerous 1–3 mm nodules randomly distributed throughout both lungs. In patients with HIV, the radiographic features of TB tend to vary based on the degree of immunosuppression.[2]

In cases of abdominal TB, CT imaging may show asymmetric thickening of the ileocecal valve and medial wall of the cecum, as well as enlarged lymph nodes. Other abdominal signs include hepatosplenomegaly with rim-enhancing lesions, peritoneal thickening, omental caking, and ascites. TB spondylitis often presents with a psoas abscess and disc space involvement.[2]

Lymphadenopathy in TB frequently shows peripheral enhancement in enlarged lymph nodes with central low-density areas after contrast administration, indicative of central caseation or liquefaction necrosis with surrounding granulation tissue.[2] Genital tuberculosis (GTB), found in approximately 1% of all TB cases, typically affects the fallopian tubes (which can lead to tubo-ovarian abscesses) in nearly 100% of cases, with the endometrium (50%) and ovaries (20%) being less frequently involved. External genital infections occur in fewer than 5% of cases.[3]

MRI features of CNS tuberculomas vary depending on whether they are caseating or noncaseating. Caseating tuberculomas tend to be isointense or hypointense on T2-weighted images and show rim enhancement. Abscesses may appear as single cavities with rim enhancement or as multiple cavities with peripheral enhancement.[3] Detailed imaging characteristics of CNS TB have been covered in prior case discussions.

REFERENCES

1. Khan FY. Review of literature on disseminated tuberculosis with emphasis on the focused diagnostic workup. J Family Community Med. 2019;26(2):83-91.
2. Feng F, Xia G, Shi Y, et al. Radiological characterization of disseminated tuberculosis in patients with AIDS. Radiology of Infectious Diseases. 2016;3(1):1-8.
3. Ilmer M, Bergauer F, Friese K, et al. Genital tuberculosis as the cause of tuboovarian abscess in an immunosuppressed patient. Infect Dis Obstet Gynecol. 2009;2009:745060.

52 Otogenic Brain Abscesses

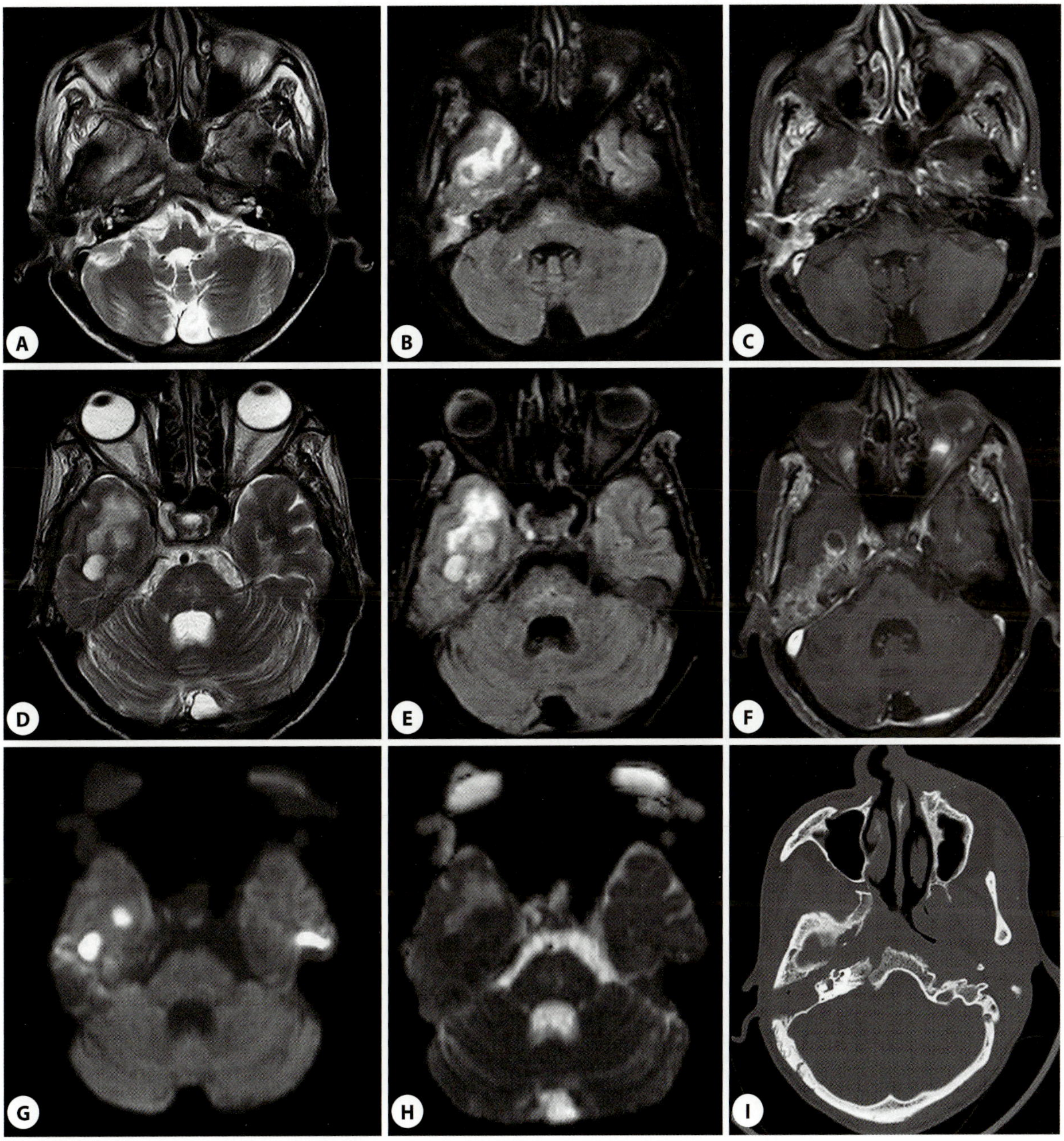

CLINICAL BACKGROUND

Known patient of right chronic suppurative otitis media (CSOM) and postmastoidectomy, came with right sided headache.

IMAGING FINDINGS

- Postoperative changes noted in right mastoid air cells and middle ear cavity **(Figs. 1A to I)**.
- T2/FLAIR hyperintensities seen within middle ear cavity showing postcontrast enhancement.
- Multiloculated T2/FLAIR hyperintense, peripherally enhancing collection noted in right temporal lobe and surrounding edema. MR-spectroscopy shows reduced NAA with lipid lactate and choline peak. The collection shows diffusion restriction.
- Focal pachymeningeal thickening and enhancement in right temporal lobe.
- Erosions in petrous apex of right temporal bone, clivus, carotid canal and tegmen tympanum on CT screening. Bony ossicles and tympanic segment of facial canal not visualized.

DISCUSSION

Otitis media (OM) is a frequently encountered ear condition in both children and adults. It is divided into three main categories: Acute otitis media (AOM), chronic otitis media (COM), and otitis media with effusion (OME). CSOM, a subtype of COM, is marked by persistent middle ear discharge, often linked to a perforated eardrum and may occur with or without cholesteatoma. OM can lead to complications that are either extracranial or intracranial, with brain abscesses being the second most common intracranial complication following meningitis.[1]

The infection can spread to the brain either through defects in the bony tegmen tympani or through infected blood clots traveling via emissary veins to a venous sinus. In otogenic brain abscesses, the areas most commonly affected are the adjacent medial section of the temporal lobe and the lateral part of the cerebellum. CT scans are typically used to diagnose suspected cholesteatoma, and signs include a mass-like soft tissue lesion in Prussak's space, extending into the lateral epitympanic recess. In some cases, bone structures like the ossicles, tegmen tympani, and semicircular canals may show signs of destruction.[2,3]

Brain abscesses from OM develop in four distinct stages:

1. Early cerebritis
2. Late cerebritis
3. Early capsule formation
4. Late capsule formation

On MRI, the cerebritis stages usually show low signals on T1-weighted images (T1WI) and high signals on T2-weighted images (T2WI), often accompanied by patchy enhancement. As the abscess forms a capsule, MRI will show a hyperintense core, hypointense border, and surrounding vasogenic edema on T2WI with defined ring-like enhancement. Diffusion-weighted imaging (DWI) typically reveals central high signals with reduced apparent diffusion coefficient (ADC) values. Additionally, a dual rim sign (an inner hyperintense line within a low-intensity rim) may be visible on T2* GRE and susceptibility-weighted imaging (SWI).[3]

Although otogenic brain abscesses are not common, they can result from untreated or inadequately managed suppurative otitis media, necessitating a careful diagnostic approach. A combination of proper imaging and collaboration among healthcare professionals is key to accurate diagnosis and effective treatment.

REFERENCES

1. Duarte MJ, Kozin ED, Barshak MB, et al. Otogenic brain abscesses: A systematic review. Laryngoscope Investig Otolaryngol. 2018;3(3):198-208.
2. Choi J, Choi J Il, Kim SD. Management of otogenic brain abscess using the transmastoid approach. J Korean Neurosurg Soc. 2014;55(3):178-80.
3. Watanabe KI, Hatano GY, Fukada N, et al. Brain abscess secondary to middle ear cholesteatoma: A report of two cases. Auris Nasus Larynx. 2004;31(4):433-7.

53 TB Meningoencephalitis with LETM

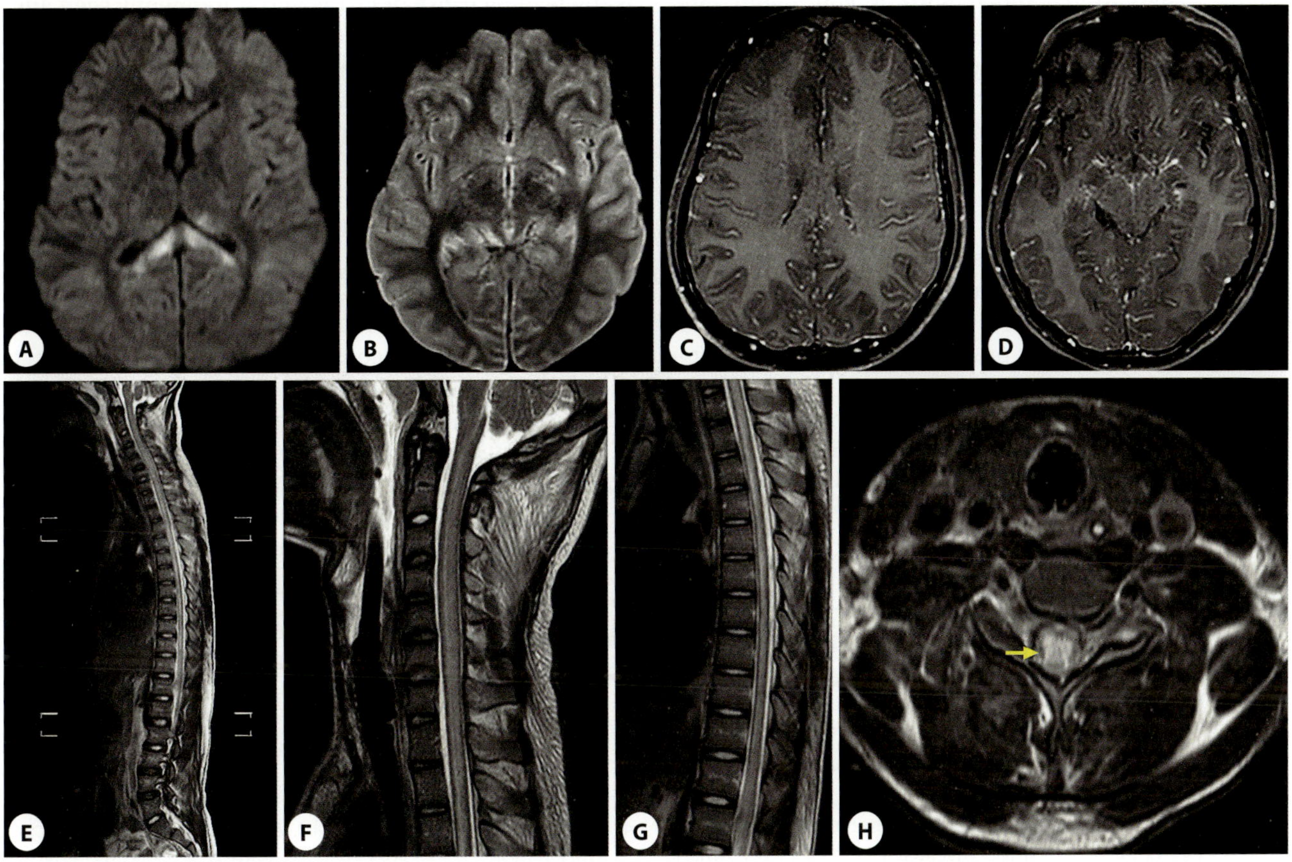

CLINICAL BACKGROUND

A 13-year-old boy came with headache, back pain, and upper arm weakness.

IMAGING FINDINGS

- Diffusion/FLAIR hyperintensities noted in posterior aspect of corpus callosum involving splenium, bilateral hippocampus, left thalamus and temporal lobe **(Figs. 1A to H)**.
- FLAIR hyperintensity in bilateral cerebral sulci with abnormal/nodular leptomeningeal thickening/ postcontrast enhancement seen.
- Long segment T2/STIR hyperintense signals noted involving entire spinal cord occupying > 2/3rd of the cross-sectional area (yellow arrow) causing diffuse enlargement of spinal cord.

DISCUSSION

Tuberculous meningitis is the most frequent central nervous system (CNS) complication of tuberculosis, accounting for 95% of cases, followed by cerebral tuberculoma and tuberculous abscess. Less common manifestations include calvarial tuberculosis, tuberculous pachymeningitis, and spinal arachnoiditis, while intramedullary spinal tuberculosis is considered rare.[1] Longitudinal extensive transverse myelitis (LETM) is a form of acute transverse myelitis (ATM) that can affect individuals of all ages. The most frequently observed cause is neuromyelitis optica (NMO), but infectious diseases, metabolic disorders, post-infectious myelitis (PIM), radiation-induced myelitis, arteriovenous (AV) dural fistula, acute disseminated encephalomyelitis (ADEM), paraneoplastic syndromes, and autoimmune conditions have also been noted. Tuberculous myelitis, a rare form of myelitis, typically affects the dorsal spinal cord, and LETM is an uncommon presentation in *Mycobacterium tuberculosis* infections.[1,2]

LETM is identified on spinal magnetic resonance imaging (MRI) as a lesion extending over three or more vertebral segments. Imaging features often include spinal cord swelling, T1 hypointense and T2 hyperintense signals within the cord, sometimes accompanied by heterogeneous or ring-like enhancement. In tuberculous cases, meningeal enhancement—characterized by linear or nodular enhancement of the meninges—typically appears at the basal subarachnoid cisterns, with dense gelatinous leptomeningeal exudates being a common finding.[3]

Neuromyelitis optica spectrum disorder (NMOSD) is the leading cause of LETM and is frequently seen after optic neuritis in pediatric patients. LETM can coexist with tuberculosis, and it has been hypothesized that the tubercular-exposed lymphocytes have a propensity to target myelin, with myelin essential protein acting as a shared antigen. In some cases, anti-AQP4 antibodies and oligoclonal bands, which are typically associated with neuromyelitis optica (NMO) and multiple sclerosis (MS), respectively, may be absent.[3,4]

Although tuberculous infection of the CNS most commonly affects the brain, spinal cord involvement can occur as a secondary consequence. Myelitis that affects the entire spinal cord is an unusual presentation, with only a few cases reported. This case highlights the importance of early detection and intervention to prevent severe complications like LETM. Clinicians should maintain a high index of suspicion for spinal cord involvement in cases of CNS tuberculosis to mitigate associated morbidity.[3]

REFERENCES

1. Jain RS, Kumar S, Tejwani S. A rare association of tuberculous longitudinally extensive transverse myelitis (LETM) with brain tuberculoma. Springerplus. 2015;4:476.
2. Cicia, Nociti V, Bianco A, et al. "Neurosarcoidosis presenting as longitudinally extensive myelitis: Diagnostic assessment, differential diagnosis, and therapeutic approach. Translational Neuroscience. 2022;13(1):191-7.
3. Amaral DM, Parreira T, Sampaio M. Longitudinally extensive transverse myelitis and meningitis due to a rare infectious cause. BMJ Case Rep. 2015;2015.
4. Ranjan S, Dev R, Keisham MD. A sporadic case of holocord tuberculous transverse myelitis with arachnoiditis. Egypt J Radiol Nucl Med. 2022;53:252.

54 Cerebral Abscess in Tetralogy of Fallot

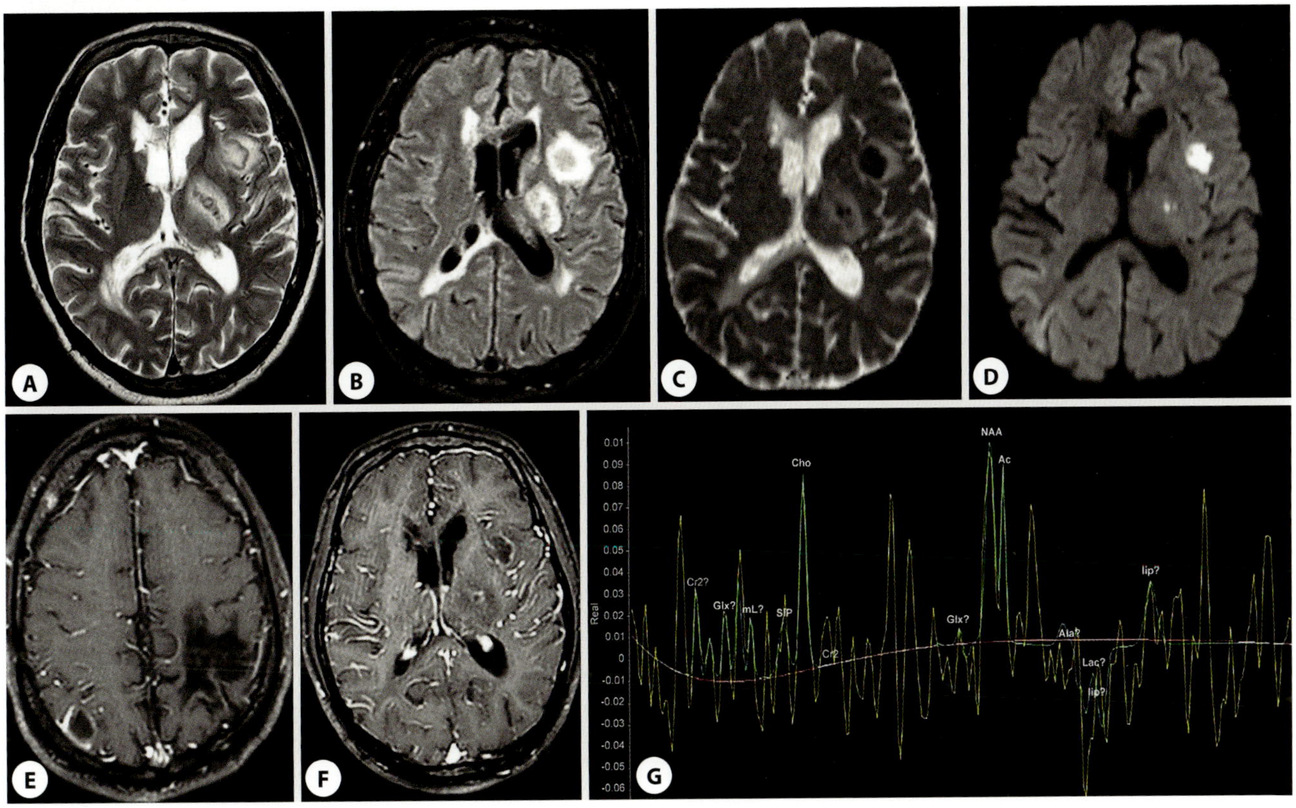

CLINICAL BACKGROUND

A 50-year-old known patient of congenital heart disease, came with headache and giddiness.

IMAGING FINDINGS

Multiple conglomerated, peripherally enhancing T1 hypointense, T2/FLAIR heterointense, predominantly hyperintense lesions showing diffusion restriction noted in left corona radiata, capsulo-thalamic region extending into left cerebral peduncle and right posterior parietal lobe with surrounding parenchymal edema **(Figs. 1A to G)**.

- Focal pachymeningeal thickening/enhancement in right parietal convexity.
- MRS shows elevated lipid lactate peak.

DISCUSSION

Brain abscesses, though rare, are serious complications that occur in 5–18.7% of individuals with cyanotic congenital heart disease (CCHD). CCHD is characterized by a right-to-left shunt that bypasses the pulmonary circulation, leading to hypoxia and cyanosis. Tetralogy of Fallot (TOF) is the most common form of CCHD and comprises four significant cardiac defects, resulting in cyanosis during childhood. Complications from untreated TOF can include developmental delays, slower growth, and a heightened risk of severe infective endocarditis.

Additionally, brain abscesses, while uncommon, have been noted as a presenting symptom in certain cases.[1]

Several factors contribute to the development of brain abscesses in patients with CCHD. Since blood flow bypasses the lungs, it is not filtered by the alveolar phagocytes, which increases the likelihood of pathogens entering the bloodstream and reaching the brain. Furthermore, areas of the brain may suffer from reduced perfusion due to significant hypoxemia and metabolic acidosis from secondary polycythemia, creating favorable conditions for pathogen colonization. Hematogenous spread of infection often leads to multiple cerebral abscesses. Brain abscesses are found to be two to three times more common in males than in females. Although they are infrequently seen, these abscesses can have severe consequences, especially in individuals in their forties. In patients with CCHD, cerebral abscesses are commonly attributed to infections from non-hemolytic streptococci, particularly *Streptococcus Milleri*.[1,2]

MRI can help distinguish cerebral abscesses from rim-enhancing tumors. Key imaging features include a smooth inner margin of the enhancing rim on contrast-enhanced scans, the presence of satellite lesions, and a dark rim on T2-weighted images. In diffusion-weighted imaging (DWI), cerebral abscesses typically show restricted diffusion, as indicated by lower apparent diffusion coefficient (ADC) values compared to adjacent healthy tissue and tumors. However, it can be challenging to differentiate abscesses from neoplasms based solely on conventional MRI findings. In such instances, dynamic susceptibility contrast perfusion MRI may provide a more reliable method for differentiating high-grade tumors from abscesses.[3]

For abscesses less than 2 cm in diameter, patients who are neurologically stable can often be managed with empirical medical treatment and regular imaging for monitoring. Conversely, invasive procedures such as craniotomy and excision carry significant mortality risks, potentially as high as 71%, and are usually reserved for cases with progressive abscesses that do not respond to conventional treatment.[4]

REFERENCES

1. NNF Begum, FR Sarker, M Begum, et al. Management of a critical case of double outlet right ventricle (DORV) and cerebral abscess by multiple interventions. JAFMC Bangladesh. 2016;11:(2016):81-4.
2. H Alvis Miranda, SM Castellar-Leones, MA Elzain, et al. Brain abscess: current management. J Neurosci Rural Pract. 2013;4(1) S67-81.
3. Holmes TM, Petrella JR, Provenzale JM. Distinction Between Cerebral Abscesses and High-Grade Neoplasms by Dynamic Susceptibility Contrast Perfusion MRI. AJR Am J Roentgenol. 2004;183(5):1247-52.
4. M Ashraf, S Ahmed, S Ahmad, et al. Burr hole aspiration of brain abscess in children with cyanotic heart disease. J Coll Physicians Surg Pak. 2017;27:483-5.

55 Scimitar Syndrome

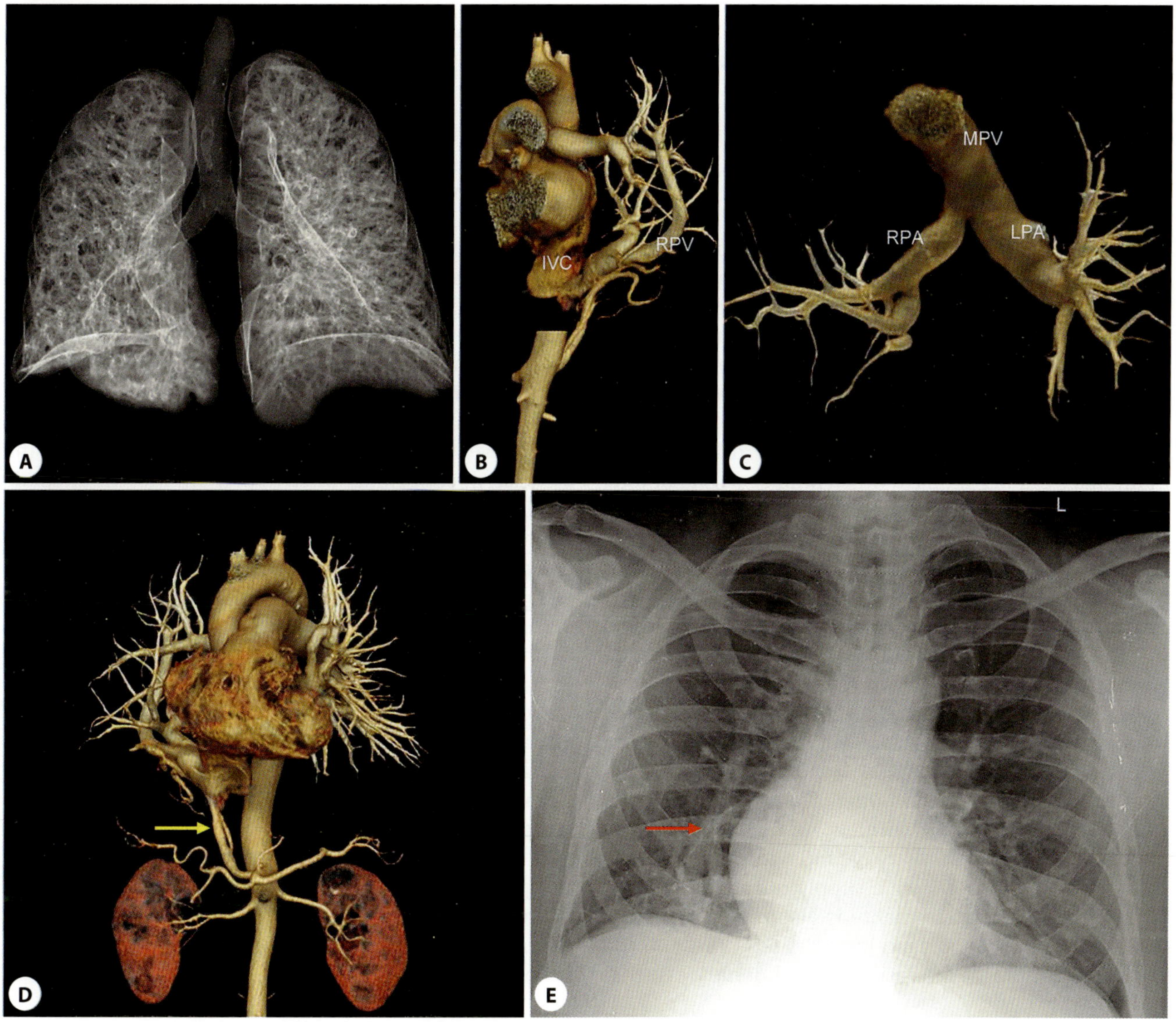

CLINICAL BACKGROUND

A 63-year-old male came with breathlessness on exertion and recurrent lower respiratory tract infection.

IMAGING FINDINGS

- Hypoplasia of right middle/lower lobe lung **(Figs. 1A to E)**.
- Right pulmonary veins noted draining into the infradiaphragmatic portion of the IVC (partial anomalous venous drainage).
- Hypoplastic right pulmonary artery.
- Anomalous arterial blood supply to the right lower lobe lung from branches of abdominal aorta (celiac axis) (yellow arrow).
- Chest X-ray (PA view) shows the "scimitar" appearance of the anomalous pulmonary vein in the right lung (red arrow) and crowding of ribs on right side.

DISCUSSION

Scimitar syndrome is a rare association of congenital cardiopulmonary anomalies, and first described in 1836, accounting for 0.5–1% of all CHD. The term 'Scimitar syndrome' was coined by Neill et al., with reference to the characteristic appearance of the anomalous right pulmonary venous confluence on the X-ray of chest. The vein is said to resemble a curved Turkish sword called a 'Scimitar'. The X-ray appearance is referred to as the 'Scimitar Sign'. The syndrome is a form of anomalous pulmonary venous drainage which implies partial or total failure of the pulmonary veins to reach the left atrium. Instead, pulmonary venous drainage is anomalously connected to the systemic vein/s, typically to SVC or inferior vena cava or directly to the right atrium.[1,2]

The characteristic components of this syndrome include anomalous arterial blood supply from the abdominal aorta without sequestration and anomalous pulmonary venous drainage into infradiaphragmatic inferior vena cava (Scimitar vein), right pulmonary artery hypoplasia and right sided lung hypoplasia. The most common components of the congenital pulmonary venolobar syndrome are hypogenetic lung and anomalous pulmonary venous return. To note, isolated anomalous systemic supply to the lower lobes without bronchial abnormality is also reported. In few cases in whom hypoplastic lung tissue is present, the proximal portion of the ipsilateral pulmonary artery is absent; however, the peripheral pulmonary arteries are present.[3,4]

According to Felson et al.[5] the anomalous pulmonary vein often drains into the inferior vena cava below the right hemidiaphragm. Less commonly partial anomalous pulmonary venous return drains into the supra-hepatic portion of the inferior vena cava, hepatic veins, portal vein, azygous vein, coronary sinus, or right atrium. Drainage of the anomalous vein into the supra-hepatic portion of the inferior vena cava or right atrium may be a clue to the associated congenital interruption of the intrahepatic portion of the inferior vena cava. When partial anomalous pulmonary venous return drains to a systemic vein or to the right atrium, there is a left-to-right shunt, which is usually asymptomatic unless the shunt is 2:1 or greater. On occasion, the partial anomalous pulmonary venous return drains to the left atrium and when it occurs; the anomalous vein is called a "meandering" pulmonary vein.[5]

Various imaging modalities contribute diagnostic information in patients with congenital heart disease. CT and MRI are especially useful in demonstrating extracardiac anatomy. Echocardiography continues to be the preferred modality for imaging intracardiac anatomy and hemodynamics. The combined use of advanced postprocessing graphic workstations, allows improved delineation of the complex and variable anatomic abnormalities seen in patients with congenital pulmonary venolobar syndrome.

REFERENCES

1. V Grech, R Xuereb, M Xuereb, et al. Late presentation and successful treatment of classical scimitar syndrome. Images Paediatr Cardiol. 2003;16:49-62.
2. F Sehgal, A Loughran-Fowlds. Scimitar syndrome. Indian J Paediatr. 2005;72:249-51.
3. SF KO, SH Ng, TY Lee. Anomalous systemic arterialization to normal basal segments of the left lower lobe: helical CT and CT angiographic findings. J Comput Assist Tomogr. 2000;24:971-6.
4. PW Morgan, DW Foley, SJ Erickson. Proximal interruption of a main pulmonary artery with transpleural collateral vessels: CT and magnetic resonance appearances. J Comput Assist Tomogr. 1991;15:311-3.
5. Felson B. Chest roentgenology Saunders, Philadelphia,1973.

56 Minimal Aortic Injury

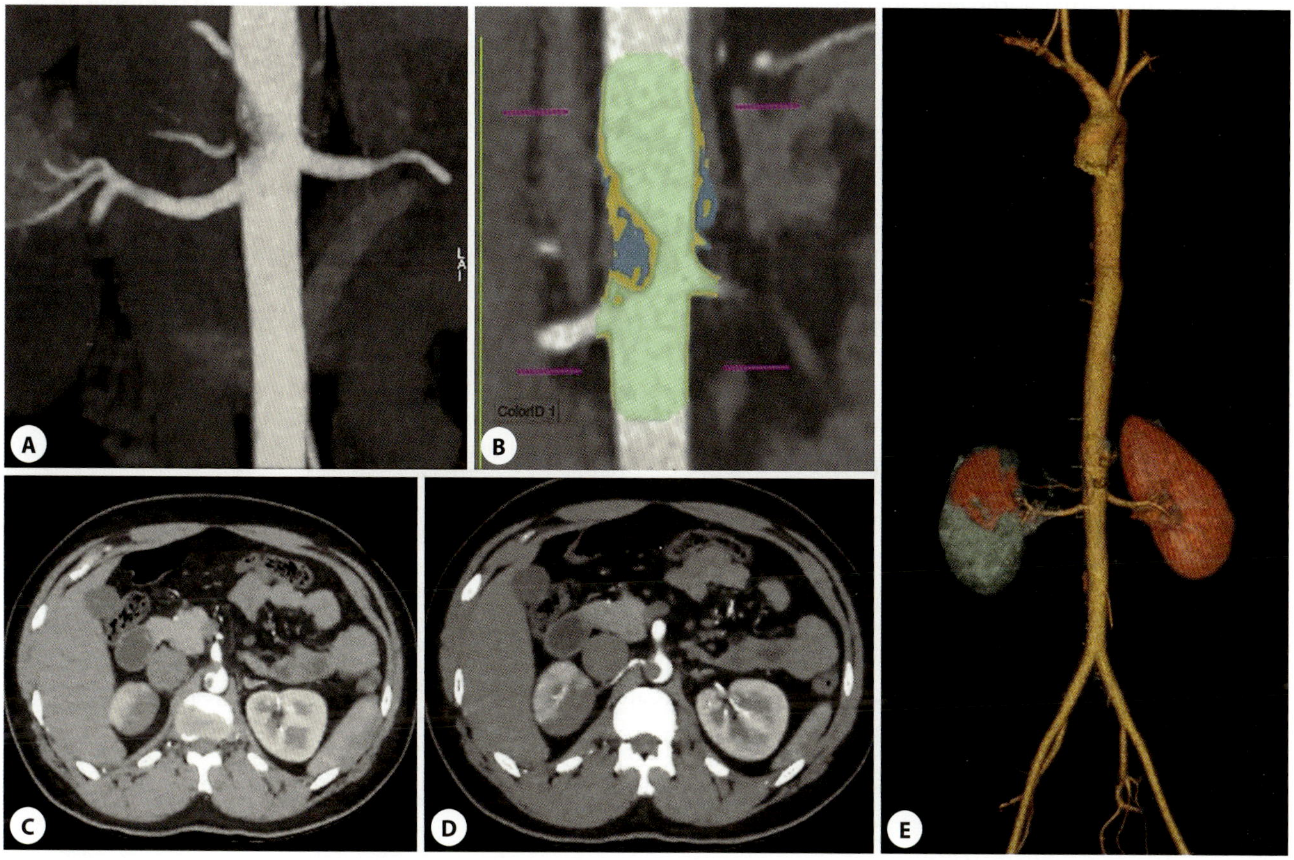

CLINICAL BACKGROUND

A 27-year-old male came with history of RTA and abdominal pain.

IMAGING FINDINGS

- Minimal asymmetric wall thickening and multifocal intraluminal partial filling defects (attached thrombus) seen in suprarenal portion of abdominal aorta, extending into accessory right renal artery, ostium of right main renal artery, origin of superior mesenteric and celiac arteries. Multifocal right renal infarcts **(Figs. 1A to E)**.
- No contrast extravasation or pseudoaneurysm.

DISCUSSION[1]

The term "minimal aortic injury" (MAI) has gained traction in evaluating patients with blunt trauma, reflecting advancements in multidetector CT imaging. MAI refers to a milder form of blunt traumatic aortic injury (BTAI) that generally resolves or stabilizes with medical management. BTAI is classified based on the presence or absence of external aortic wall abnormalities, such as pseudoaneurysms, into minimal aortic injury (MAI) and significant aortic injury (SAI).

MAI is characterized as a "sub-centimeter intimomedial abnormality without any external contour deformity," which includes small intimal tears and intramural hematomas. While small intimal tears (SVS grade I) have long been associated with MAI, the more recent inclusion of intramural hematomas (SVS grade II) in this classification is supported by contemporary management-based systems like the Vancouver and Harborview classifications.

The isthmus of the descending thoracic aorta is the most frequently affected site in MAI, occurring in approximately two-thirds of patients with BTAI who present to hospitals. A smaller percentage of cases involve the ascending aorta (8–27%), aortic arch (8–18%), distal descending aorta (11-21%), and the abdominal aorta, particularly at the aortic hiatus (7–22%). The most common imaging findings of an intimal tear in MAI are a rounded or triangular intraluminal filling defect (measuring 10 mm or less in 80% of cases) and a thin focal intimal flap (seen in 15% of cases) that remains attached to the vessel wall without external contour deformity. These findings are usually located at the aortic isthmus and represent an SVS grade I injury. A small intramural hematoma (1 cm or less in thickness) is characterized by increased attenuation within the aortic wall due to bleeding from ruptured vasa vasorum or small intimal-medial tears. This condition is classified as SVS grade II injury but is included in the MAI spectrum by several surgical groups, accounting for 5% of all MAI cases. The improved identification of MAI due to advancements in CT technology and its increased application has facilitated studies involving larger patient populations in recent years.

Research indicates that spontaneous healing of MAI often occurs within 4–8 weeks, with only 10–15% of cases persisting or progressing during follow-up. The variation in reported resolution rates (from 55 to 85%) is primarily due to discrepancies in short- to mid-term follow-up data.

Society of Vascular Surgery Classification (Azzazideh et al.)		**Vancouver classification (Lemarche et al.)**		**Harborview classification (Heneghan et al.)**	
Year proposed 2009 most widely used		**Year proposed 2012 proposed advantage better reproducibility**		**Year proposed 2016 proposed advantage—tailored to guide management**	
Grade	**Description**	**Grade**	**Description**	**Grade**	**Description**
I	Intimal tear/flap	I	Thrombus/flap/IMH < 1 cm	Minimal	Thrombus/flap/IMH < 1 cm w/o contour abnormality
II	Intramural hematoma (IMH)	II	Thrombus/Flap/IMH > 1 cm	Moderate	External contour abnormality or flap > 1 cm
III	Pseudoaneurysm (PSA)	III	PSA without extravasation		
IV	Free rupture	IV	Contrast extravasation	Severe	Extravasation, left subclavian artery hematoma > 1.5 cm

REFERENCE

1. Kapoor H, Lee JT, Orr NT, et al. Minimal Aortic Injury: Mecha-nisms, Imaging Manifestations, Natural History, and Management. RadioGraphics. 2020;40:1834-47.

57 Aggressive Giant Cell Tumor

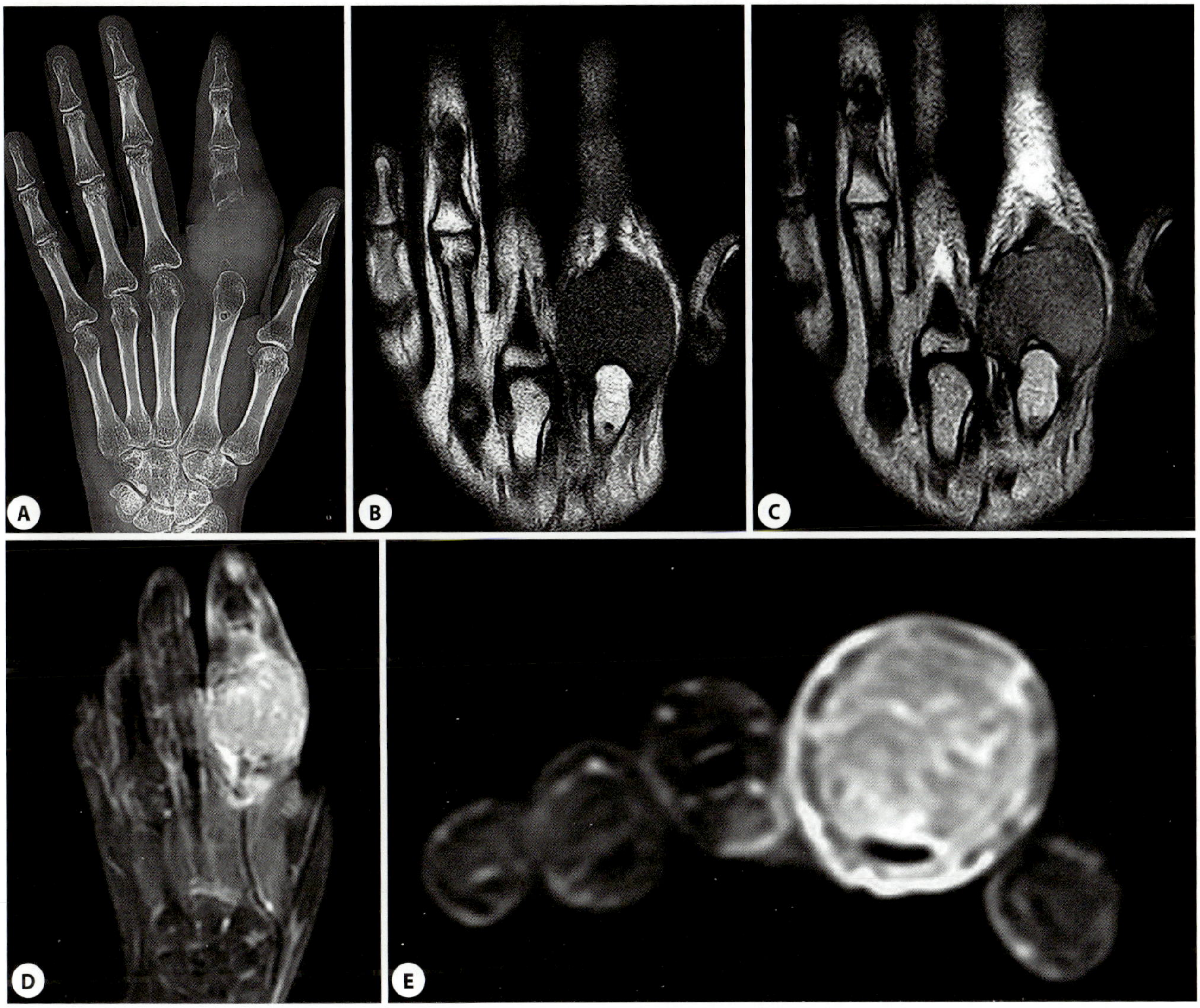

CLINICAL BACKGROUND

A 17-year-old girl came with swelling in the left-hand index finger for past 1 year, which increasing in size for past 3 months, associated with pain.

IMAGING FINDINGS

Ill-defined expansile osteolytic lesion with T1/T2 isointense soft tissue component noted involving base and shaft of proximal phalanx of index finger (epi-metaphyseal region). The lesion shows mild diffusion restriction and postcontrast enhancement **(Figs. 1A to E)**.

DISCUSSION

Giant cell tumor (GCT) of the bones of the hand has some special features as compared to GCT at other sites. GCT of the metacarpal bones is rare. It occurs predominantly in the younger age-groups and displays more aggressive behavior. The metaphyseal region of the metacarpal is reported to be the common site for GCT. GCTs recur more rapidly in the hand than at other locations. The incidence of multicentric foci for GCTs of hand is 18%, indicating that a bone scan should be part of the routine workup in these tumors.[1]

On conventional radiographs and CT, GCT is typically seen as an eccentric, epi-metaphyseal osteolytic lesion, with well-defined nonsclerotic border and extension underneath the subchondral articular bone in closed physes. GCT may also show aggressive features consisting of poorly demarcated margins, cortical thinning and destruction and soft tissue extension. CT may be useful in evaluating cortical bone integrity, absence of matrix mineralization and demonstration of pathologic fracture. GCT of the hand tends to be less eccentric and more centrally located.[2]

MRI can help determine the precise intramedullary and soft-tissue extent of the lesion. Generally, GCT has a low-to-intermediate signal on T1WI and a heterogeneous-high signal on T2WI. However, due to intratumoral hemosiderin or fibrosis, the signal may be low on T2WI. The lesion enhances after intravenous gadolinium contrast administration, reflecting the increased vascular supply. Fluid-fluid levels, consistent with secondary formation of aneurysmal bone cysts, are seen in 14% of cases.[2,3]

Rarely, GCT is associated with histologically benign lung metastases or undergoes malignant degeneration (sarcomatous transformation)—which may be an osteosarcoma, fibrosarcoma, or undifferentiated pleomorphic sarcoma (historically known as malignant fibrous histiocytoma). The findings that should alert the radiologist to think of malignant transformation in GCTB are areas of new cortex destruction, a new soft tissue mass, and new tumor localizations i.e., (nonpulmonary) metastases.[4]

There are subtypes of osteosarcoma that may mimic GCT. For instance, both telangiectatic osteosarcoma and giant cell–rich osteosarcoma is often expansile and typically do not produce the extensive osteoid matrix seen in conventional osteosarcomas. Like GCT, telangiectatic osteosarcoma often demonstrates fluid-fluid levels at MRI. Fibroblastic osteosarcoma also does not typically demonstrate osteoid matrix at imaging; however, central areas of low signal intensity may be seen within the lesion. All three subtypes of osteosarcoma can be included in the differential diagnosis for an aggressive GCT of bone.[2]

REFERENCES

1. Saikia KC, Bhuyan SK, Ahmed F, et al. Giant cell tumor of the metacarpal bones. Indian J Orthop. 2011;45(5):475-8.
2. Chakarun CJ, Forrester DM, Gottsegen CJ, et al. Giant cell tumor of bone: Review, Mimics and new developments in treatment. RadioGraphics. 2013;1:197-211.
3. Pereira HM, Marchiori E, Severo A. Magnetic resonance imaging aspects of giant-cell tumours of bone. J Med Imaging Radiat Oncol. 2014;58(6):674-8.
4. SV Domovitov, JH Healey. "Primary malignant giant-cell tumor of bone has high survival rate. Annals of Surgical Oncology. 2010;17(3):694-701.

58 Giant Superior Vena Cava Aneurysm

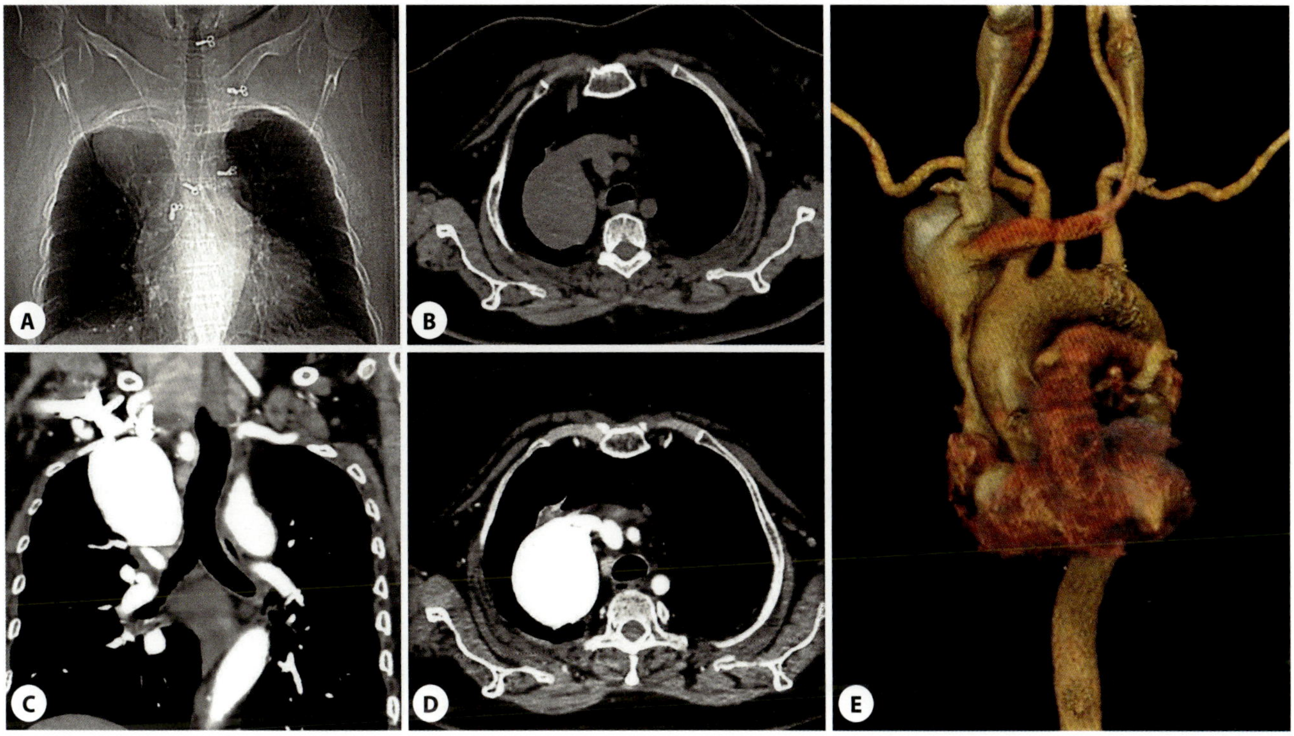

CLINICAL BACKGROUND

A 79-year-old male came with right chest discomfort.

IMAGING FINDINGS

Large saccular aneurysm seen arising from proximal portion of the SVC in right posterolateral wall, involving the confluence of both innominate veins and related posteriorly to the confluence. Superiorly the aneurysm extends up to level of I rib and inferiorly up to level of draining of azygous vein **(Figs. 1A to E)**.

DISCUSSION

Superior vena cava (SVC) aneurysms are an uncommon cause of mediastinal widening identified incidentally on chest X-rays. These aneurysms can be classified into two morphological types: Fusiform and saccular, with fusiform being the predominant form. Although the precise mechanisms behind the formation of SVC aneurysms are not fully understood, several potential causes have been proposed, including congenital abnormalities, inflammation, infection, mechanical trauma, and pathological deficiencies in the adventitia of the SVC's longitudinal muscle wall.[1]

Vein aneurysms are a particularly rare medical phenomenon. In 1963, Abbot and Leight established a classification system for aneurysms, categorizing them into four groups: Congenital, acquired, pseudoaneurysms, and arteriovenous aneurysms. The fusiform aneurysm comprises the majority of these cases and may occur as solitary lesions or in conjunction with cystic hygromas and angiomas. For asymptomatic patients with an aneurysm diameter of less than 40 mm, conservative management—including anti-plaque therapy and regular imaging—may be appropriate. However, aneurysms that exceed 40 mm, are growing, symptomatic, or contain thrombus necessitate radical surgical intervention. To date, only 27 cases of aneurysms originating from mediastinal systemic veins have been reported, with SVC aneurysms being the most common type. The first documented case appeared in 1950.[2]

While angiography has traditionally been the standard diagnostic method for SVC aneurysms, most recent cases have been diagnosed through contrast-enhanced computed tomography (CECT), with or without three-dimensional reconstruction. A CECT scan revealing a mediastinal lesion that shows a similar contrast enhancement pattern to the SVC can help distinguish it from other vascular mass lesions in the mediastinum. For larger saccular SVC aneurysms, even in asymptomatic cases, prophylactic surgical resection is often recommended.[3]

REFERENCES

1. Jacobson AM, Ailiani RG, Paramesh V. A Rare Case of Superior Vena Cava Saccular Aneurysm. CASE (Phila). 2019;3(6):246-9.
2. Janczak D, Skiba J, Gemel M, et al. Giant saccular superior vena cava aneurysm—a rare and difficult clinical case. J Thorac Dis. 2016;8(3):E247-9.
3. Panduranga P, Thomas E, Al-Maskari S, et al. Giant superior vena caval aneurysm in a post-Glenn patient. ICVTS. 2012;14(6): 878-9.

59 Cephalic Arch Stenosis: Post AVF

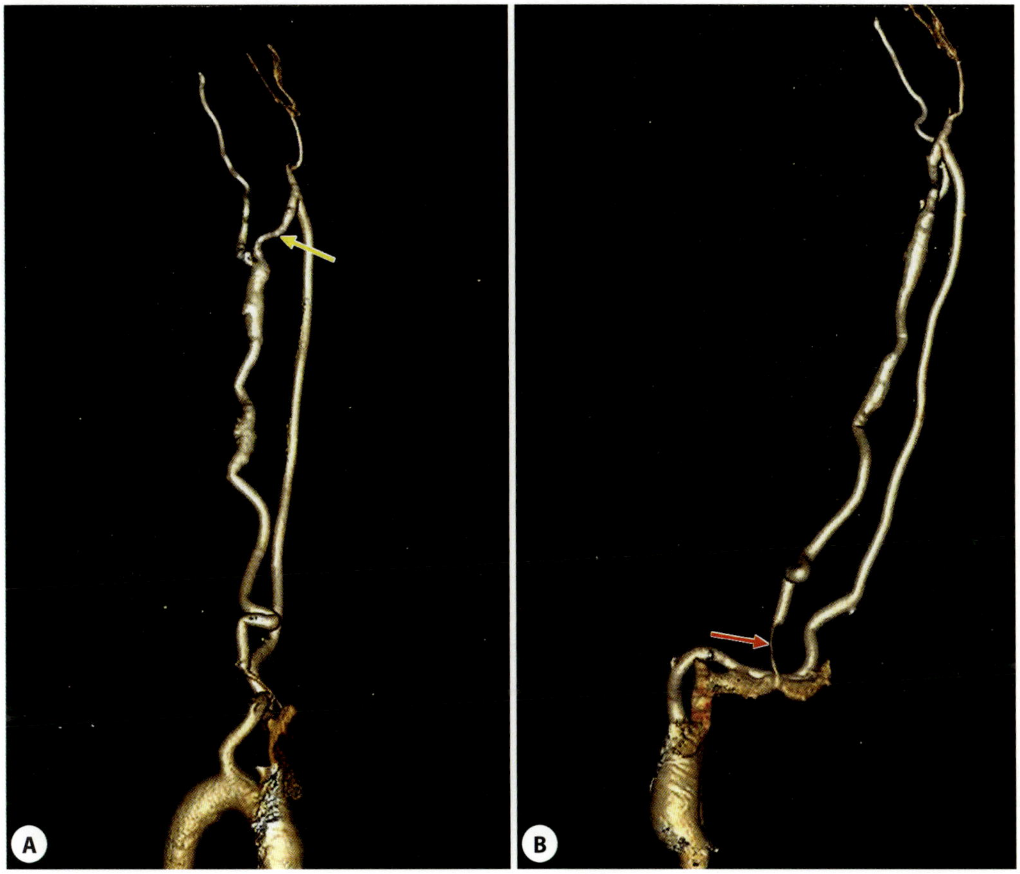

CLINICAL BACKGROUND

A 48-year-old female, known patient of CKD came with brachiocephalic fistula dysfunction.

IMAGING FINDINGS

Diffuse luminal narrowing in the central perpendicular portion of the cephalic vein (as it transverse the deltopectoral groove) and joins the axillary vein (red arrow).

Brachiocephalic fistula at elbow. Cephalic vein appears dilated and tortuous in arm and forearm region/ fistula site appears patent (yellow arrow) **(Figs. 1A and B)**.

DISCUSSION

The cephalic arch is the last section of the cephalic vein before it drains into the first part of the axillary vein. This region is a common site for vascular access dysfunction due to its unique anatomical characteristics. The actual incidence of cephalic arch stenosis (CAS) may be underestimated because of patient selection biases, which often lead to the diagnosis of clinically significant CAS while leaving subclinical cases unnoticed.[1]

CAS is more frequently observed in brachiocephalic fistulas (BCFs) compared to radiocephalic fistulas (RCFs). This lower prevalence in RCFs can be attributed to the presence of alternative outflow veins, such as the basilic and median cubital veins, which allow for better blood drainage, unlike in BCFs where the cephalic vein serves as the main vessel. Although the pathophysiology of CAS is not fully understood, several potential mechanisms have been proposed. These include altered blood flow dynamics, extrinsic compression from surrounding fascia and the pectoralis major muscle, the anatomical structure of the cephalic arch, the entry angle of the cephalic vein into the axillary vein, as well as turbulence resulting from multiple valves.[2]

Doppler ultrasound can indicate increased blood flow velocities at the cephalic arch, with some studies recommending a threshold velocity of 4 m/s at an insonation angle of 60° or a peak systolic velocity ratio exceeding three when comparing the stenosed segment to an adjacent normal segment as criteria for considering intervention. Nonetheless, computed tomography (CT) angiography is highly effective in accurately demonstrating cephalic arch stenosis, including its precise location, length, and severity, while also ruling out any abnormalities in the central veins of the neck and chest.[2]

Currently, percutaneous balloon angioplasty, with or without stenting, is viewed as the primary management option for venous stenosis in patients undergoing hemodialysis. Although angioplasty is frequently attempted, the presence of resilient stenosis may necessitate the placement of stents. Once stents are deployed, they can lead to intimal hyperplasia within the stent and subsequently result in further stenosis and access failure. Surgical treatment for CAS is reserved for recurrent cases that do not respond to angioplasty. One surgical option, cephalic vein transposition, involves ligating the cephalic vein at the deltopectoral groove and relocating the remaining segment to the distal axillary vein. Alternatively, an interposition graft may be surgically moved from the cephalic vein to the jugular vein, bypassing the axillary vein.[1,2]

REFERENCES

1. Echefu G, Shivangi S, Dukkipati R, et al. Contemporary review of management techniques for cephalic arch stenosis in hemodialysis. Ren Fail. 2023;45(1):2176166.
2. Sarala S, Sangeetha B, Mahapatra VS, et al. Cephalic Arch Stenosis: Location of Stenosis in Indian Hemodialysis Patients. Indian J Nephrol. 2018;28(4):273-7.

60

Intraconal Orbital Dermoid Cyst

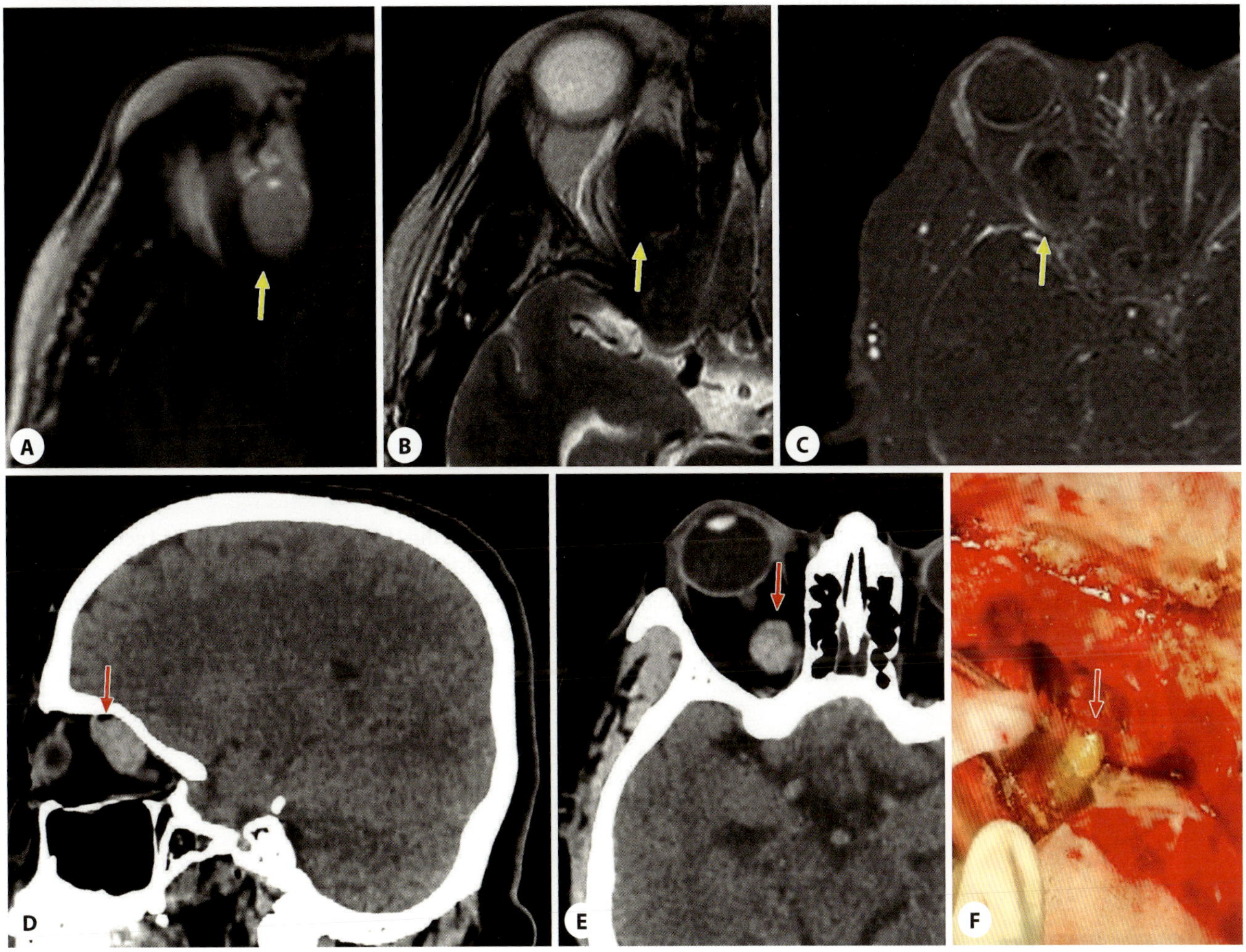

CLINICAL BACKGROUND

A 39-year-old male presented with right eye proptosis.

IMAGING FINDINGS

Evidence of well-defined T1 hyperintense/T2 hypointense lesion (yellow arrows) with moderate postcontrast enhancement and small internal fat attenuating area noted (red arrow) in intra-conal portion of the right orbit, superomedial aspect of right orbit abutting the superior rectus, superior oblique and levator palpebrae superioris muscles and optic nerve/mild proptosis of right globe. No evidence of diffusion restriction or blooming within the lesion. No evidence of orbit wall erosions. Intraoperative image is shown **(Figs. 1A to F)**.

DISCUSSION

A dermoid cyst is a noncancerous soft tissue growth that originates from embryonic epithelium along the body's suture lines. These cysts account for about 2% of all orbital tumors. They can be classified based on their position relative to the musculofascial cone as either extraconal or intraconal, with intraconal dermoid cysts being particularly rare, comprising only 0.5–0.6% of the total. Most orbital dermoids are found in the superficial compartment of the eye and are typically identified in childhood, although cases in adults, like the one presented here, do occur.[1]

Most patients with these cysts are asymptomatic, presenting primarily with a painless swelling around the eye due to their superficial location. However, an intraconal dermoid may exhibit various symptoms depending on the pressure it exerts on nearby neuromuscular structures. Intraocular pain may arise from inflammatory reactions within the dermoid cyst, potentially resulting from chronic inflammation.[1,2]

Radiological imaging plays a crucial role in diagnosing orbital dermoids, as fine needle aspiration is not always feasible—especially with deep-seated masses where neurovascular injury could occur. On contrast-enhanced CT scans, these cysts typically appear as well-defined cystic lesions with surrounding hyperostosis and peripheral calcification. Contrast-enhanced MRI is particularly effective in identifying the fat component and provides superior soft tissue resolution. It excels over CT scans in detailing the anatomy of the lesion, including its extent and its relationship with adjacent neuromuscular structures and the orbital rim. MRI is also beneficial for identifying complications, such as hemorrhage or rupture of the cyst.[1,3]

The definitive treatment for intraconal dermoid cysts is surgical excision, typically performed via an orbital incision. With advancements in endoscopic sinus surgery techniques, these lesions can often be removed through a transnasal endoscopic approach, which minimizes intraoperative and postoperative complications.

REFERENCES

1. Samal S, Sable MN, Pradhan S, et al. Intraconal orbital dermoid cyst: a rare location. Autops Case Rep. 2021;25:11.
2. Shields JA, Kaden IH, Eagle RC Jr, et al. Orbital dermoid cysts: clinicopathologic correlations, classification, and management: the 1997 Josephine E. Schueler Lecture. Ophthal Plast Reconstr Surg. 1997;13(4):265-76.
3. Nugent RA, Lapointe JS, Rootman J, et al. Orbital dermoids: features on CT. Radiology. 1987;165(2):475–8.

61 Leptomeningeal Carcinomatosis—Carcinoma Breast

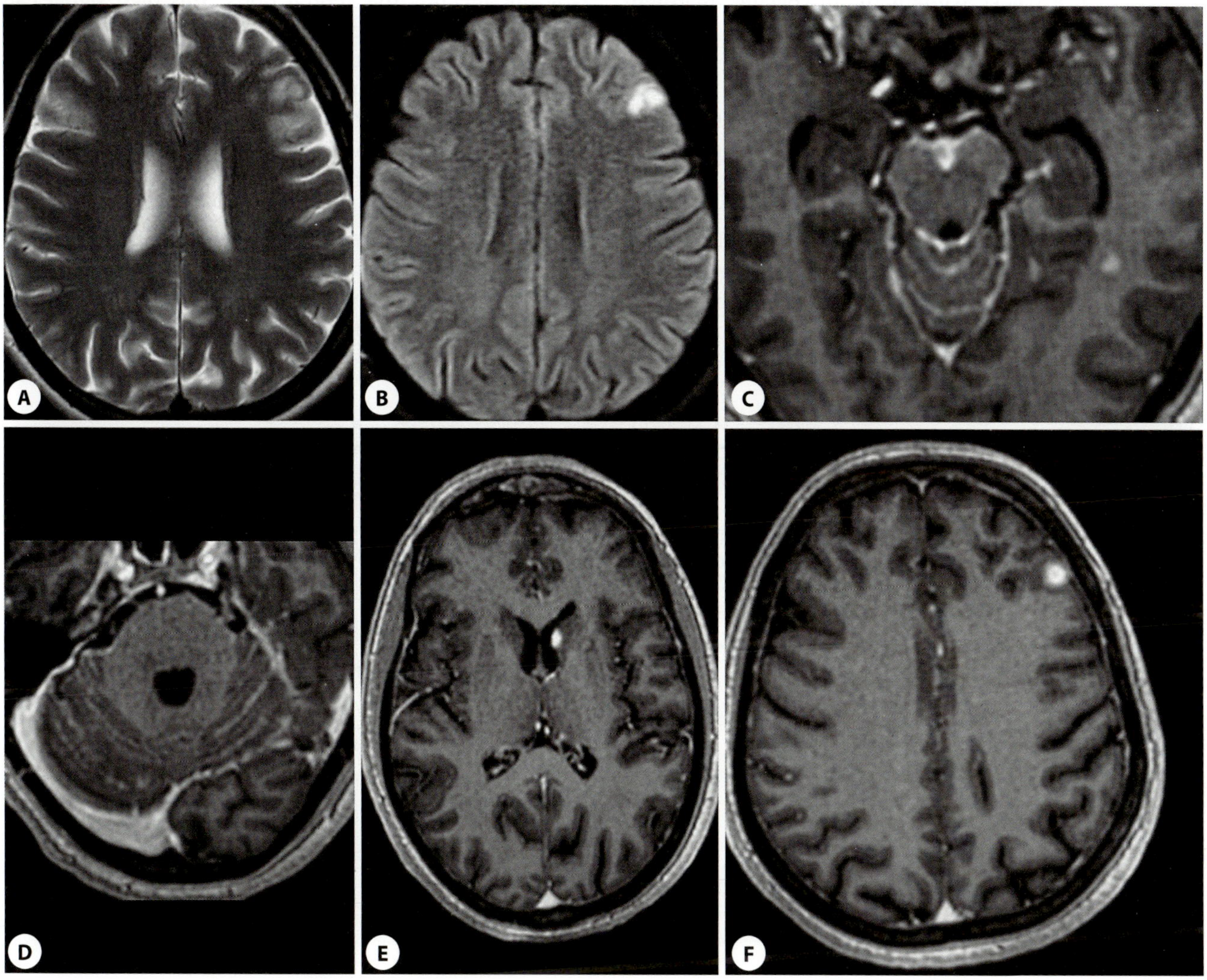

CLINICAL BACKGROUND

A 49-year-old female, known patient of carcinoma left breast, came with headache and giddiness.

IMAGING FINDINGS

Intra-axial T2/FLAIR hyperintense lesion measuring—(1.0 × 1.2 cm) noted in left frontal sub cortical white matter. Another similar lesion noted in subependymal location of frontal horn of left lateral ventricle and in left temporal lobe white matter. The lesions show homogeneous postcontrast enhancement/on MRS, choline peak with reduced NAA noted.

Nodular leptomeningeal enhancement noted around basal cistern and bilateral cerebellar folia **(Figs. 1A to F)**.

DISCUSSION

Leptomeningeal carcinomatosis (LC) is a devastating complication of cancer, and the incidence of LC in patients with solid tumors has increased in the past decade. The clinical presentation of LC depends primarily on the location of involvement and is variable and nonspecific. Median survival of this fatal complication is low and is limited to 6–8 weeks without tumor-specific treatment. Neuroimaging is an imperative procedure for detecting LC; about 70–80% of patients with leptomeningeal disease present abnormalities on image scans.[1]

The characteristic MRI abnormalities of LC include focal or diffuse sulcal enhancement, linear ependymal enhancement, cranial nerve or nerve root enhancement, leptomeningeal enhancing nodules of the brain or spinal cord, and hydrocephalus.[1] The classical So-called "sugar coating" or zuckerguss (German for sugar icing) refers to the appearance of diffuse linear/sheetlike leptomeningeal contrast enhancement in the brain or spinal cord due to drop metastasis or leptomeningeal carcinomatosis. It is seen both as a result of CNS involvement from distant primaries as well as direct spread from CNS malignancies.[1,2]

The bloomy rind sign is a radiological sign appreciated on MRI brain that is rarely but characteristically described in these patients. It describes the appearance of a curvilinear T2/FLAIR hyperintensity on the surface of brainstem typically affecting the ventral pons. This high signal can also be appreciated on DWI, with corresponding low signal on ADC, but notably does not correspond with any accompanying contrast (gadolinium) enhancement. This 'layer' of T2/FLAIR hyperintensity, against the normal signal has been likened to the bloomy rind coating the surface on certain cheeses. The etiology of the sign is unclear, with proposed theories including tumor infiltration, microinfarction, or effects from cytotoxic edema.[2]

To conclude, LC is rare but fatal complication of tumor metastasis which has poor prognosis and imaging plays a vital role in diagnosis, although CSF cytology remains gold standard.

REFERENCES

1. Liu C, Zhang Y, Li Y, et al. A rare magnetic resonance imaging pattern of leptomeningeal carcinomatosis: a case description. Quant Imaging Med Surg. 2021;11(7):3367-70.
2. Gaillard F, Rasuli B, Sharma R, et al. Leptomeningeal metastases. Reference article, Radiopaedia.org (Accessed on 11 May 2024) https://doi.org/10.53347/rID-1579

62

Cervical Rib with Subclavian Artery Pseudoaneurysm—Thoracic Outlet Obstruction Syndrome with Distal Emboli

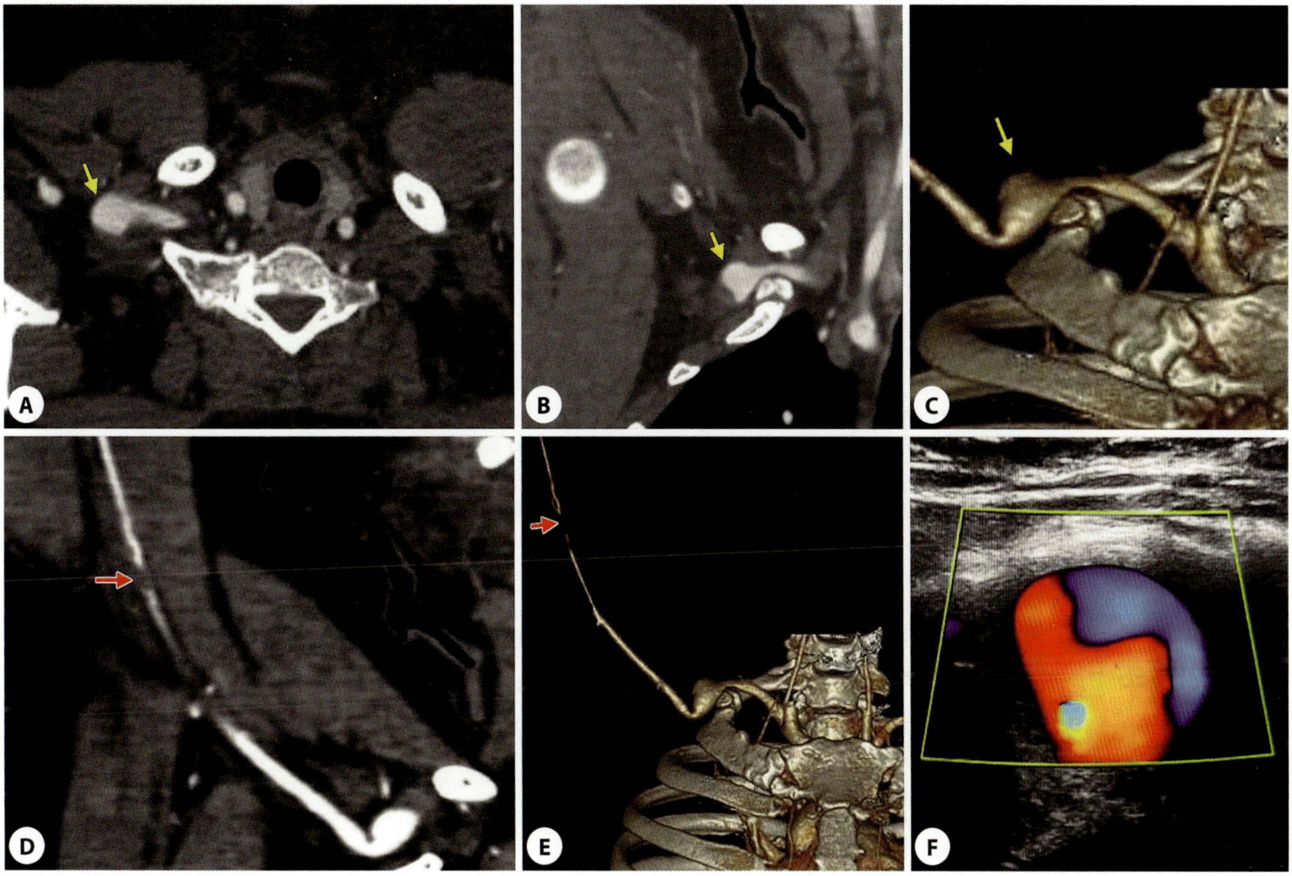

CLINICAL BACKGROUND

A 40-year-old female, known patient of right brachial artery thrombosis came with pain and numbness in right upper limb.

IMAGING FINDINGS

Focal short segment saccular dilatation noted in the distal portion of subclavian artery, at the level of cervical (C7) rib (yellow arrows). Mild irregular wall thickening seen in its posterior aspect and normal distal flow in axillary artery (could represent partial thrombosis) **(Figs. 1A to F)**.

Short segment occlusion with absent contrast opacification (red arrows) in mid portion of brachial artery with collaterals supplying ulnar artery (known patient of complete distal brachial artery thrombosis)/poor contrast opacification seen in the distal ulnar artery with poor formation of palmer arches and digital arteries.

Ultrasound screening shows yin-yang sign at aneurysmal site, monophasic flow in radial and ulnar arteries/ low velocity flow—consistent with proximal (brachial artery) occlusion.

DISCUSSION

The thoracic outlet comprises three anatomical spaces: The scalene triangle, costoclavicular space, and subcoracoid pectoralis minor space. When the ipsilateral arm is abducted, these spaces can become narrowed. Thoracic outlet syndrome (TOS) is characterized by the compression of neurovascular structures resulting from anatomical predispositions, which can be either congenital or acquired. TOS is classified into three types:

1. Neurogenic: This type occurs due to the compression of the brachial plexus at the scalene triangle and/or the retropectoral space.
2. Venous: This type results from compression at the anterior costoclavicular junction.
3. Arterial: This is caused by compression of the subclavian artery, often due to the presence of a cervical rib.[1,2]

The estimated prevalence of neurogenic TOS is approximately 3 per 100,000 individuals, whereas venous TOS is estimated at about 1 per 100,000. Neurogenic thoracic outlet syndrome is the most common form, accounting for around 90% of cases, followed by venous TOS. Arterial thoracic outlet syndrome is the least prevalent, occurring in only 1–2% of patients. Compression of the subclavian artery may lead to the development of an aneurysm, which can be prestenotic or poststenotic. Persistent compression can damage the artery's intima, resulting in atheroma formation, which can precipitate anterograde or retrograde thromboembolic events.[1,2]

Chest X-rays are typically employed to exclude bony abnormalities. For diagnosing thoracic outlet syndrome, both CT scans and MRI are preferred modalities. Magnetic resonance angiography (MRA) is often favored over CT due to its superior tissue contrast and capability to assess veins and nerves. The primary objective of these imaging techniques is to identify the underlying causes of TOS, which may be anatomical or pathological. Common etiologies include cervical ribs, muscle hypertrophy, trauma, and repetitive movements. Patients with arterial TOS frequently present with a cervical rib, anomalies of the first rib, or fractures of the first rib or clavicle.[1–3]

Vascular TOS is identified when there is a reduction of more than 30% in the subclavian artery diameter or more than 50% narrowing of the subclavian vein. To avoid streak artifacts, it is essential to use contrast material on the opposite side. Imaging findings associated with arterial TOS may include the formation of aneurysms or pseudoaneurysms of the axillo-subclavian artery, arterial thrombosis, and focal stenosis of the subclavian artery on the side of compression. Although aneurysmal dilation is a less frequently reported complication, it remains a potential concern.[2,3]

REFERENCES

1. CA Raptis, S Sridhar, RW Thompson, et al. Imaging of the patient with thoracic outlet syndrome. Radiographics. 2016;36(4): 984-1000.
2. S Poyyamoli, E Swamiappan, J Gandhi. Non-aortic vascular findings on chest CT angiogram: including arch vessels and bronchial arteries. Cardiovasc Diagn Ther. 2019;9(1):S59-S73.
3. MA Ghouri, N Gupta, AP Bhat, et al. CT and MR imaging of the upper extremity vasculature: pearls, pitfalls, and challenges. Cardiovasc Diagn Ther. 2019;9:S152-S173.

63

Cerebellar Hemangioblastoma

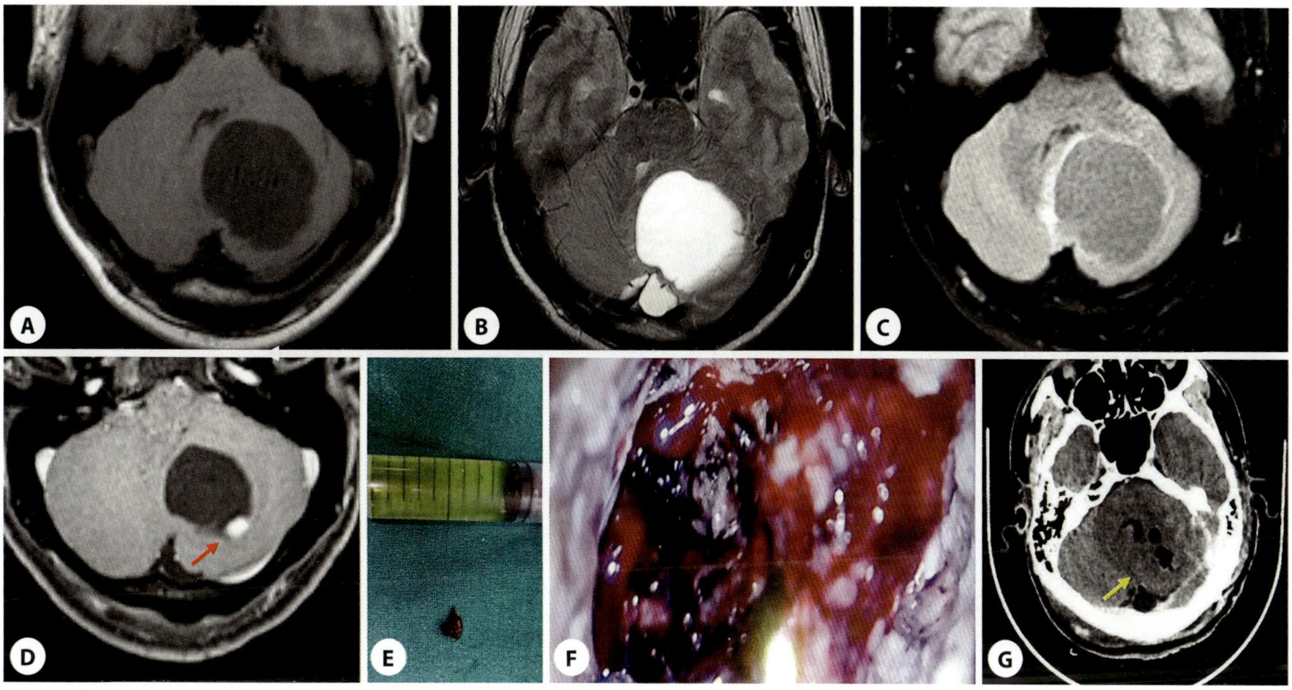

CLINICAL BACKGROUND

A 28-year-old male came with headache and altered mental status.

IMAGING FINDINGS

Large well defined T1 hypointense and T2 hyperintense cystic lesion seen occupying left superior cerebellar hemisphere. The lesion shows incomplete suppression on FLAIR sequence.

T2 hypointense mural nodule seen in posterior inferior aspect of cystic component (red arrow), showing avid enhancement on postcontrast study. No wall enhancement seen.

No evidence of diffusion restriction or blooming artifact within the lesion. The lesion is causing mass effect on fourth ventricle and dorsal aspect of brainstem with acute obstructive hydrocephalus involving bilateral lateral and third ventricle. Mild diffuse cerebral edema.

Intraoperative and postoperative (yellow arrow) images are shown in **(Figs. 1A to G)**.

DISCUSSION

Hemangioblastomas (HBs) are classified as grade I, mesenchymal, and nonmeningothelial tumors according to the World Health Organization's classification of central nervous system tumors. They represent 1.5–2.5% of all intracranial neoplasms and 7–12% of posterior fossa tumors. Additionally, HBs are most frequently present in the cerebellar hemisphere and in individuals in their third to fifth decades of life. Moreover, 20% of cases are associated with von Hippel-Lindau (VHL) disease.[1]

On conventional magnetic resonance imaging (MRI), HBs typically appear as mural nodules with an adjacent nonenhancing surrounding cyst or solid and internal and/or peripheral vessels located in the cerebellum. However, they sometimes cannot be reliably distinguished from other tumors by conventional MRI, especially pilocytic astrocytomas (PAs) in adolescents and metastatic brain tumors (metastasis) in adults, because of their similar imaging findings and locations.[1]

Traditionally, HBs have been classified into four morphologic patterns based on macroscopic pathology. A cyst with a mural nodule type was the most common (60%), followed by a solid tumor type (26%) and a solid tumor with internal small cysts (9%), whereas a simple cyst type was the least common (5%). In our cases, an enhanced mural nodule with an adjacent nonenhanced surrounding cyst showed the common conventional MR pattern.

The differential diagnoses of cerebellar HBs include pilocytic astrocytoma and metastasis.

Table 1: Comparisons of general imaging features of hemangioblastomas, pilocytic astrocytomas, and metastatic tumors on conventional and advanced MRI.[1]

	Hemangioblastomas	Pilocytic astrocytomas	Metastatic tumors
Age	Adults	Children	Adults
Morphology	Cyst with a mural nodule, solid, cyst, solid and cyst	Cyst with a mural nodule, solid	Solid with necrosis
Number	Single	Single	Multiple > single
Flow voids	+	–	+
rCBV	Prominent increased	Mild increased	Mild to prominent increased
ADC	Increased	Iso to increased	Decreased to mild increased
Lip/Lac	+ (Lip)	+ (Lac)	+(Lip/Lac)
Cho	– or +	++	++
NAA	–	+	–

REFERENCE

1. Matsusue E, Inoue C, Tabuchi S, et al. Advanced magnetic resonance imaging findings of cerebellar hemangioblastomas: A report of three cases and a literature review. Acta Radiol Open. 2022;11(2):20584601221077074.

64 Post Varicella—Pediatric Stroke

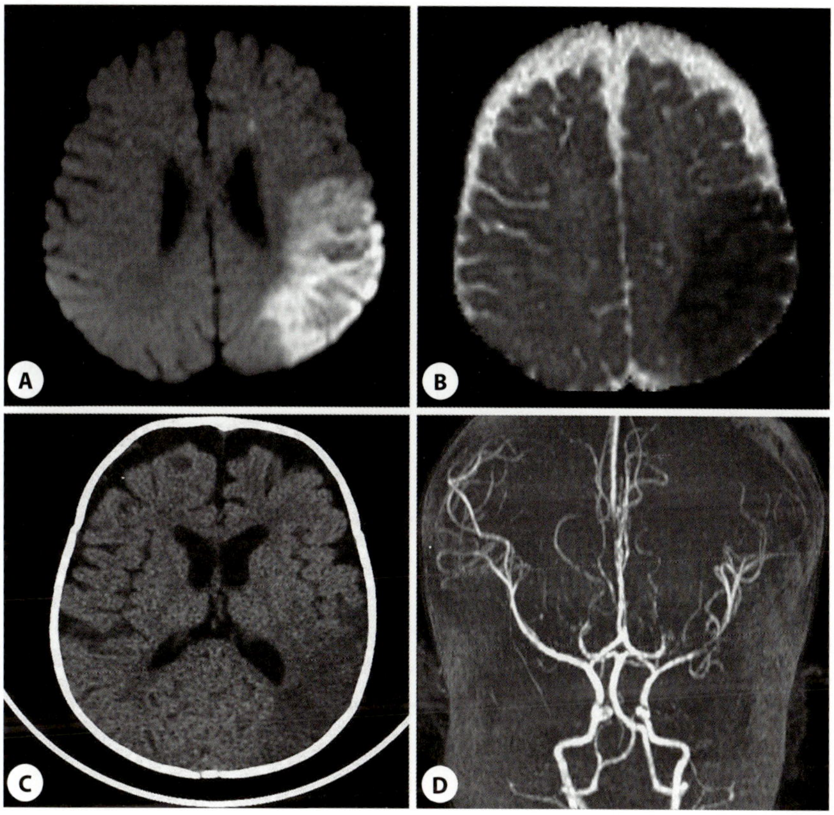

CLINICAL BACKGROUND

A 2-year-old child, known patient of recent varicella infection, came with altered mental status.

IMAGING FINDINGS

Diffusion restriction area noted in left fronto-parieto-temporal cortex. MRA shows short segment, irregular luminal narrowing with poor flow related signal in distal portion of M1 segment of left MCA with preserved distal collateral flow **(Figs. 1A to D)**.

DISCUSSION

Varicella zoster virus (VZV) is classified as a neurotropic alpha herpes virus. The primary infection, which usually occurs during childhood, leads to varicella (chickenpox). Following this initial infection, the virus remains dormant in the cranial nerve ganglia, dorsal root ganglia, and autonomic ganglia throughout the neuraxis. The primary mechanism behind post-varicella angiopathy is that VZV can disseminate along the ophthalmic branch of the trigeminal nerve, resulting in granulomatous angiitis.[1]

Among infectious agents, VZV is a significant cause of central nervous system vasculopathy and strokes in pediatric patients. The exact mechanisms underlying VZV-associated strokes remain unclear. However, post-varicella strokes are generally linked to angiopathy, predominantly affecting the proximal segment of the middle cerebral artery and leading to basal ganglia strokes. Although less common, involvement of the posterior circulation can also occur, particularly in young, immunocompetent children.[1-3]

Literature indicates that the risk of stroke is highest within the first 6 months following VZV infection, with a significant reduction in risk observed 12 months post-infection. Nevertheless, there is mounting evidence of virologically confirmed post-varicella angiopathy (PVA) and post-VZV strokes occurring even after extended intervals from the initial infection. Notably, there have been anecdotal reports of post-varicella strokes arising as long as 4 years after the infection.[3]

Late-onset inflammatory VZV-related focal cerebral arteriopathy can be identified using high-resolution vessel wall MRI, with confirmation from cerebrospinal fluid analysis showing a VZV-specific antibody index. This type of cerebral vasculitis typically exhibits a concentric, diffuse, and smooth pattern of enhancement, contrasting with atherosclerotic lesions, which are rare in children and usually demonstrate eccentric, focal, and irregular enhancement. Currently, there are no clear guidelines regarding the timing of neuroradiological follow-ups for patients experiencing VZV-related strokes.[3]

REFERENCES

1. Bala A, Bhardwaj P, Garg V, et al. Post varicella angiopathy as a cause of pediatric stroke: a case report. International Journal of Science & Healthcare Research. 2021;6(2):36-9.
2. Monteventi O, Chabrier S, Fluss J. Prise en charge diagnostique et thérapeutique actuelle des accidents vasculaires cérébraux post-varicelleux chez l'enfant: revue de la littérature [Current management of post-varicella stroke in children: a literature review]. Arch Pediatr. 2013;20(8):883-9.
3. Bertamino M, Signa S, Vagelli G, et al. An atypical case of post-varicella stroke in a child presenting with hemichorea followed by late-onset inflammatory focal cerebral arteriopathy. Quant Imaging Med Surg. 2021;11(1):463-71.

65 Solitary Fibrous Tumor of Pleura

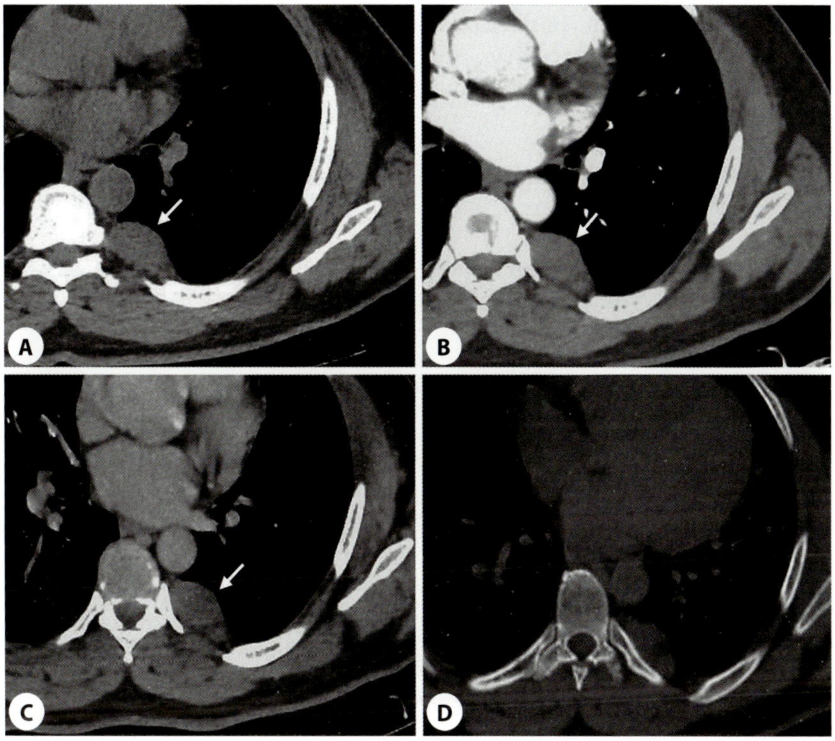

CLINICAL BACKGROUND

A 57-year-old male, came with chest discomfort.

IMAGING FINDINGS

Solitary, well defined, broad extrapulmonary pleural based soft tissue dense lesion noted in posterolateral aspect at VII intercostal space, on left side with minimal subpleural atelectasis. The lesion shows mild homogeneous postcontrast enhancement. No evidence of rib erosion **(Figs. 1A to D)**.

DISCUSSION

Solitary fibrous tumor of the pleura (SFTP), first recognized as a distinct clinical entity by Klemperer and Rabin in 1931, is a type of mesenchymal tumor primarily involving the pleura but also occurring in various thoracic and extrathoracic locations. Typically, SFTP presents as a peripheral mass that lies adjacent to the pleural surface, connected by a broad base or a pedicle that permits mobility. These tumors can be benign or malignant.[1] Many patients are asymptomatic at diagnosis, and SFTP is often detected incidentally on routine chest X-rays. For those with symptoms, the most frequent complaints include chest pain, cough, and dyspnea.[2]

When small, SFTP is usually characterized on CT scans as a homogeneous, well-defined, noninvasive, lobular soft-tissue mass, often located next to the chest wall and forming an obtuse angle with the pleural surface. The "incomplete border sign" is helpful in distinguishing extrapleural SFTPs from lung masses. However, larger tumors or those originating from the mediastinal aspect of the parietal pleura may resemble primary pulmonary or mediastinal masses. Intense enhancement observed in an SFTP is often attributed to its high vascularity.[1]

Larger SFTPs tend to be heterogeneous and might not display CT characteristics typical of focal pleural tumors. These lesions generally create acute angles with the adjacent pleural surface, potentially leading to misdiagnosis as peripheral lung cancer. Intralesional calcifications—whether punctate, linear, or coarse—are commonly associated with areas of necrosis and are more visible in larger tumors. In cases involving sizable masses with calcification, postcontrast enhancement is usually intense and heterogeneous, featuring central regions of low attenuation. This intralesional geographic pattern has been linked to myxoid changes and areas of hemorrhage, necrosis, or cystic degeneration.[1]

The characteristic well-circumscribed appearance of an SFTP typically helps differentiate it from malignant pleural mesothelioma, which generally presents as multiple scattered pleural masses or a more diffuse mass encasing the lung.[1]

REFERENCES

1. Cardinale L, Ardissone F, Garetto I, et al. Imaging of benign solitary fibrous tumor of the pleura: a pictorial essay. Rare Tumors. 2010;2(1):e1.
2. You YH, Liu RT, Zhang Y. A large solitary fibrous tumour of the pleura: a case report and review of the literature. J Int Med Res. 2018;46(4):1672-77.

66 Scalp Arteriovenous Malformations

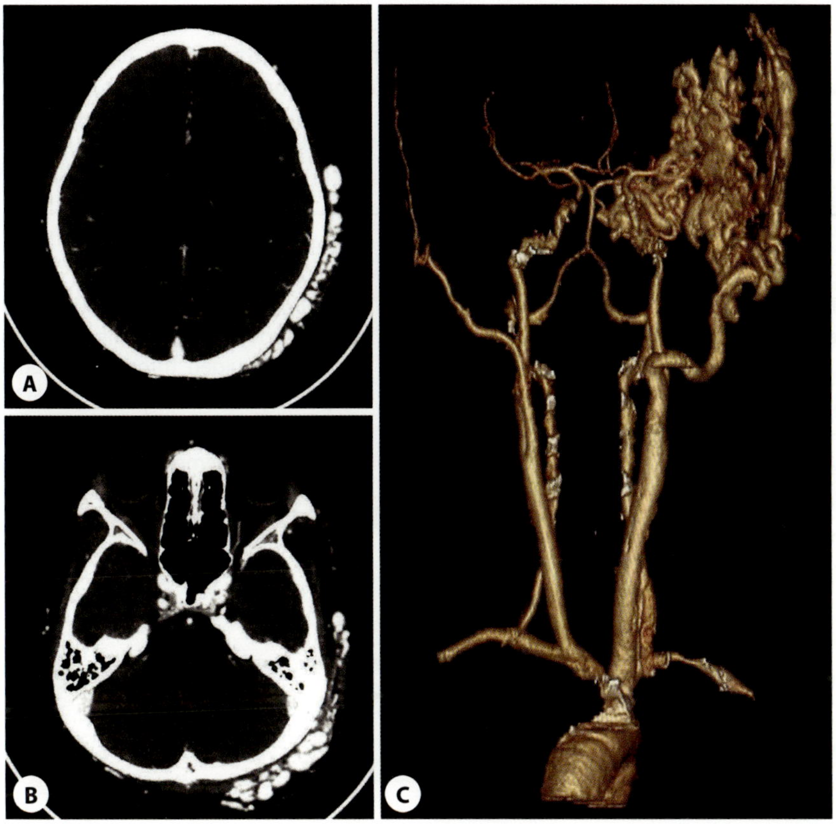

CLINICAL BACKGROUND

An 18-year-old female came with severe headache.

IMAGING FINDINGS

Multiple serpiginous dilated scalp vessels noted in left fronto-parietal and occipital regions, showing feeding branches from ipsilateral left external carotid artery/draining into left internal jugular vein through numerus dilated extracranial veins. No intracranial communication **(Figs. 1A to C)**.

DISCUSSION

Arteriovenous malformations (AVMs) in the scalp are relatively uncommon compared to other vascular anomalies such as hemangiomas and venous malformations in subcutaneous or cervicofacial areas. Scalp AVMs constitute only 8.1% of all AVM cases and can arise either from trauma or spontaneously. They represent an abnormal connection between feeding arteries and draining veins without an intervening capillary bed. Typically, scalp AVMs are identified during late childhood, adolescence, or early adulthood, often leading to significant esthetic and social challenges, or they may be triggered by factors such as trauma, pregnancy, or puberty.[1,2]

The first documented case of an AVM was by William Hunter in 1757, after which various terms, including aneurysmal serpentinum, aneurysm cirsoides, plexiform angioma, arteriovenous fistula, and AVM, have been used to describe these vascular malformations of the scalp.[3] Symptoms and signs associated with scalp AVMs can include pain, throbbing headaches, a bruit, hemorrhage, and psychomotor retardation. Larger lesions may also lead to scalp necrosis.[4]

CT angiography (CTA) is the preferred noninvasive imaging technique, capable of revealing multiple, tortuous dilated vessels with arterial feeders and early draining veins. It can also assess any calvarial bony defects, intracranial extension, or communication before any intervention. Various treatment options are available for scalp AVMs, and a personalized approach is crucial. A minimally invasive treatment option includes a combination of ultrasound-guided thrombin injection (UGTI) and transarterial coil embolization, which eliminates the need for surgical excision. In cases where endovascular therapy is challenging or unfeasible, surgical excision proves highly beneficial. Additionally, temporarily clipping the feeding arteries allows for the complete excision of large AVMs with minimal blood loss, providing a definitive cure.[5,6]

REFERENCES

1. Mohamed WN, Abdullah NN, Muda AS. Scalp arteriovenous malformation: A case report. Malays J Med Sci. 2008;15(3):55-7.
2. PV Worm, LG Ruschel, MR Roxo, and R. Camelo, Giant scalp arteriovenous malformation. Rev Assoc Med Bras. 62;828-30.
3. Ghoddusi Johari H, Shahriarirad R, Erfani A, et al. High Flow Scalp Arteriovenous Malformation: A Case Report. World J Plast Surg. 2020;9(2):228-31.
4. Nagasaka S, Fukushima T, Goto K, et al. Treatment of scalp arteriovenous malformation. Neurosurgery. 1996;38(4):671-7.
5. I Nishijima, R Ikemura, M Gushiken, et al. Nonsurgical treatment of scalp arteriovenous malformation using a combination of ultrasound-guided thrombin injection and transarterial coil embolization. J of Vasc Sur. 2012;55(3):833-6.
6. SB Gangadharaswamy, N. Maulyavantham Nagaraj, and BS Pai, Surgical management of scalp arteriovenous malformations using a novel surgical technique—Case series. Int J Surg Case Rep. 2017;37:250-3.

67 Adhesive Capsulitis

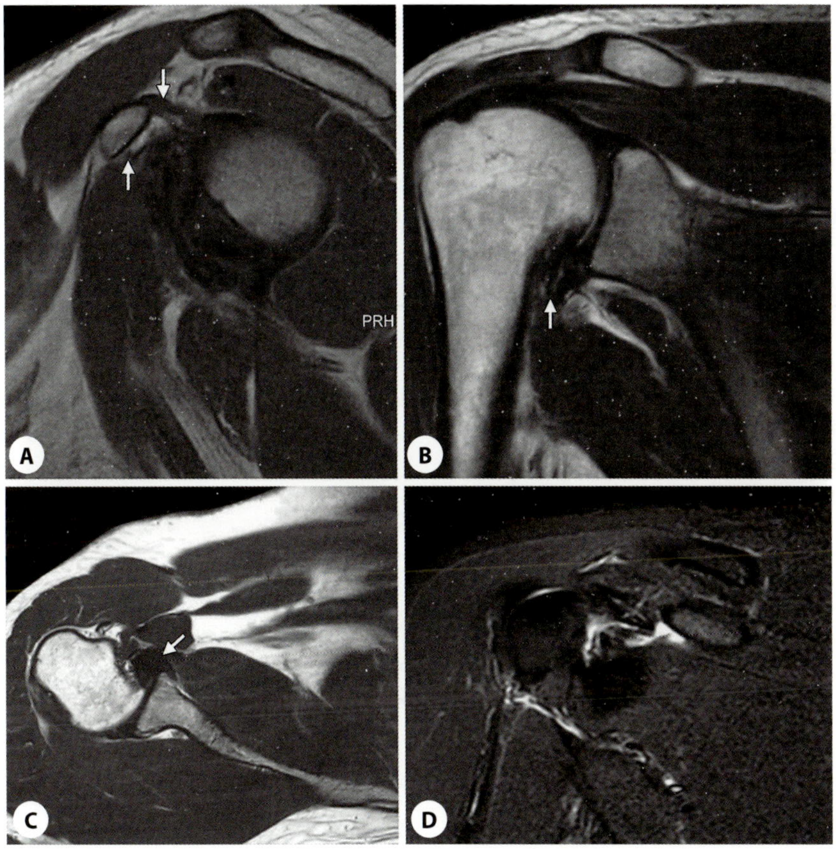

CLINICAL BACKGROUND

A 28-year-old male came with post-traumatic right shoulder pain for past 1 year.

IMAGING FINDINGS

Thickening of coracohumeral ligament and inferior glenohumeral ligament with obliteration of T1 hyperintense signal in subcoracoid fat. Associated soft tissue edema in rotator cuff interval. Mild joint effusion noted **(Figs. 1A to D)**.

DISCUSSION

Adhesive capsulitis, commonly known as "frozen shoulder," is an inflammatory condition affecting the glenohumeral joint's synovium and capsule, leading to restricted range of motion. It is most frequently observed in women aged 40–60 years. Primary or idiopathic adhesive capsulitis occurs without any prior trauma, while secondary adhesive capsulitis, also referred to as post-traumatic arthritis, develops due to previous injuries, low-level repetitive trauma, surgical procedures, or rheumatologic conditions.[1]

Although the underlying mechanisms are not completely understood, adhesive capsulitis is thought to begin as an inflammatory hypervascular synovitis, which triggers a progressive fibroblastic response in the surrounding capsule. This process results in thickening and contraction of the capsule. MRI is particularly useful for visualizing the rotator interval and the axillary recess, both of which are commonly affected by this condition. The rotator interval is located between the supraspinatus muscle and tendon posterosuperiorly and the subscapularis muscle and tendon anteroinferiorly. It comprises the coracohumeral ligament and the superior glenohumeral ligament.[2]

The clinical course of adhesive capsulitis is typically described in three or four stages:

1. First stage (Painful stage)
2. Second stage (Freezing stage)
3. Third stage (Frozen stage)
4. Fourth stage (Thawing stage)

MRI findings suggestive of adhesive capsulitis include soft tissue thickening in the rotator interval, which may surround the coracohumeral and superior glenohumeral ligaments, as well as thickening adjacent to the biceps anchor. A thickened inferior glenohumeral ligament, measuring more than 4 mm, is often visible in the axillary pouch. Additionally, there may be a loss of definition of the inferior capsule due to edema and synovitis. The subcoracoid fat triangle, a fat-filled space bounded by the coracohumeral ligament, the joint capsule, and the subscapularis muscle, can be effaced by hypointense synovium, which is referred to as the "subcoracoid triangle sign".[2,3]

REFERENCES

1. Hannafin JA, DiCarlo ED, Wickiewicz TL, et al. Adhesive capsulitis: capsular fibroplasias of the Glenohumeral joint. J Shoulder Elbow Surg. 1994;3(S):5.
2. Carillon Y, Noel E, Fantino O, et al. Magnetic resonance imaging findings in idiopathic adhesive capsulitis of the shoulder. Rev Rhum Engl Ed. 1999;66(4):201-6.
3. Connell D, Padmanabhan R, Buchbinder R. Adhesive capsulitis: role of MR imaging in differential diagnosis. European Radiology. 2002;12(8):2100-6.

68 Acute Traumatic Aortic Injury

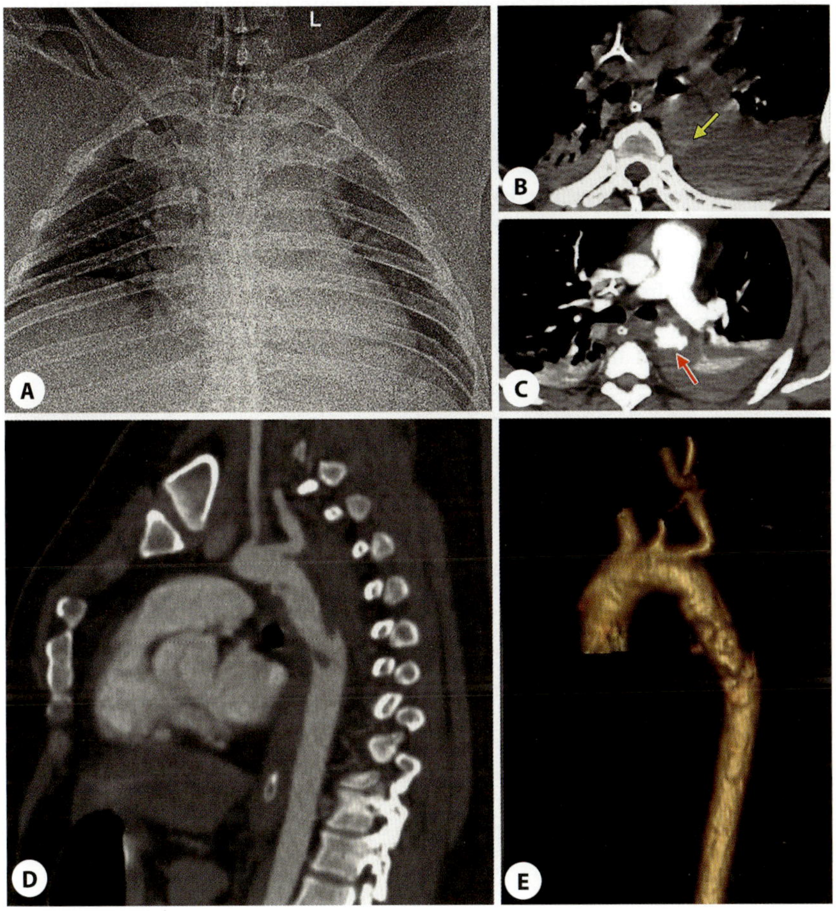

CLINICAL BACKGROUND

A 25-year-old RTA male patient presented with altered hemodynamic status and respiratory distress.

IMAGING FINDINGS

Chest radiograph shows mediastinal widening. CT angiogram shows intimal tear with intramural hematoma (yellow arrow)/associated wall irregularity and thickening in proximal descending aorta (red arrow) from distal to origin of left subclavian artery (aortic isthmus), intramural thrombus extending from aortic isthmus to descending thoracic aorta. No evidence of active contrast extravasation or pseudoaneurysm or aortic dissection **(Figs. 1A to E)**.

Left moderate hemothorax with underlying lung collapse/right minimal hemothorax with lower lobe segmental collapse.

DISCUSSION

Acute traumatic aortic injuries are associated with significant mortality rates, with fatal outcomes occurring in 80–90% of cases at the time of admission. Although these injuries are relatively uncommon, they often present with nonspecific clinical signs. Blunt trauma, particularly from high-velocity impacts such as motor vehicle collisions, is the leading cause, accounting for 70% of cases. The most frequently imaged site of acute traumatic aortic injury is the aortic isthmus, located just distal to the origin of the left subclavian artery, due to the aorta's relative immobility at the ligamentum arteriosum.[1]

Radiographic indicators of acute traumatic injury to the thoracic aorta include a widened mediastinum measuring over 8 cm or more than 25% of the thoracic width at the level of the aortic knob. Other signs include loss of the aortic knob or aortopulmonary window contour, depression of the left mainstem bronchus (more than 40° from the horizontal), and the presence of a left apical pleural cap due to bleeding along the reflection of the left subclavian artery.[2]

On CT angiography, direct signs of injury to the aortic wall—categorized by the degree of intimal, medial, and adventitial damage—include the presence of an intimal flap, intraluminal and mural thrombus, focal wall outpouching, aortic dissection, abnormal aortic contours, sudden changes in aortic caliber (termed aortic "pseudocoarctation"), and periaortic contrast extravasation. Indirect signs encompass periaortic hematoma, which can present as a mediastinal hematoma in the thorax and retroperitoneal hematoma in the abdomen.[1]

Minimal aortic injury (MAI) corresponds to Society for Vascular Surgery (SVS) grade 1 and 2 injuries. A grade 2 injury typically involves an intimal tear, intraluminal or intramural thrombus (or both) measuring less than 1 cm, without any external contour abnormalities or only minimal mediastinal hematoma. These injuries generally have a favorable prognosis and may be managed nonoperatively with close follow-up, as they are known to heal spontaneously.[1]

REFERENCES

1. Gupta S, Kumar A, Kaur T, et al. Current updates in acute traumatic aortic injury: radiologic diagnosis and management. Clin Exp Emerg Med. 2022;9(2):73-83.
2. Raptis CA, Hammer MM, Raman KG, et al. Acute traumatic aortic injury: practical considerations for the diagnostic radiologist. J Thorac Imaging. 2015;30:202-13.

69 As with Chalk-Stick Fracture

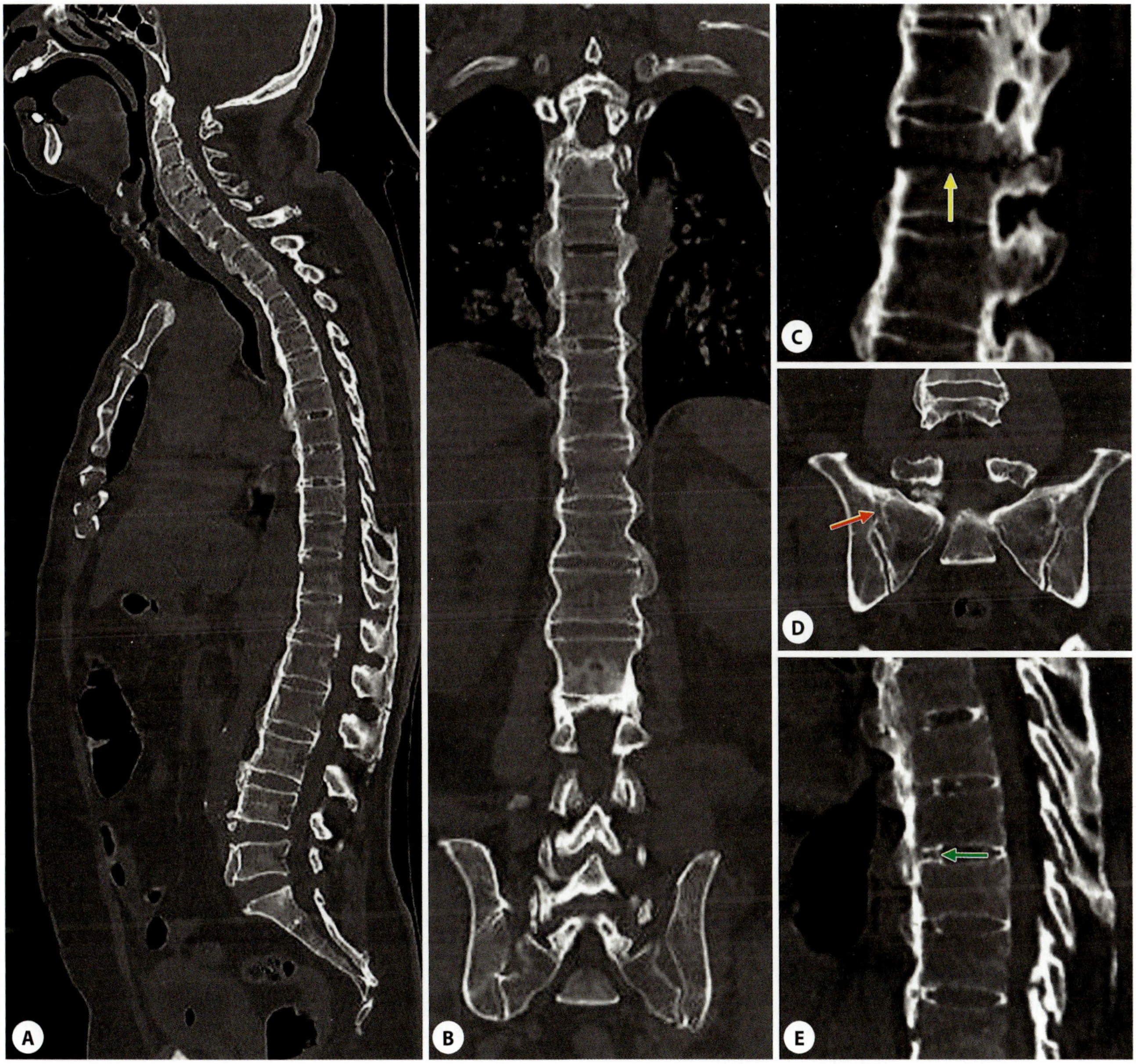

CLINICAL BACKGROUND

A 65-year-old known ankylosing spondylitis male patient came with severe back pain.

IMAGING FINDINGS

Extensive paravertebral syndesmophytic changes in entire spine. Ossification of anterior, posterior longitudinal/ supraspinous ligaments **(Figs. 1A to E)**.

Ossification of intervertebral disc noted at multiple levels (green arrow). Ankylosis of bilateral SI-joints (red arrow). Fracture line seen traversing the D11 vertebral body (yellow arrow) and involving posterior elements on left side.

DISCUSSION

Ankylosing spondylitis (AS) is a chronic inflammatory disease characterized mainly by spinal ankylosis, inflammation and, ultimately, fusion of the sacroiliac joints and the rest of spine. Osteoporosis is a common comorbidity in AS and, when superimposed on the fused spine, it results in a higher prevalence of spinal fractures. A type of fracture typically seen in patients with AS are the chalk-stick fractures. These are fractures affecting the vertebrae, the intervertebral disc and the other spinal segments. They are also called carrot stick fractures and typically occur in a fused spine, even following minor trauma.[1]

A key feature of AS is bilateral and symmetric sacroiliac involvement; however, early in the disease, the pattern may be unilateral and asymmetric. Active disease, on MRI, is characterized by inflammation, with subchondral bone marrow edema that is low signal intensity on T1-weighted and hyperintense on STIR/T2 images, and by gadolinium contrast enhancement. Chronic disease is characterized by the enchondral bone formation of the healing response and is low signal intensity on T1 and T2-weighted images, and includes subchondral sclerosis, joint space narrowing, bone bridging and ankylosis.[2]

In spine, syndesmophytes (typically vertical) are visible as thin, vertically oriented osseous outgrowths along the vertebral body margins that may result in bridging of the vertebral bodies. The disc space is usually preserved. Facet and uncovertebral joint may show erosions and subchondral sclerosis manifested by subchondral bone marrow and adjacent soft tissue edema and enhancement in active stages on MRI.[3]

Romanus lesions (also known as marginal spondylitis and the "MRI corner sign") are manifested by vertebral body corner erosions and bone formation characterized by fluffy amorphous bone sclerosis, forming so-called "shiny corners." The process results in a squared appearance of the vertebral body with loss of anterior concavity. Discovertebral lesions, the so-called andersson lesions, are the same as Romanus lesions but are more central in location at the discovertebral junction. Erosions are seen later on CT. Enthesitis of the posterior ligamentous attachments is manifested by erosions, calcifications and ossification.[3]

Chalk-stick or carrot stick fractures—complication of AS are typically horizontal, through the disc or vertebral body, and involve all three columns. The fracture may extend as tears of the posterior ligaments rather than involve the neural arch.[4]

REFERENCES

1. Katsimpari C, Koutsoviti S, Mpalanika A, et al. Spontaneous Chalk-Stick Fracture in Ankylosing Spondylitis: A Case Report. Mediterr J Rheumatol. 2022;33(3):346-8.
2. Bredella M, Steinbach L, Morgan S, et al. MRI of the sacroiliac joints in patients with moderate to severe ankylosing spondylitis. Am J Roentgenol. 2006;187:1420-6.
3. Lacout A, Rousselin B, Pelage JP. CT and MRI of spine and sacroiliac involvement in spondyloarthropathy. Am J Roentgenol. 2008; 191:1016-23.
4. Wang Y, Teng M, Chang C, et al. Imaging manifestations of spinal fractures in ankylosing spondylitis. Am J Neuroradiol. 2005;26: 2067-76.

70 Diversion Colitis

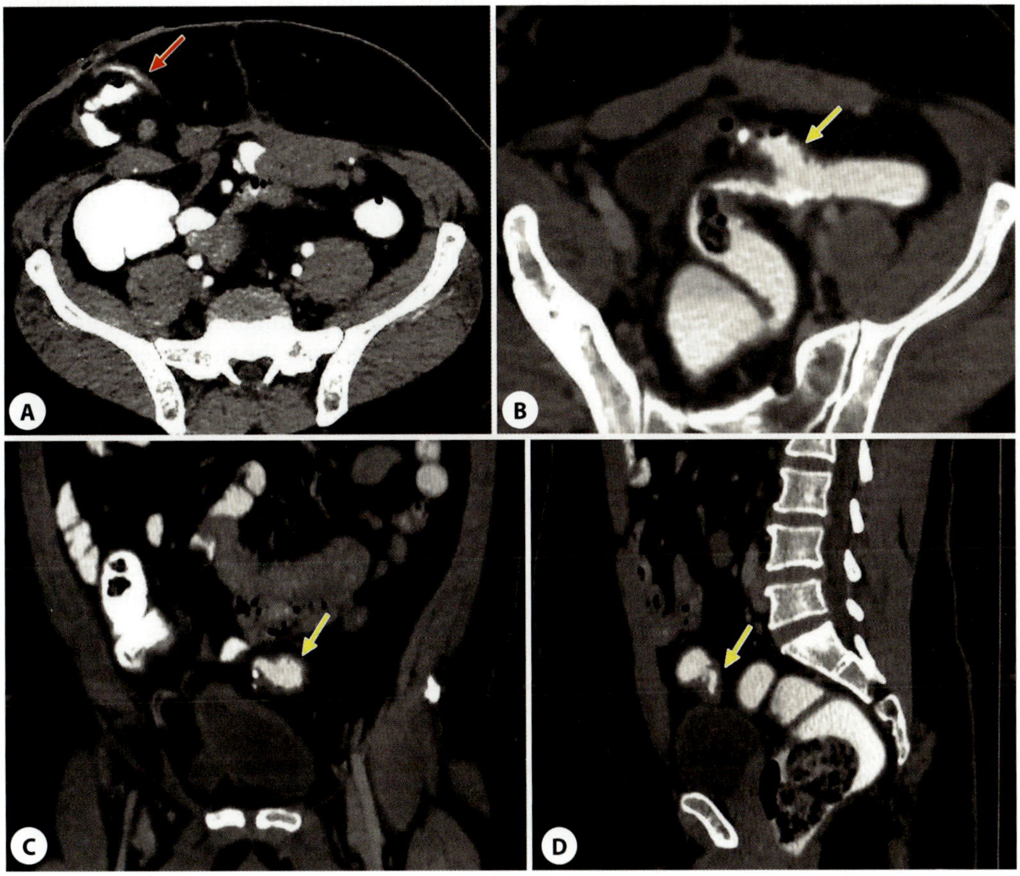

CLINICAL BACKGROUND

A 45-year-old male, known ileostomy patient came with lower abdomen pain.

IMAGING FINDINGS

Short segment circumferential irregular wall thickening (yellow arrow) noted at recto- sigmoid anastomotic site causing mild luminal narrowing/adjacent mesenteric fat stranding and hyperemia noted **(Figs. 1A to D)**.

- Ileostomy defect noted in right para umbilical region (red arrow).
- Subcentimetric periaortic and left para-aortic lymphnodes noted.

DISCUSSION

Diversion colitis was first identified by Morson et al. in 1974 and is characterized by inflammation of the mucosa in the defunctioned segment of the colon following colostomy or ileostomy. The exact mechanisms behind diversion colitis remain unclear. Glotzer proposed that it may arise from factors such as bacterial overgrowth, the presence of harmful bacteria, nutritional deficiencies, toxins, or disruptions in the symbiotic relationship between luminal bacteria and the mucosal layer. More recently, ischemia has also been suggested as a potential cause of diversion colitis.[1]

While most patients are asymptomatic, approximately one-third may present with symptoms related to diversion colitis, including abdominal discomfort, tenesmus, anorectal pain, mucous discharge, and rectal bleeding. The most prevalent symptoms include bloody, serous, or mucous discharge, which occurs in about 40% of patients, and abdominal pain along with tenesmus, reported in around 15% of cases.[1]

Double-contrast barium enema examinations have shown various features, including diffuse mucosal nodularity, inflammatory pseudopolyps, punctate ulcerations, and, in more chronic cases, a diffuse granular appearance of the mucosa. Multidetector CT scans reveal nonspecific colitis features, such as long-segment diffuse circumferential wall thickening accompanied by surrounding fat stranding; the involved mucosa may also resemble that seen in ulcerative colitis.[2]

Treatment for diversion colitis primarily focuses on restoring bowel continuity to reinstate luminal flow, which typically alleviates symptoms and helps the bowel return to normal function. Resection is generally unnecessary, except in cases of uncontrolled perianal sepsis, perianal fistulous disease, anal incontinence, or severe symptoms related to diversion colitis.[1] It's important to note that prolonged chronic inflammation associated with diversion colitis may increase the risk of developing malignancy.[2]

REFERENCES

1. Tominaga K, Kamimura K, Takahashi K, et al. Diversion colitis and pouchitis: A mini-review. World J Gastroenterol. 2018;24(16):1734-47.
2. Weinstein S, Osei-Bonsu S, Aslam R, et al. Multidetector CT of the postoperative colon: review of normal appearances and common complications. Radiographics. 2013;33:515-32.

71

Acute Mesenteric Ischemia

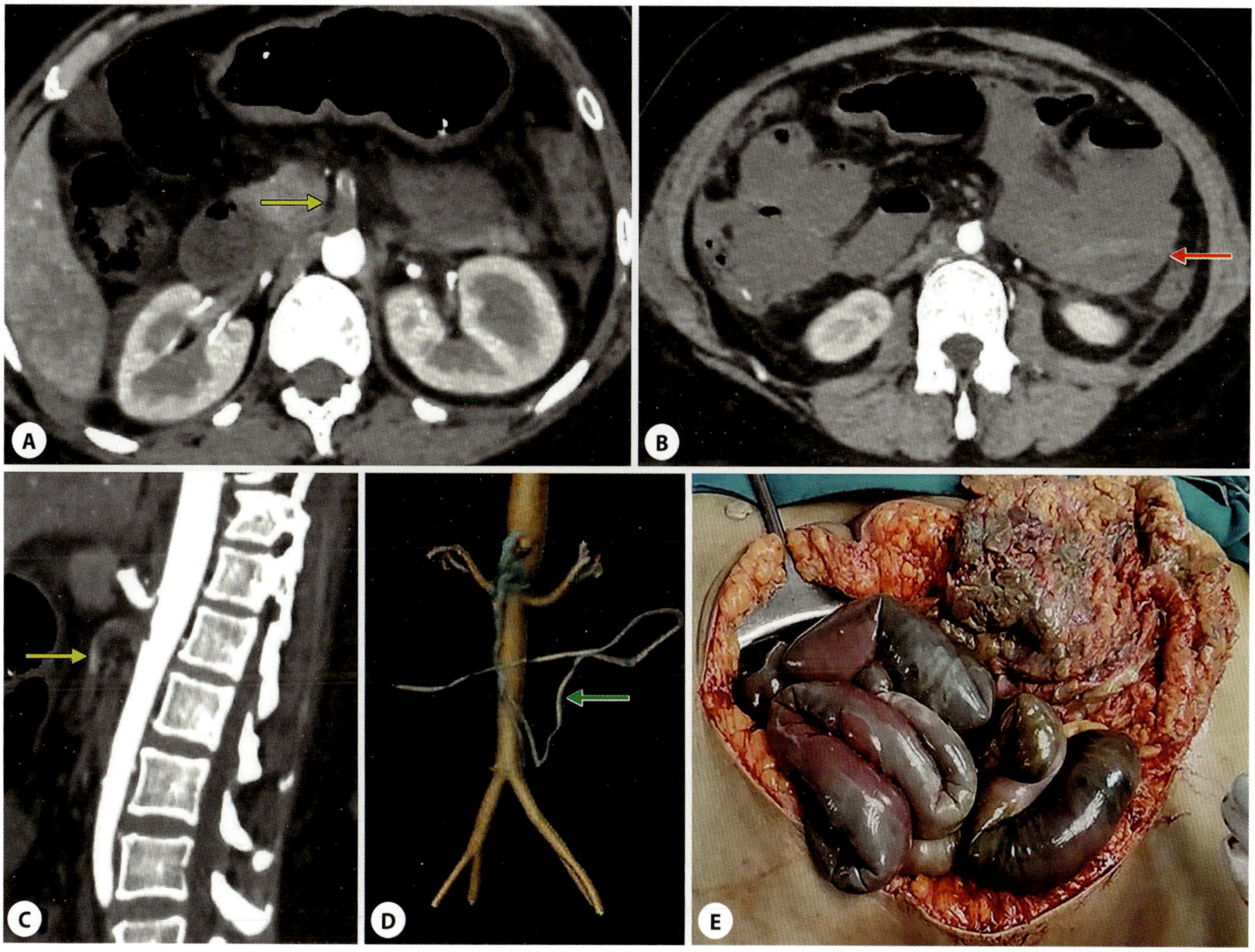

CLINICAL BACKGROUND

A 44-year-old female patient came with severe abdomen pain.

IMAGING FINDINGS

CECT abdomen shows absent contrast opacification of SMA, IMA and its branches (yellow arrow). Dilatation of jejunal and ileal loops with reduced/absent wall enhancement (red arrow)/edematous large bowel loops. Diffuse mesenteric haziness and minimal free fluid seen. Demonstrable arc of riolan seen between SMA and IMA (green arrow). Intraoperative image shows necrosed bowel loops **(Figs. 1A to E)**.

DISCUSSION

Acute mesenteric ischemia (AMI) is a critical condition characterized by a sudden decrease or cessation of blood flow to the bowel, leading to severe complications. It is considered a relatively rare abdominal emergency, comprising only 0.1% of acute surgical admissions. AMI can be classified into two main categories: Arterial and nonarterial, with arterial AMI further divided into occlusive and nonocclusive forms. The occlusive type is subcategorized into embolic and thrombotic causes.[1]

The most prevalent cause of AMI is arterial embolic disease, which accounts for up to 50% of cases and is often linked to underlying cardiovascular conditions. The superior mesenteric artery (SMA) is particularly vulnerable to emboli due to its high flow rate and narrow angle of branching from the aorta. Emboli typically lodge 3–10 cm distal to the origin of the SMA, near the take-off of the middle colic artery. This location often spares the inferior pancreaticoduodenal branches, preserving blood flow to the proximal jejunum. In contrast, thrombosis usually occurs at the ostia of mesenteric vessels, resulting in ischemia that can affect long segments of the bowel and is associated with a poor prognosis.[1,2]

In cases of arterial thromboembolic disease, a reduction or cessation of arterial blood flow leads to a lack of bowel wall enhancement on imaging. Restoration of intestinal perfusion may result in mural thickening, hyperenhancement, and stratification, resembling the changes seen in shock bowel. As ischemia progresses, it causes damage to intramural nerves and a reduction in tissue volume and muscle tone, leading to a "paper thin" appearance of the small-bowel wall—a specific but not very sensitive sign of AMI. Irreversible transmural infarction can lead to the development of pneumatosis intestinalis, portomesenteric venous gas, and intra-abdominal free air.[1,2]

CT imaging has become the primary modality for diagnosing AMI, and recent advances in imaging protocols have enhanced its effectiveness. It is crucial to recognize that vascular abnormalities can manifest before bowel changes; thus, accurate and timely diagnosis of mesenteric ischemia requires thorough examination of the mesenteric vasculature during contrast-enhanced CT, particularly in the arterial phase.[1]

REFERENCES

1. Olson MC, Bach CR, Wells ML, et al. Imaging of bowel ischemia: an update, from the AJR special series on emergency radiology. AJR Am J Roentgenol. 2023;220:173-185.
2. Bobadilla JL. Mesenteric ischemia. Surg Clin North Am. 2013; 93:925-40.

72 Budd–Chiari Syndrome due to RCC

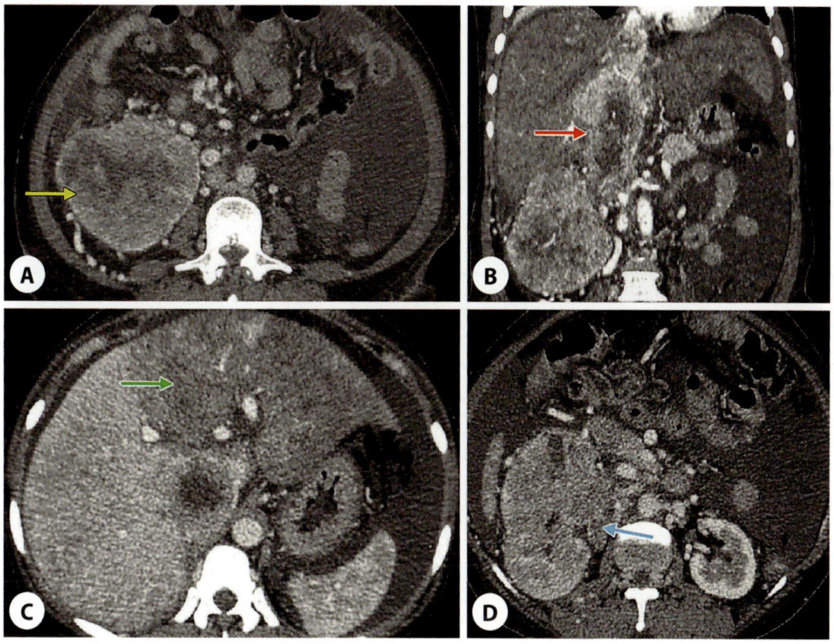

CLINICAL BACKGROUND

A 49-year-old female presented with right side abdomen pain and heaviness.

IMAGING FINDINGS

Heterogeneously enhancing exophytic mass lesion noted arising from mid/lower pole of right kidney, also involving the upper pole (yellow arrow). Filling defect noted in right renal vein (blue arrow), IVC—left renal vein confluence/enhancing component seen in IVC involving infra and supra-hepatic portions of IVC (red arrow). Indistinct left and middle hepatic veins noted with heterogeneous left lobe of liver (green arrow). Multiple venous collaterals noted in perinephric region. Moderate ascites noted/portal vein appears normal **(Figs. 1A to D)**.

DISCUSSION

Budd–Chiari syndrome (BCS) is a severe vascular liver disease defined by the presence of partial or complete impairment of hepatic venous outflow, in the absence of right heart failure or constrictive pericarditis. It classically presents with the triad of hepatomegaly, right hypochondrial pain, and ascites. Notably, only hepatic venous outflow tract obstruction of major veins can be visualized on imaging, while small hepatic veins obstruction (known as small vessel BCS) can only be diagnosed on histology. Secondary BCS represents <1% of the total cases and is linked to invasion or extrinsic compression of the hepatic veins and/or the IVC, either by benign (e.g., hydatid cysts, hemangiomas) or malignant conditions like RCC.[1]

In acute BCS, the liver is usually normal or enlarged and exhibits patchy, decreased peripheral enhancement caused by portal and sinusoidal stasis with stronger central liver enhancement a pattern called "flip-flop" or "zonal" enhancement on CT imaging. T1 weighted imaging will reveal decreased signal intensity within the liver periphery with preservation of higher signal intensity within the caudate lobe. T2-weighted sequences instead show heterogeneously increased signal intensity in the peripheral portion of the liver while the caudate lobe shows normal hypointense signal intensity.[1]

In subacute or chronic BCS, morphological changes and fibrosis occur, following the type of venous involvement. The hepatic artery is usually enlarged in chronic stages compared as is the caudate lobe vein (>3 mm). Portal vein thrombosis can develop in chronic BCS as the result of underlying thrombophilia or stagnation of portal flow caused by outflow block, resulting in portal hypertension. The other late complications include progressive hepatic fibrosis, hepatic nodules, and an increased risk of hepatocellular carcinoma (HCC).[1]

Hepatocellular carcinoma, adrenal tumors and renal cell carcinoma are the major malignant conditions capable of direct IVC invasion and venous obstruction. Hepatic vein invasion by renal cell carcinoma with inferior vena cava tumor thrombus is relatively uncommon. The BCS that results from obstruction of the suprahepatic venous drainage by the tumor could evolve toward liver fibrosis and death. Early diagnosis and surgical treatment of this condition is of prime importance.[2]

REFERENCES

1. Porrello G, Mamone G, Miraglia R. Budd-Chiari Syndrome Imaging Diagnosis: State of the Art and Future Perspectives. Diagnostics. 2023;13(13):2256.
2. Ciancio G, Soloway M. Renal cell carcinoma invading the hepatic veins. Cancer. 2001;92:1836-42.

73 Heterotopic Pregnancy with Ruptured Ectopic

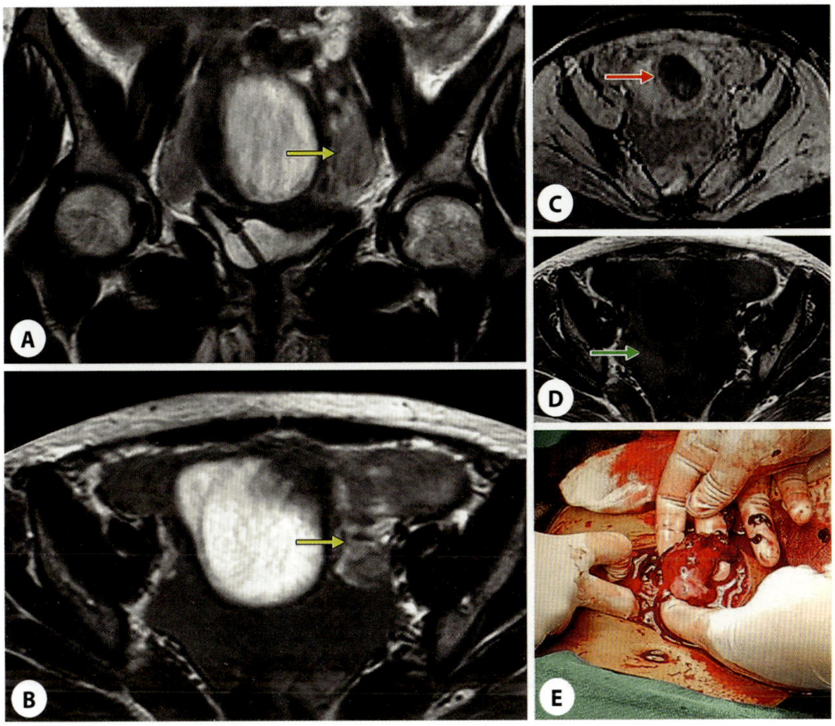

CLINICAL BACKGROUND

A 25-year-old ANC female presented with severe abdomen pain.

IMAGING FINDINGS

Intrauterine gestation with fetal pole (red arrow)/developing placenta seen in right lateral wall. T2 heterointense lesion seen in left adnexa (yellow arrow). Gross hemoperitoneum noted (green arrow). Intraoperative image shows ruptured ectopic **(Figs. 1A to E)**.

DISCUSSION

Heterotopic pregnancy is a rare gynecological condition defined by the simultaneous presence of both intrauterine and extrauterine pregnancies. The incidence of heterotopic pregnancy is estimated to be between 1 in 7,000 to 1 in 50,000 pregnancies in the general population, while the incidence is higher, ranging from 0.09 to 1.00%, among those using assisted reproductive technologies.[1]

Ruptured heterotopic pregnancy represents a rare obstetric emergency that can be challenging for inexperienced physicians to diagnose, necessitating a high degree of suspicion. Up to 70% of heterotopic pregnancies can be identified between 5 and 8 weeks of gestation. Various conditions may mimic heterotopic pregnancy, especially on ultrasound, including intrauterine pregnancy associated with corpus luteum cysts, hemorrhagic cysts, and gestation in a bicornuate uterus.

The presence of an adnexal heterogeneous mass along with peritoneal free fluid and intact solid organs can help clarify conflicting histories during abdominal ultrasound examinations. In these scenarios, high-resolution transvaginal ultrasound combined with color Doppler imaging serves as an excellent diagnostic tool, providing better visualization of the trophoblastic tissue, which typically shows high blood flow and low resistive indices. Magnetic resonance imaging (MRI) can be utilized as a problem-solving modality for further characterization and confirmation of peritoneal blood products and a ruptured ectopic mass.

Interestingly, heterotopic pregnancy can occur without any identifiable predisposing risk factors, as demonstrated in our patient. The identification of an intrauterine pregnancy does not rule out the possibility of a concurrent ectopic pregnancy; therefore, clinicians should remain vigilant for this condition during ultrasound evaluations.[2]

REFERENCES

1. Elhadidi A, Alhariri A, Hosny Garib M, et al. Ruptured Heterotopic Pregnancy: A Rare Encounter in Acute Surgical Care Settings. Cureus. 2020;12(11).
2. Kong M, Paramesparan K, Keshvala C, et al. Acute abdomen or life-threatening heterotopic pregnancy with tubal rupture: where does imaging play a role? BMJ Case Rep. 2020;13(12):e239178.

74

Diabetic Foot with Calcaneum Osteomyelitis

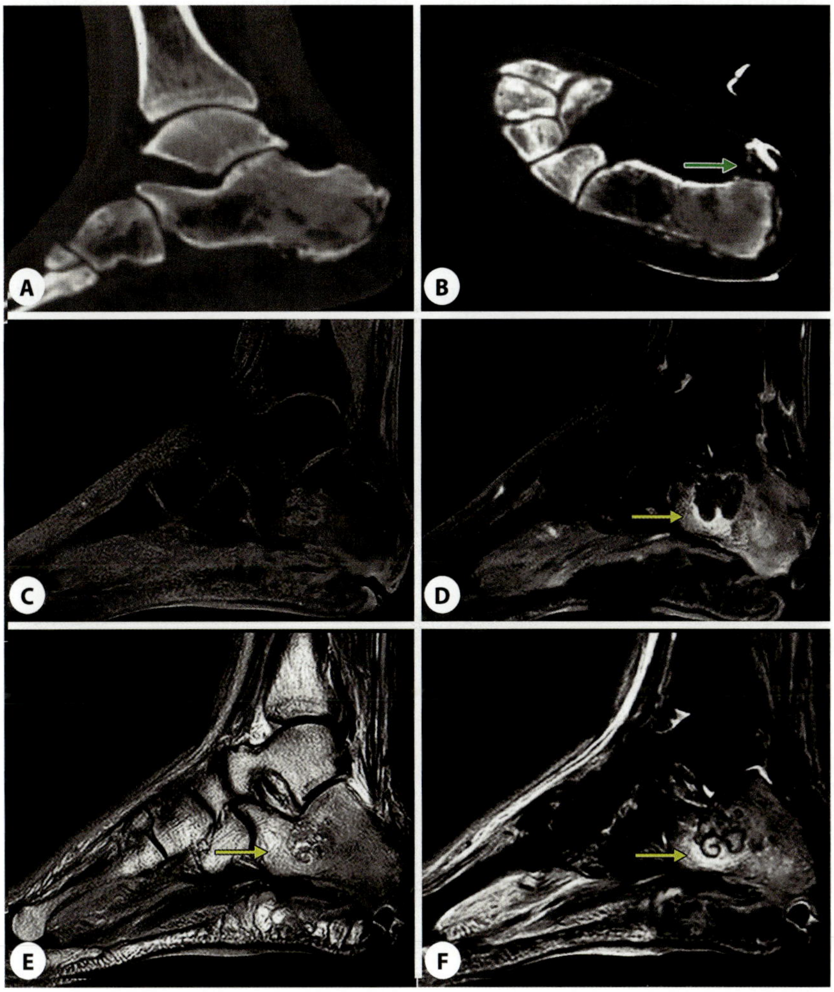

CLINICAL BACKGROUND

A 49-year-old male patient presented with severe right foot and heel pain.

IMAGING FINDINGS

Cortical erosions/destructions in calcaneum with altered bone marrow signals. Ill-defined T2/STIR heterointesne intramedullary collection with diffusion restriction and significant peripheral postcontrast enhancement s/o intramedullary abscess (yellow arrow). Plantar muscles appear bulky with severe edema **(Figs. 1A to F)**.

DISCUSSION

Osteomyelitis of the calcaneus, a relatively uncommon foot infection, is often associated with poorer outcomes compared to cellulitis or osteomyelitis affecting more distal bones. It frequently occurs in diabetic foot conditions and is notably difficult to treat, often leading to unfavorable results.[1]

In the early stages of infection (within the first 10 days), plain radiography has limited sensitivity for detecting the extent of bone involvement, although nonspecific soft tissue swelling may be observed. Bony changes, such as periosteal thickening, trabecular loss, osteopenia, and osteolytic destruction, typically become evident after at least a week. Ultrasound is a useful and efficient method, especially in children, for identifying subperiosteal spread in acute osteomyelitis due to the looser attachment of the periosteum. Signs such as periosteal elevation, fluid collections, or abscesses strongly suggest osteomyelitis.[1]

Magnetic resonance imaging (MRI) is considered the best modality for early detection of acute osteomyelitis. Bone marrow abnormalities can be identified within 3–5 days after infection begins on Fat-Sat T2-weighted imaging. MRI also provides detailed visualization of soft tissue involvement, joint effusion, abscesses, and sinus tracts. A key indicator of acute osteomyelitis is the presence of intramedullary fat globules on T1-weighted imaging, which appear as areas of high signal intensity due to necrotic fat cells released by damaged lipocytes.[1]

In subacute osteomyelitis, Brodie's abscess, typically located in the metaphysis, is seen as an oval radiolucent lesion with peripheral sclerosis on plain radiographs. The penumbra sign, which consists of a thin rim of high signal intensity on T1-weighted imaging around the abscess, is a hallmark feature. This high signal intensity is attributed to granulation tissue, which contains lipid-laden macrophages in the abscess wall. After intravenous gadolinium contrast administration, the thin vascularized rim enhances.[1]

Chronic osteomyelitis is characterized by inhomogeneous osteosclerosis and/or sequestrum formation, which represents necrotic bone, on plain radiographs. A sequestrum appears as a denser area than surrounding living bone, separated by granulation tissue and bone resorption. Sometimes, new periosteal bone or an involucrum can be observed surrounding the sequestrum. On MRI, the sequestrum is typically hypointense across all pulse sequences. After gadolinium contrast, a cloaca, or opening in the involucrum, may be visible, allowing the discharge of pus, granulation tissue, and sequestra. Sinus tracts extending from the bone to the skin surface are also well demonstrated on contrast-enhanced MRI.[1]

REFERENCE

1. Desimpel J, Posadzy M. Vanhoenacker. The many faces of osteomyelitis: A pictorial review. Journal of the Belgian Society of Radiology. 2017;101(1):24.

75 Midgut Malrotation with Bowel Ischemia

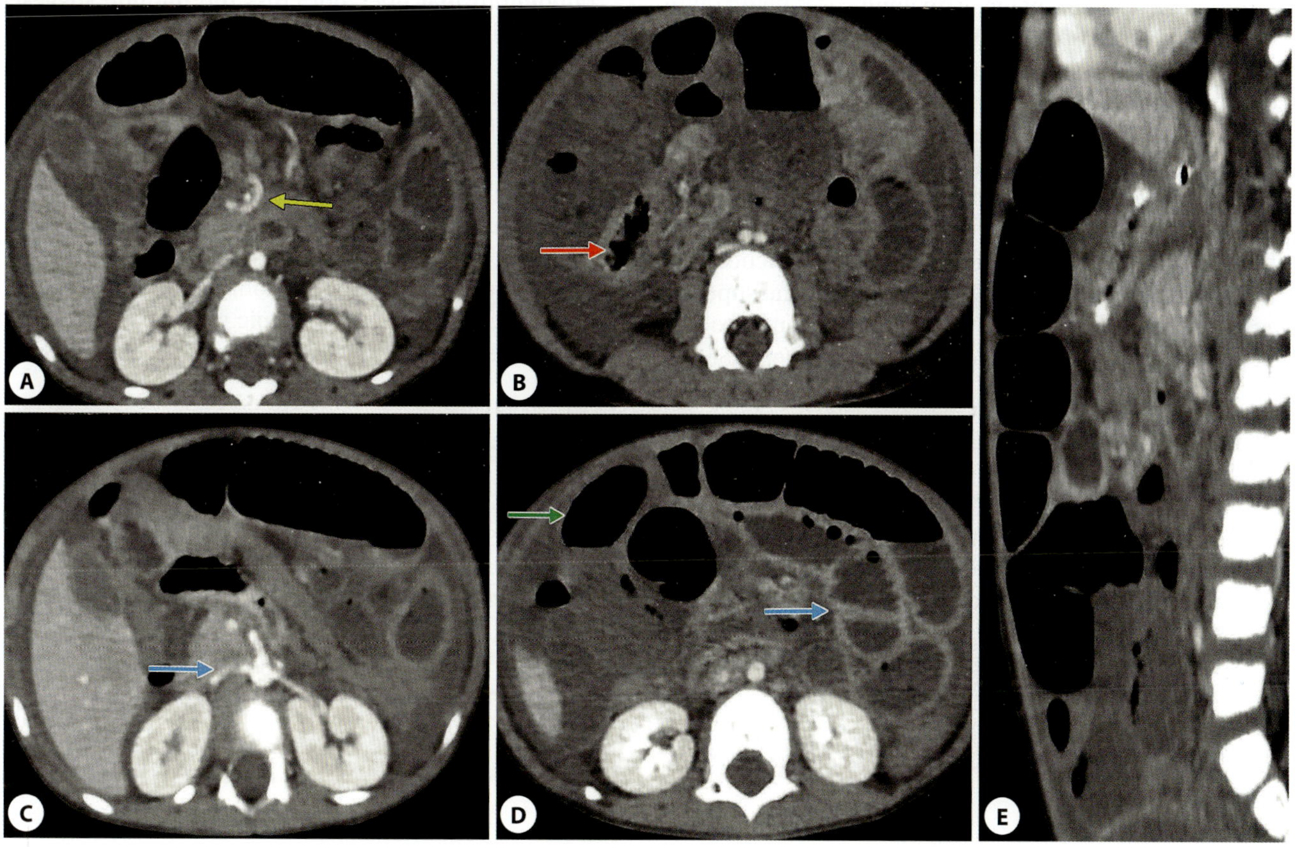

CLINICAL BACKGROUND

A 2-year-old male patient presented with severe abdomen pain.

IMAGING FINDINGS

DJ flexure not crossing midline with predominant jejunal loops on right side and suspicious whirl sign (yellow arrow). Thickened terminal ileum, cecum with moderate dilatation of small bowel loops and fluid collection/air pockets in RIF (red arrow) **(Figs. 1A to E)**.

Significantly reduced postcontrast enhancement noted involving a long segment of small bowel (green arrow). Collapsed IVC with moderate ascites and hyper-enhancing small bowel loops complex (blue arrow).

DISCUSSION

Intestinal malrotation occurs when the midgut fails to rotate properly around the superior mesenteric vessels during embryonic development. This incomplete or halted rotation leads to a narrow-based mesentery, increasing the risk of midgut twisting, which can cause obstruction and necrosis. The majority of malrotation cases present within the first month of life, with adult cases being quite rare, occurring in about 0.2–0.5% of the population.[1]

Various imaging modalities such as plain radiography, contrast-enhanced upper gastrointestinal studies, ultrasonography, and computed tomography (CT) scans are useful for diagnosing malrotation. A characteristic radiological feature is the "corkscrew sign," which is seen as the dilatation of different duodenal segments and the abnormal positioning of the duodenojejunal junction due to the folding of the jejunum. On ultrasound, the superior mesenteric vein (SMV) is often seen positioned to the left or in front of the superior mesenteric artery (SMA), and Doppler ultrasound may reveal the "whirlpool sign," indicating the SMV rotating around the SMA, a hallmark of malrotation.[2]

In contrast-enhanced CT (CECT) scans of the abdomen, several key imaging findings should be assessed, including:

- Whether the duodenum crosses the midline (a duodenum that does not cross the midline suggests nonrotation; if it crosses and then returns to the right, it indicates partial rotation; crossing without folding back suggests malrotation),
- The location of the jejunum,
- The position of the cecum,
- The relationship between the SMA and SMV,
- The presence of the whirlpool sign.[3]

Surgical correction, typically by Ladd's procedure, is the standard treatment for malrotation, whether performed urgently or electively. Laparoscopic surgery is becoming an increasingly favored approach for uncomplicated cases.

REFERENCES

1. Zengin A, Uçar Bi, Düzgün ŞA, et al. Adult midgut malrotation presented with acute bowel obstruction and ischemia. International Journal of Surgery Case Reports. 2016;22:5-7.
2. Gamblin TC, Stephens RE, Johnson RK, et al. Adult malrotation: a case report and review of the literature. Current Surgery. 2003;60(5):517-20.
3. Xiong Z, Shen Y, Morelli, JN, et al. CT facilitates improved diagnosis of adult intestinal malrotation: a 7-year retrospective study based on 332 cases. Insights into Imaging. 2021;12:58.

76 Unhappy Triad of O'Donoghue

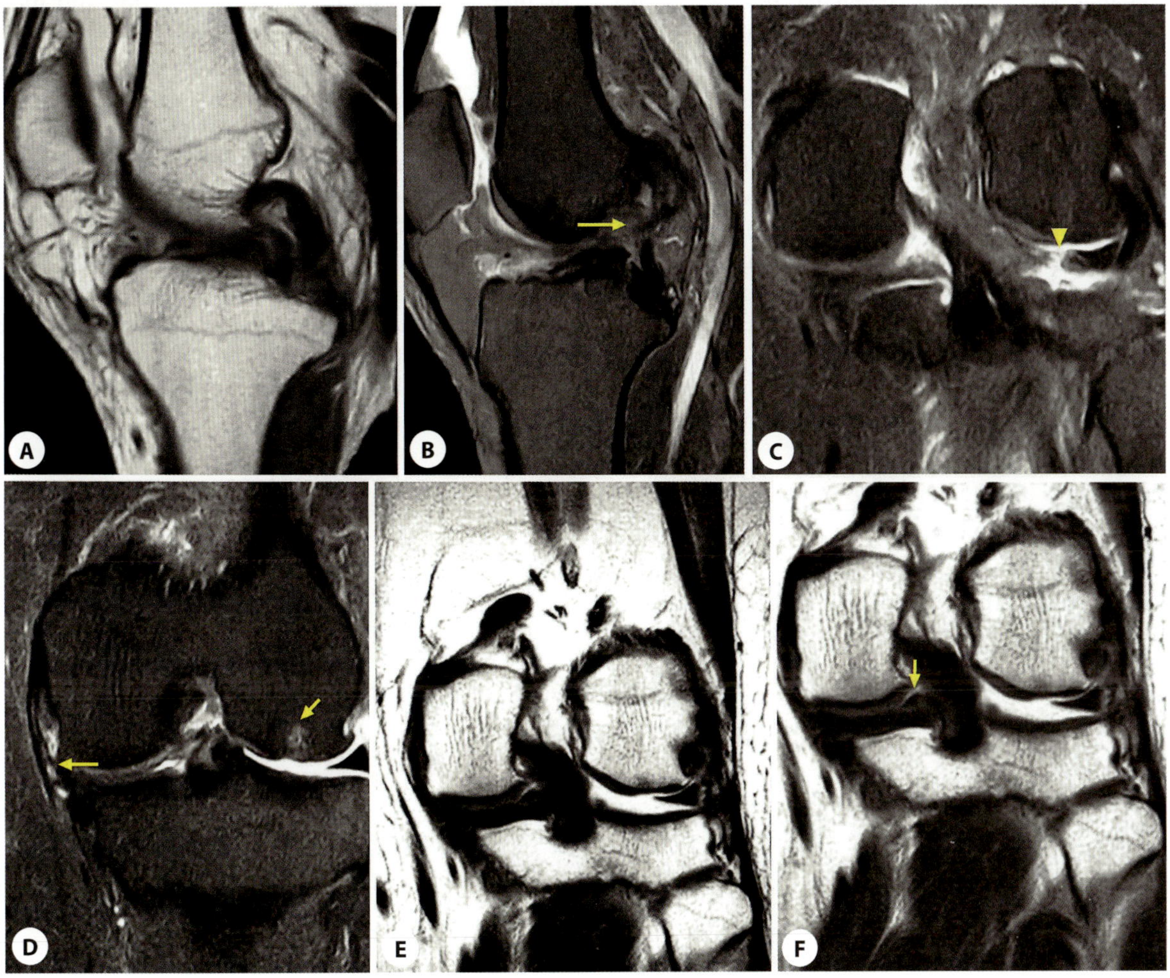

CLINICAL BACKGROUND

A 41-year-old male presented with severe knee pain, after recent RTA.

IMAGING FINDINGS

Complete disruption of ACL fibers seen. Radial tear in posterior horn of lateral meniscus/bucket handle tear noted in posterior horn of medial meniscus with "double PCL" sign **(Figs 1A to F)**.

T2/STIR hyperintensity noted involving femoral attachment of lateral collateral ligament. Moderate knee joint effusion noted extending into suprapatellar bursa. Degenerative osteoarthritic changes with significantly reduced medial joint space, causing thinning of medial meniscus. Fissuring noted in articulating cartilage of lateral femoral condyle with adjacent bone marrow edema/contusions. Minimal bone marrow edema/contusions noted in lateral tibial plateau.

DISCUSSION

In 1936, Campbell first described a "combination" knee injury, which involved damage to the anterior cruciate ligament (ACL), medial collateral ligament (MCL), and medial meniscus (MM). However, it was not until O'Donoghue 1950 report that this specific triad was highlighted, with approximately a quarter of all acute sports-related knee injuries involving the ACL, MCL, and MM. Interestingly, lateral meniscus injuries are now thought to be more frequently associated with ACL and MCL tears, raising the question: Medial meniscus or lateral meniscus, triad or tetrad?[1]

Magnetic resonance imaging (MRI) is the preferred imaging modality for identifying traumatic knee tears, especially for meniscus and ACL injuries, which are among the most frequent in the knee joint. Although there is no universal classification system for meniscus tears, they are most commonly described as horizontal, longitudinal, radial, root, complex, displaced, or bucket-handle tears. One notable sign is the "double PCL sign," which occurs when a displaced fragment from a bucket-handle tear of the medial meniscus lies in front of and parallel to the posterior cruciate ligament (PCL).[2]

ACL tears can be either partial or complete. Partial tears vary in severity, ranging from minor damage affecting only a few fibers to near-complete tears. These can affect both or just one of the ACL bundles. Partial tears are identified by increased signal intensity, fiber laxity, and increased concavity (or bowing) of the ACL, but intact fibers indicate the tear is not full-thickness. However, around 80% of ACL tears are complete, with the majority occurring in the middle third of the ligament (90%), while others occur near the femoral (7%) or tibial (3%) attachments.[3]

The key indication of an ACL tear is fiber discontinuity. In complete ACL tears, the "empty notch sign" is a common finding on coronal MRI scans. In acute or subacute cases, the ACL appears thickened and edematous, with increased signal intensity on T2 or intermediate-weighted sequences. MRI has proven to be highly accurate in diagnosing ACL tears, with more than 90% accuracy, sensitivity, and specificity.[3]

REFERENCES

1. Hoveidaei AH, Sattarpour R, Dadgostar H, et al. Unhappy triad of the knee: What are the current concepts and opinions? World J Orthop. 2023;14(5):268-74.
2. Pakdemirli E, Cesur T, Bozkurt İ. MRI in the Diagnosis of Bucket Handle Tears: What Is the Current Situation? Cureus. 2023;15(8).
3. Ng WH, Griffith JF, Hung EH, et al. Imaging of the anterior cruciate ligament. World J Orthop. 2011;2(8):75-84.

77 Seminal Vesiculitis

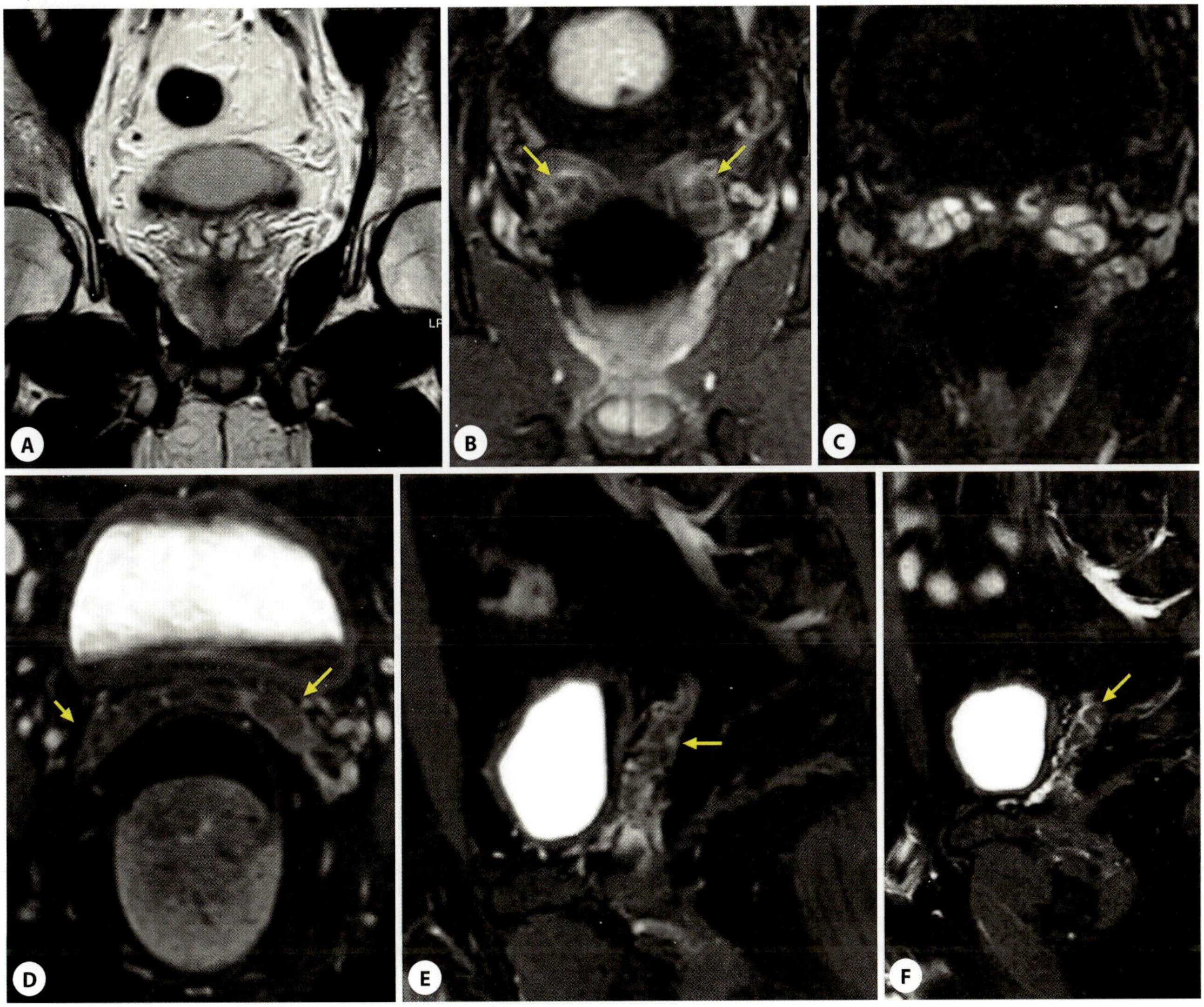

CLINICAL BACKGROUND

A 37-year-old male presented with secondary infertility.

IMAGING FINDINGS

Mild cystic dilatation of bilateral seminal vesicle (maximum diameter 7–8 mm) with mild wall thickening and enhancement on postcontrast study **(Figs. 1A to F)**.

DISCUSSION

The seminal vesicles (SV) are a pair of accessory glands in the male reproductive system, located extraperitoneally between the bladder and rectum. The vas deferens (VD), which are continuous with the epididymal tail, terminate and form bilateral outpouchings.[1]

Genitourinary tuberculosis is a prevalent form of extrapulmonary tuberculosis. Approximately two-thirds of reproductive system tuberculosis cases are linked with urinary system tuberculosis, though it can also manifest independently. Tuberculosis in the male reproductive system may affect the prostate, seminal vesicles, vas deferens, epididymis, testes, and penis. Among these, epididymal and prostatic tuberculosis are the most common, while seminal vesiculitis is often discovered during evaluations for prostatic and urinary tuberculosis.[2]

Seminal vesiculitis, whether acute or chronic, is typically secondary to an infection that also involves the prostate. Urethritis and prostatitis are frequent clinical conditions managed by urologists, and research suggests that seminal vesiculitis can be present in up to 24% of patients with other genitourinary infections, such as gonococcal urethritis.[1]

On imaging, vesiculitis typically presents with distinct features on ultrasound, CT, or MRI, such as diffuse thickening of the SV walls and septal enhancement on postcontrast CT or MRI. In regions where tuberculosis and schistosomiasis are endemic, these should be considered as potential causes. During the acute or subacute phase, cystic dilation of the SVs may occur, while in the chronic phase, they may appear shrunken with decreased signal intensity on T1- and T2-weighted MRI. If active inflammation is present, the T2 signal will be higher than fat, and T1 signal may increase if there is a hemorrhagic component. In cases of long-standing tuberculosis, calcifications may be seen in the burned-out lesions.[1,2]

REFERENCES

1. Reddy MN, Verma S. Lesions of the Seminal Vesicles and their MRI Characteristics. J Clin Imaging Sci. 2014;4:61.
2. Kim B, Kawashima A, Ryu JA, et al. Imaging of the seminal vesicle and vas deferens. RadioGraphics 2009;29(4):1105–21.

78

TB Spondylodiscitis with Bilateral Psoas Abscess: Pigtail Drainage of Psoas Abscess

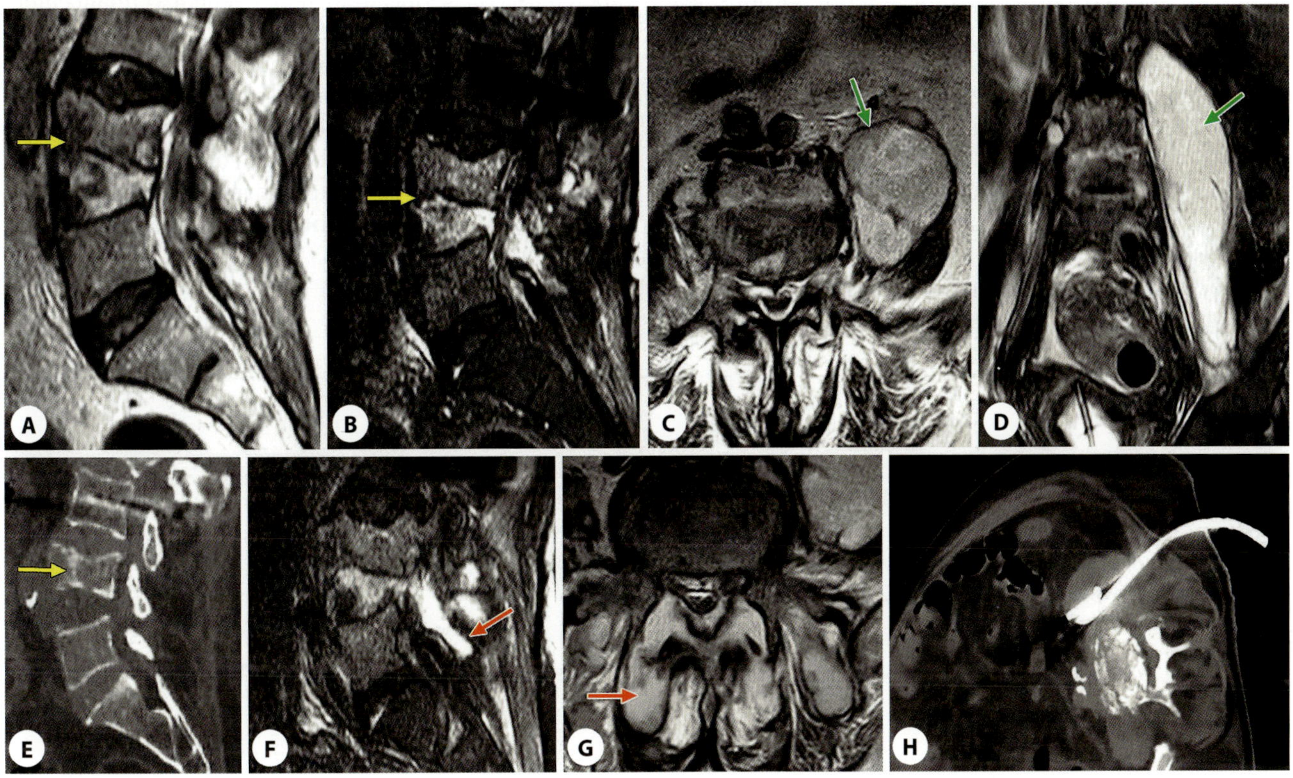

CLINICAL BACKGROUND

A 75-year-old male patient came with severe back pain.

IMAGING FINDINGS

Anterior wedge compression fracture of L4 vertebral body and endplate erosions with marrow edema. Severe disc edema at L4-L5 level and mild marrow edema at L5 vertebral body (yellow arrow) **(Figs. 1A to H)**.

- Multiloculated T2/STIR hyperintense collection seen in bilateral (Left >> Right) psoas muscles (green arrow).
- T2/STIR hyperintense collection in bilateral posterior paravertebral muscles at L4-L5 level, extending into posterior epidural space (red arrow).
- Image of pigtail drainage for psoas abscess also added.

DISCUSSION

Tuberculous spondylitis, also known as Pott disease, is a condition in which *Mycobacterium tuberculosis* causes destruction of the vertebral body and intervertebral disc. It typically presents with an insidious onset, manifesting as back pain, stiffness, localized tenderness, fever, and malaise. The thoracic and lumbar vertebrae are most frequently affected, particularly the anterior portions near the superior and inferior endplates.[1]

The involvement of the anterior vertebrae often leads to the development of a gibbus deformity. Vertebral destruction typically begins as fragmentary damage, followed by lytic destruction. Other common features include paraspinal masses, epidural and psoas abscesses, and collapse of the intervertebral disc spaces. Abscesses can extend widely and may become calcified, which helps differentiate them from nontuberculous abscesses that rarely calcify.[1]

Differentiating between tuberculous and pyogenic spondylitis can be challenging due to overlapping imaging features. However, tuberculosis is more likely if there are associated lesions in other organs (e.g., lungs or urinary tract), if the spine is involved at multiple levels, or if there is a gibbus deformity. Recent MRI studies suggest that tuberculosis causes localized, heterogeneous enhancement of the vertebral body, compared to the diffuse, homogeneous enhancement seen in pyogenic spondylitis.[2]

Treatment of psoas abscesses typically involves a combination of medical therapy and abscess drainage. As shown in this case, percutaneous drainage is an effective and less invasive alternative to surgical drainage, complementing medical therapy for managing large tuberculous psoas abscesses.[3]

REFERENCES

1. Sinnan T, Al-Khawari H, Ismail M, et al. Spinal tuberculosis: CT and MRI features. Ann Saudi Med. 2004;24(6):437-41.
2. Chang MC, Wu HTA, Lee CH, et al. Tuberculous spondylitis and pyogenic spondylitis: comparative magnetic resonance imaging features. Spine. 2006;31(7):782-8.
3. Pombo F, Martín-Egaña R, Cela A, et al. Percutaneous catheter drainage of tuberculous abscesses. Acta Radiol. 1993;34(4): 366-8.

79 Mid Aortic Syndrome

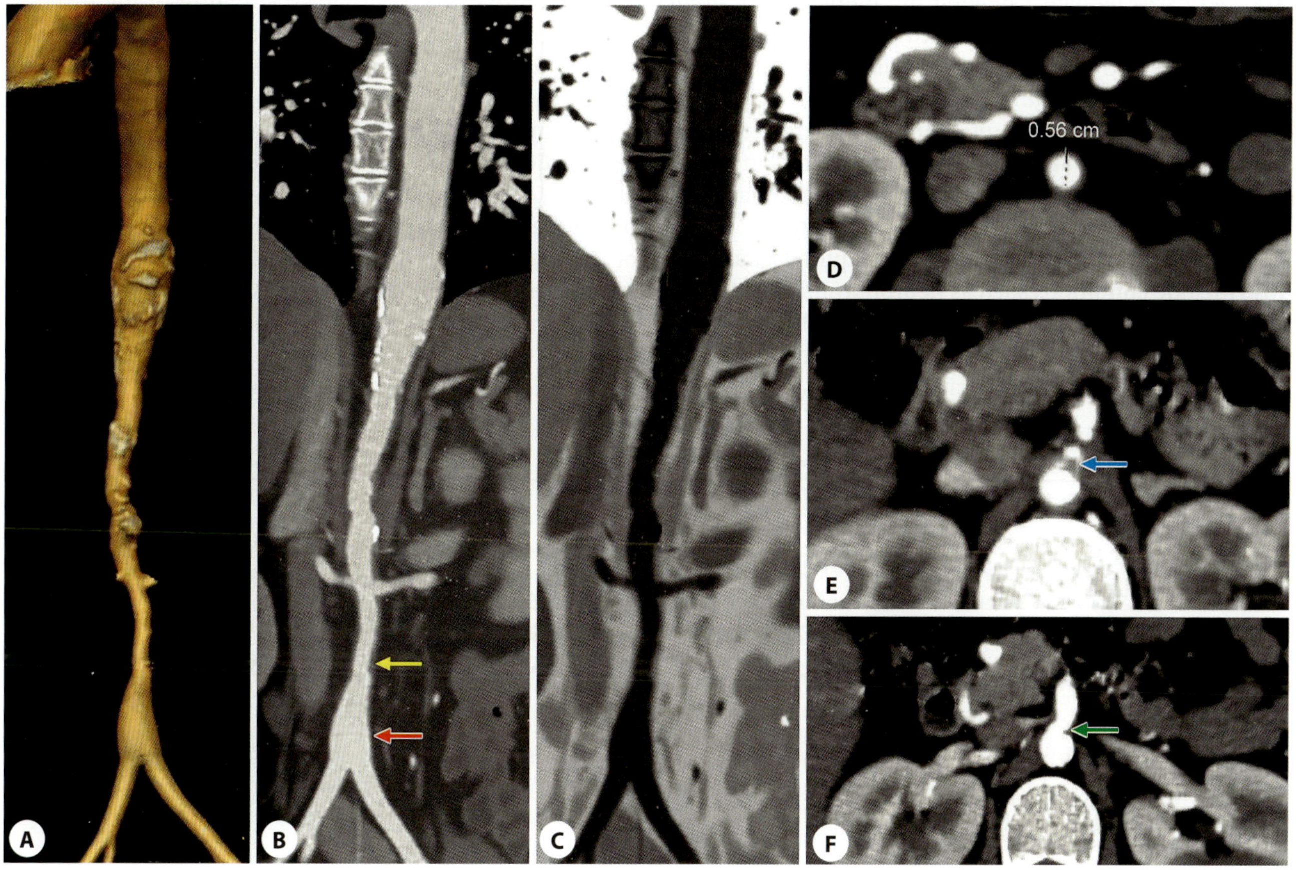

CLINICAL BACKGROUND

A 35-year-old female patient came with severe uncontrolled hypertension.

IMAGING FINDINGS

- CT aortic angiogram show diffuse multifocal wall calcification and thickening of aorta with contour irregularity/ irregular luminal narrowing **(Figs. 1A to F)**.
- Long segment and irregular narrowing of abdominal aorta from distal descending thoracic to abdominal aorta, just before its bifurcation, from D11 to L3 levels, narrowest diameter measures (5–6 mm) at L2-L3 level (yellow arrow). Aortic bifurcation and iliac arteries appear normal (red arrow).
- Non-calcified plaque, at ostium of celiac trunk causing moderate luminal narrowing (50–60%) (blue arrow).
- Mild irregular narrowing and kinking at ostium of superior mesenteric artery causing mild luminal narrowing (20–30%) (green arrow). Except for mild wall thickening, bilateral renal ostium/renal arteries show normal contrast opacification.

DISCUSSION

Middle aortic syndrome (MAS) is a rare vascular condition characterized by segmental narrowing of the abdominal aorta or distal descending thoracic aorta. This stenosis is often accompanied by narrowing of the origins of major aortic branches, particularly the renal and visceral arteries. MAS can be congenital or acquired, with fewer than 700 reported cases globally,[1] making up about 0.5–2% of all aortic stenosis cases in children and young adults.[2]

MAS can lead to significant complications due to the restricted blood flow through the aorta and its visceral branches. The exact cause of MAS remains unclear, but around 64% of cases are considered idiopathic. Congenital MAS is typically linked to developmental anomalies in the fusion and maturation of the paired embryonic dorsal aortas, often identified early in life. Acquired causes of MAS include conditions such as neurofibromatosis type 1, Williams syndrome, Alagille syndrome, fibromuscular dysplasia, retroperitoneal fibrosis, mucopolysaccharidosis, and arteritis like Takayasu arteritis.[3]

Previously, catheter angiography was the preferred method for diagnosing idiopathic MAS, but it can now be effectively diagnosed using computed tomography angiography (CTA) or magnetic resonance angiography (MRA). In cases of infrarenal MAS, patients often present with vague abdominal discomfort, sometimes without hypertensive symptoms. Early treatment and monitoring are crucial due to the progressive nature of the disease, which can eventually lead to life-threatening hypertension. Differentiating MAS from conditions like Takayasu arteritis can be challenging.[3]

Treatment of MAS often involves surgical or endovascular intervention to reduce blood pressure and relieve symptoms, although specific guidelines for invasive management are not well-established. Factors such as the location and length of the stenosis, and the degree of involvement of visceral vessels, influence treatment decisions. Multidisciplinary management is required, with individualized treatment plans based on the severity of symptoms, response to medical therapy, and extent of end-organ damage.[3]

REFERENCES

1. Rumman RK, Nickel C, Matsuda-Abedini M, et al. Disease beyond the arch: a systematic review of middle aortic syndrome in childhood. Am J Hypertens. 2015;28(7):833-46.
2. Cohen JR, Birnbaum E. Coarctation of the abdominal aorta. J Vasc Surg. 1988; 8:160-4.
3. Zurcher K, Towbin RB, Schaefer CM, et al. Middle Aortic Syndrome. Appl Radiol. 2021;50(6):21-3.

80 C-section Scar Dehiscence

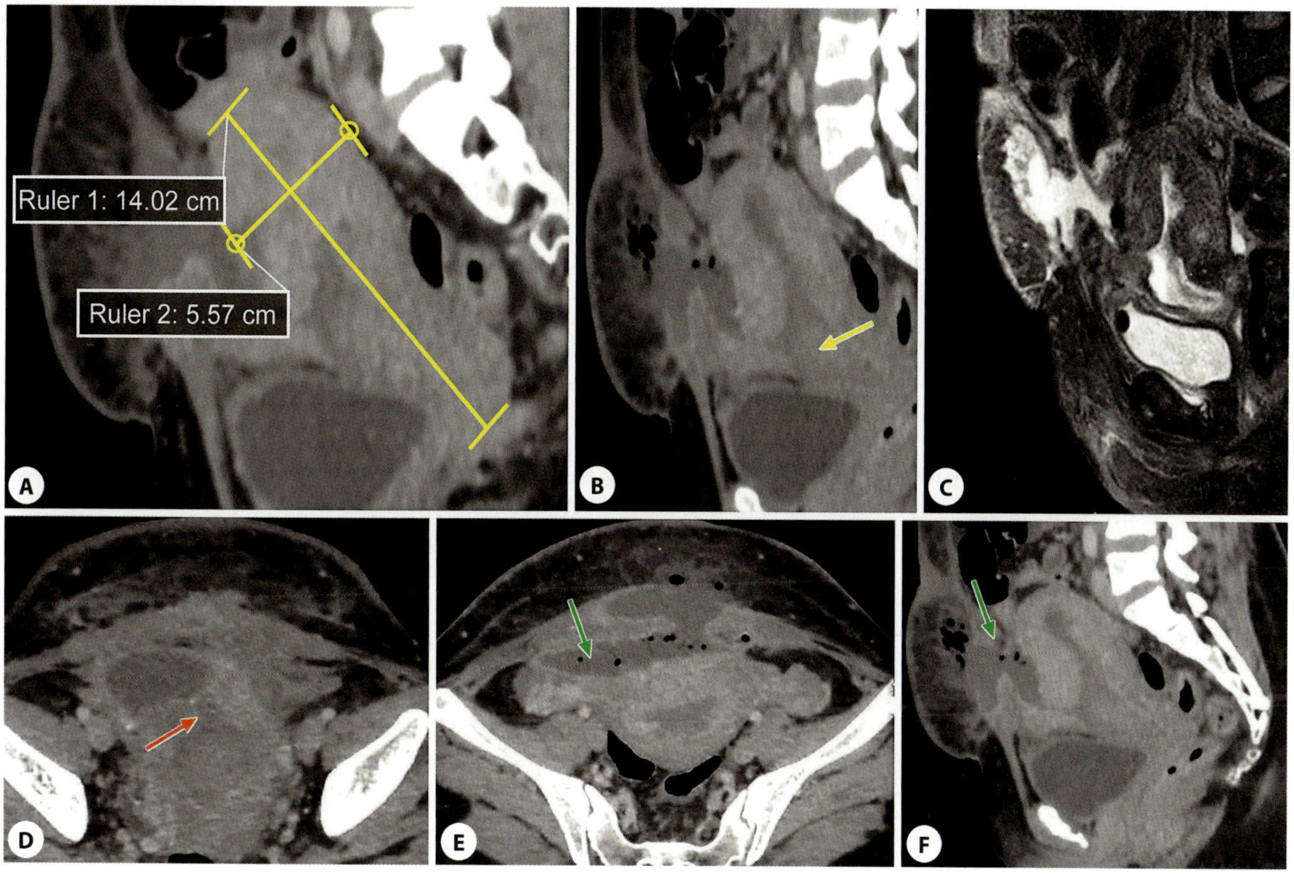

CLINICAL BACKGROUND

A 28-year-old female, postoperative follow-up patient of LSCS came with severe abdominal pain.

IMAGING FINDINGS

- Uterus appear bulky—postpartum status/endometrium appears thickened with hyperdense content noted in lower uterine cavity (yellow arrow). (Likely blood product) **(Figs. 1A to F)**.
- Suspicious defect in anterior myometrium (measures 1.8 cm) at the site of cesarean section site (red arrow).
- Ill-defined loculated collection with air pockets seen anterior to uterus. Inflammatory adhesions with adjacent bowel and anterior abdominal wall (green arrow). The collection noted extending into rectus muscle and subcutaneous plane of lower anterior abdominal wall. Bilateral rectus muscles appear bulky with intramuscular with adjacent inflammatory fat strandings noted.
- The collection shows peripheral enhancement on postcontrast study.

DISCUSSION

Postpartum uterine dehiscence is defined as the separation of the incision line following a cesarean section, characterized by disruption of both the endometrium and myometrium, while the uterine serosa remains intact.[1] This complication is rare, occurring in approximately 0.06–3.8% of cases.[2] Despite its low incidence, it is a significant cause of maternal mortality, and its detection has become more frequent due to the rising rates of cesarean deliveries.[3] Several risk factors for uterine dehiscence include diabetes, emergency surgery, infection, multiparity, suture technique, hematoma at the uterine incision site, and retrovesical hematoma.[2,4]

The clinical presentation of uterine dehiscence can be subtle, often manifesting as nonspecific abdominal pain, which may be easily misinterpreted and lead to delayed diagnosis. Thus, it is essential to consider this differential diagnosis, with imaging playing a crucial role in establishing it.

Ultrasonography (US) should be the first-line imaging modality for evaluating postpartum complications, as it can assist in assessing the uterine incision. While US can identify indirect signs of dehiscence, such as free fluid, collections, or hematomas, it may not reliably differentiate between uterine dehiscence and the normal appearance of the incision.[2,5] When US findings are inconclusive, computed tomography (CT) scans with multiplanar reconstructions can provide additional information, particularly in emergency situations. Magnetic resonance imaging (MRI) has superior diagnostic yield compared to CT, enabling simultaneous visualization of the cervix and anterior uterine wall, which allows for better assessment of serosal integrity.

REFERENCES

1. Hatstat LM. Sonographic Assessment of Uterine Dehiscence During Pregnancy in Women With a History of Cesarean Section: A Case Series. Journal of Diagnostic Medical Sonography. 2016;32(5):283-6.
2. El-Agwany AS. Conservative Management of Infected Postpartum Uterine Dehiscence after Cesarean Section. J Med Ultrasound. 2018; 26(1):59-61.
3. Nagaya K, Fetters MD, Ishikawa M, et al. Causes of maternal mortality in Japan. JAMA. 2000 May;283(20):2661-7.
4. Wagner MS, Bédard MJ. Postpartum uterine wound dehiscence: a case report. J Obstet Gynaecol Can. 2006;28(8):713-5.
5. Shaamash AH, Ahmed AGM, Abdel Latef MM, et al. Routine postpartum ultrasonography in the prediction of puerperal uterine complications. Int J Gynaecol Obstet. 2007;98(2):93-9.

81

Hepatic Arterioportal Shunt with Giant IMV in CLD

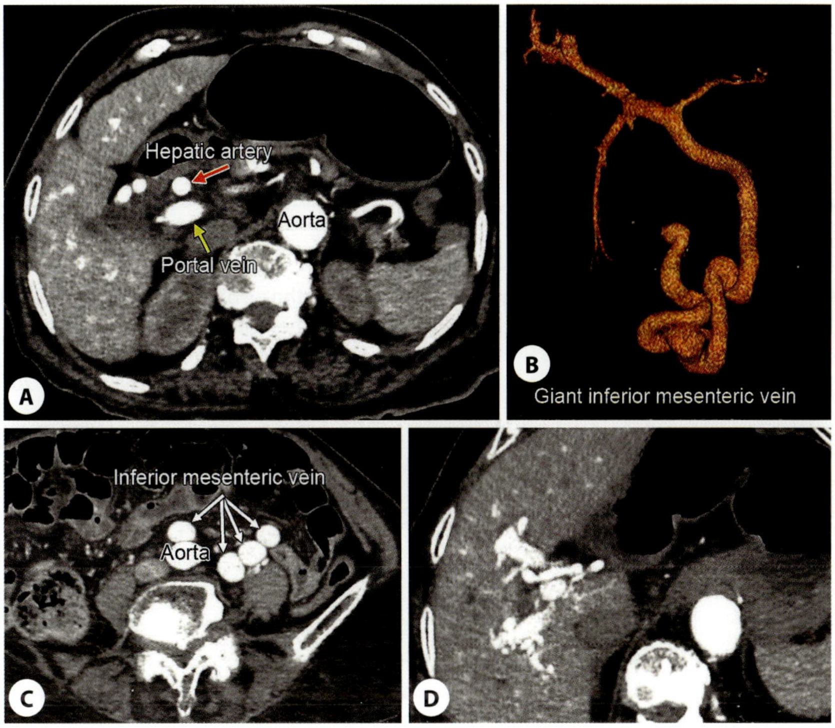

CLINICAL BACKGROUND

A 91-year-old female patient came with nonspecific abdominal pain.

IMAGING FINDINGS

Liver shows altered parenchymal attenuation with surface nodularity/multiple nonenhancing hypodense lesion noted in both lobes of liver **(Figs. 1A to D)**.

- Early portal venous filling with dilatation of hepatic artery (could represent arterioportal shunt).
- Gross dilatation of inferior mesenteric vein and tortuosity.

DISCUSSION

Liver cirrhosis results from chronic hepatocellular injury, necrosis, and fibroblast activation, leading to altered hepatic hemodynamics characterized by increased hepatic arterial flow and decreased portal venous flow to the liver. Cirrhosis is a recognized cause of nontumorous hepatic arterioportal shunt (HAPS), with literature indicating that angiography can reveal nontumorous HAPS in up to 13% of patients with liver cirrhosis.[1]

Nontumorous HAPS associated with liver cirrhosis is thought to occur due to secondary occlusion of small hepatic venules, causing retrograde filling of small portal vein branches via an arterioportal anastomotic route (trans-sinusoidal route). In this scenario, the portal vein acts as a draining vessel rather than a supplying one, leading to a compensatory increase in hepatic arterial flow to sustain liver perfusion. Radiologically, this condition presents as diffusely inhomogeneous parenchymal enhancement, strongly suggestive of advanced cirrhosis.[1]

The inferior mesenteric vein (IMV) is a tributary of the portal vein that collects blood from the large intestine, sigmoid colon, and rectum. It typically connects with the splenic vein before draining into the portal vein but may also directly join the superior mesenteric vein (SMV) or connect at the confluence of the SMV and splenic vein. Varices of the inferior mesenteric vein can occur due to portal hypertension and may be isolated or associated with other portosystemic collaterals.[1]

In our case, two peculiarities were noted:

1. The presence of a giant isolated inferior mesenteric vein with an anomalous insertion, where the IMV connected to the superior mesenteric vein before draining into the portal vein.[2]
2. Despite the liver exhibiting signs of cirrhosis and HAPS, the superior mesenteric vein, splenic vein, and portal vein were neither enlarged nor varicosed, and there were no obvious signs of splenic enlargement.[2]

REFERENCES

1. Wang Q, Koniaris LG, Milgrom DP, et al. CT and MRI imaging and interpretation of hepatic arterioportal shunts. Transl Gastroenterol Hepatol. 2019;21;4:34.
2. Jayarathna MJS, Udayakumara S, Dhanushkar R, et al. Isolated giant mesenteric vein and anomalous inferior mesenteric vein insertion in the presence of cirrhosis – A cadaveric case report. Sri Lanka Anatomy Journal (SLAJ). 2021;5(II):30-4.

82 Peristomal Varices

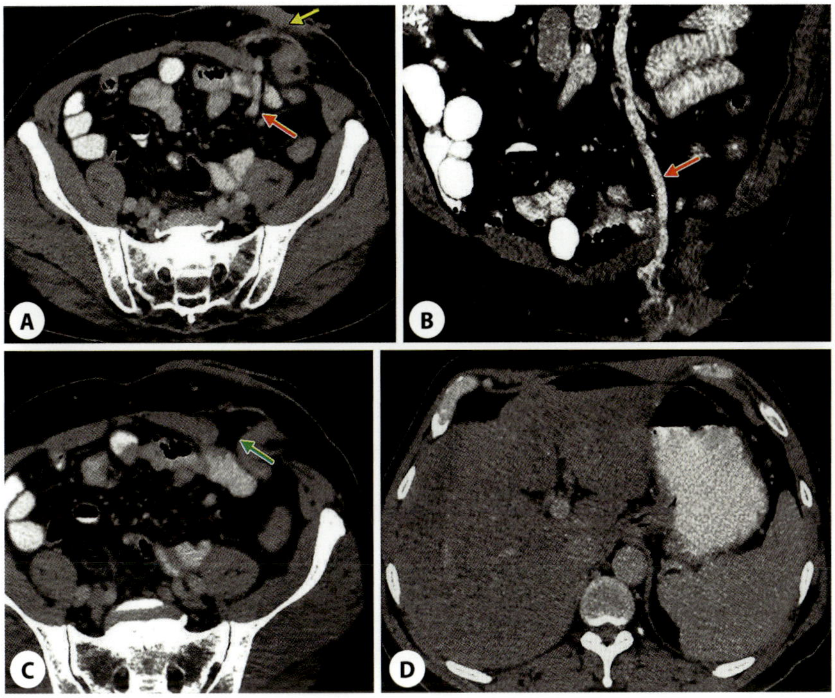

CLINICAL BACKGROUND

A 49-year-old male postoperative follow up patient of carcinoma lower rectum/postcolostomy came with complaints of bleed at colostomy site.

IMAGING FINDINGS

Colostomy site noted in left iliac fossa with descending colon within it. Dilated venous branches of inferior mesenteric vein at the colostomy site (red arrow) and soft tissue thickening (yellow arrow) **(Figs. 1A to D)**.

- Parastomal hernia noted, with fat as herniating content (green arrow).
- Hepatomegaly with contour irregularity and splenomegaly noted

DISCUSSION

Ectopic varices are defined as varices located outside the esophageal or gastric mucosa and account for up to 5% of all variceal bleeding. Similar to esophageal and gastric varices, ectopic varices are commonly associated with portal hypertension and can lead to clinically significant hemorrhage. Patients with portal hypertension who undergo surgical enterostomy formation are particularly prone to developing peristomal ectopic varices, which have a high tendency to bleed. The estimated mortality rate from these peristomal variceal bleeds is 3–4% per episode.[1]

The formation of an abdominal wall stoma does not inherently pose a significant risk for the development of peristomal varices; however, the presence of liver disease and portal hypertension, combined with an abdominal wall stoma—as seen in our patient—greatly increases this risk. The specific etiology and severity of the liver disease, along with the reasons for creating a small bowel or colonic stoma, may influence the likelihood of variceal development.[1]

Given that portal hypertension is the primary factor responsible for the bleeding, it is prudent to consider decompressing the portal venous system using transjugular intrahepatic portosystemic shunt (TIPS), provided that pre- and postsinusoidal causes of portal hypertension have been ruled out. Another successful approach for treating symptomatic peristomal varices has been through a percutaneous transhepatic route, which provides direct access to the portal system through the liver parenchyma without creating portosystemic shunting. Although this technique has proven effective, it carries a considerable risk of bleeding, especially in patients with underlying liver disease and often elevated international normalized ratio (INR). Direct percutaneous puncture of the intra-abdominal varix, followed by embolization, has also been reported as a safe and effective alternative.[1]

REFERENCE

1. Ryan W, Dako F, Cohen G, et al. Direct Percutaneous Embolization of Peristomal Ileostomy Varices in an Emergency Setting. Case Rep Radiol. 2018;2018:6239183.

83 Bilateral Atretic Transverse Sinuses with Persistent Occipital Sinus and Emissary Condylar Vein

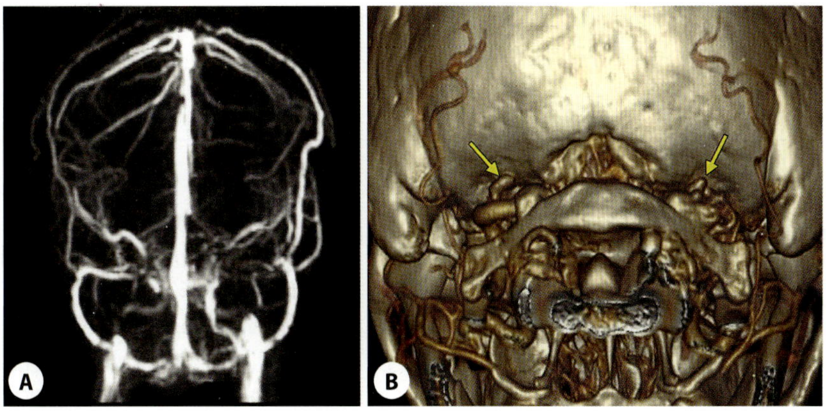

CLINICAL BACKGROUND

A 49-year-old male patient came with nonspecific headache.

IMAGING FINDINGS

Small calibre bilateral transverse sinus with poor contrast opacification and occipital sinus draining bilaterally into IJV/note made of bilateral emissary condylar veins (yellow arrows)/no evidence of acute DVT in visualized dural venous sinus **(Figs. 1A and B)**.

DISCUSSION

The persistent occipital sinus, often associated with absent transverse or sigmoid sinuses, is a rare anatomical variant found in fewer than 10% of individuals. This sinus connects the marginal sinus to the torcula and is the smallest among all cerebral dural venous sinuses. While it is commonly observed in neonates, it typically diminishes during adulthood. Its significance in surgical procedures is noteworthy, particularly when planning approaches for lesions in the posterior fossa, including retrosigmoid surgeries.[1]

Originating as a small venous channel from the primitive torchla and the medial portions of the transverse sinuses, the occipital sinus is most prominent around 5 months of gestation. After this period, it gradually decreases in size and is only found in a minority of the population at birth. The sinus may follow variable pathways, usually descending from the torcula to the marginal veins near the foramen magnum before draining into the suboccipital veins, paravertebral venous plexus, or jugular veins.[2]

Due to its connection with the posterior internal vertebral plexus, the occipital sinus receives a small volume of blood from the spine and spinal cord, classifying it as an emissary vein. This sinus serves as an alternative venous drainage route from the vertebral column when the internal jugular vein's return is compromised. In cases where the transverse sinus is absent, the occipital sinus becomes the main venous drainage pathway from the brain.[3]

Patients with a persistent occipital sinus are generally asymptomatic, and no gender preference has been noted. Conventional CT imaging is not useful for diagnosis; however, CT venography can reveal the anomaly with clear anatomical representation. Conventional T1 and T2-weighted MR images may show a signal void in the area of the occipital sinus, while gradient imaging indicates a loss of signal void. MR venography is the preferred diagnostic modality, as it provides detailed anatomical information and drainage routes, as well as highlights other associated venous anomalies.[4]

Since this entity is usually incidental, no specific management is required except for addressing other pathological conditions, such as venous thrombosis or occlusion. Nevertheless, a patent occipital sinus with an absent transverse sinus is a significant clinical consideration. This finding emphasizes the need for an experienced neurosurgical team if a posterior fossa approach is being planned.[2-4]

Radiologists should be familiar with the persistent occipital sinus and its imaging characteristics, ensuring that they report patent sinuses in cases of posterior fossa abnormalities. Such knowledge is essential for adjusting surgical plans during posterior fossa procedures to prevent catastrophic bleeding, brain swelling, and neurosurgical complications arising from sinus injury.[4,5]

REFERENCES

1. Manjunath KY. Anomalies of transverse and sigmoid sinuses associated with contracted jugular foraminifera. Indian J Otolaryngol Head Neck Surg. 2004;56(02):108-14.
2. Satyarthee GD, Jain G. Indication of surgical management of vestibular schwannoma in the older age group: mysteries still unresolved. World Neurosurg. 2017;101:803-4.
3. Widjaja E, Griffith PD. Intracranial MR venography in children: Normal anatomy and variations. AJNR Am J Neuroradiol. 2004;25(09):1557-62.
4. Jana Vascovic. Occipital sinus. Kenhub.com 2022.
5. Guru DS, Luis RM, Amit A. Persistent enlarged occipital sinus with absent unilateral transverse sinus. J Neurosci Rural Pract. 2019;10:519-21.

84 Pediatric Abdominal Mass: Inflammatory Myofibroblastic Tumor

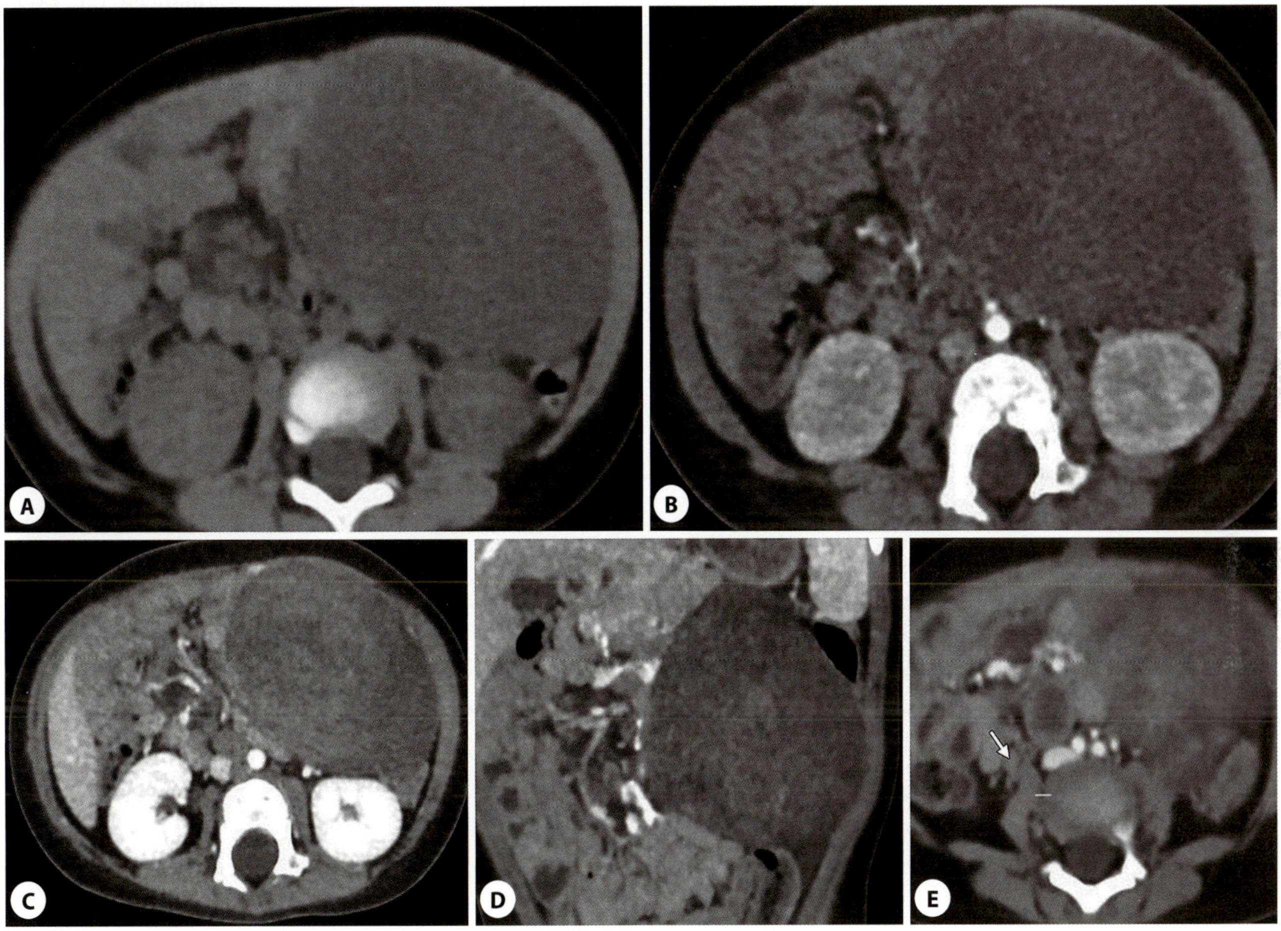

CLINICAL BACKGROUND

A 9-month-old male baby brought with abdominal distension and palpable abdominal mass.

IMAGING FINDINGS

Evidence of large well defined soft tissue dense in intraperitoneal compartment left paramedian aspect of abdomen, inferior to stomach. The lesion seen indenting the distal body/tail region of pancreas and abutting the anterior pararenal fascia/left psoas muscle posteriorly. Medially, the lesion noted displacing the adjacent small bowel loops and laterally displacing the colon. Anteriorly, the lesion seen abutting the parietal peritoneum/anterior abdominal wall with loss of fat plane **(Figs. 1A to E)**.

- Heterogeneous postcontrast enhancement of the lesion noted.
- Multiple enlarged mesenteric lymphnodes noted along the branches of SMA and SMV (white arrow).

DISCUSSION

An inflammatory myofibroblastic tumor (IMT), also known as an inflammatory pseudotumor, is a rare inflammatory lesion resembling a sarcoma, consisting of spindle-shaped myofibroblasts and inflammatory cells. While IMTs are commonly found in the lungs and orbits, they can also appear in various other tissues and organs. They are most frequently diagnosed in children and young adults, with abdominal IMTs in children being of particular concern, as they can closely resemble malignant tumors like sarcomas, lymphomas, or metastases.[1]

The term IMT was introduced by Umiker and Iverson in 1954 due to its tendency to imitate malignancies both clinically and radiologically. Over time, various names have been used to describe these tumors, such as "inflammatory pseudotumor," "pseudosarcomatous myofibroblastic proliferation," and "inflammatory fibrosarcoma." The term inflammatory myofibroblastic tumor has become more accepted due to electron microscopy and immunohistochemistry findings.[1]

The mesentery is a common site for extrapulmonary IMTs, which often present as an abdominal mass. Symptoms such as fever, weight loss, abdominal pain, and vomiting may arise due to the tumor's compressive effects, as seen in cases like the infant in this report who presented with vomiting.

Ultrasound (US) is typically the first imaging modality used, but CT and MRI are more commonly employed for a detailed evaluation. On contrast-enhanced CT, IMTs can present as either homogeneous or heterogeneous masses with varying degrees of enhancement, often due to fibrosis. Similarly, gadolinium-enhanced MRI reveals low signal intensity on T1- and T2-weighted images, reflecting the presence of fibrotic tissue.

Although it can be challenging to differentiate an abdominal IMT from a malignancy based on imaging alone, recognizing its characteristics and conducting a biopsy can help avoid unnecessary aggressive surgery. Familiarity with the imaging features of IMTs is crucial for early identification and appropriate management before confirming malignancy.[2]

REFERENCES

1. Kim SJ, Kim WS, Cheon JE, et al. Inflammatory myofibroblastic tumors of the abdomen as mimickers of malignancy: Imaging features in nine children. AJR Am J Roentgenol. 2009;193: 1419-24.
2. Cantera JE, Alfaro MP, Rafart DC, et al. Inflammatory myofibroblastic tumours: A pictorial review. Insights Imaging. 2015;6(1):85-96.

85 Anomalous Origin of Left Vertebral Artery Supplying the Right Lower Lobe Lung Sequestration

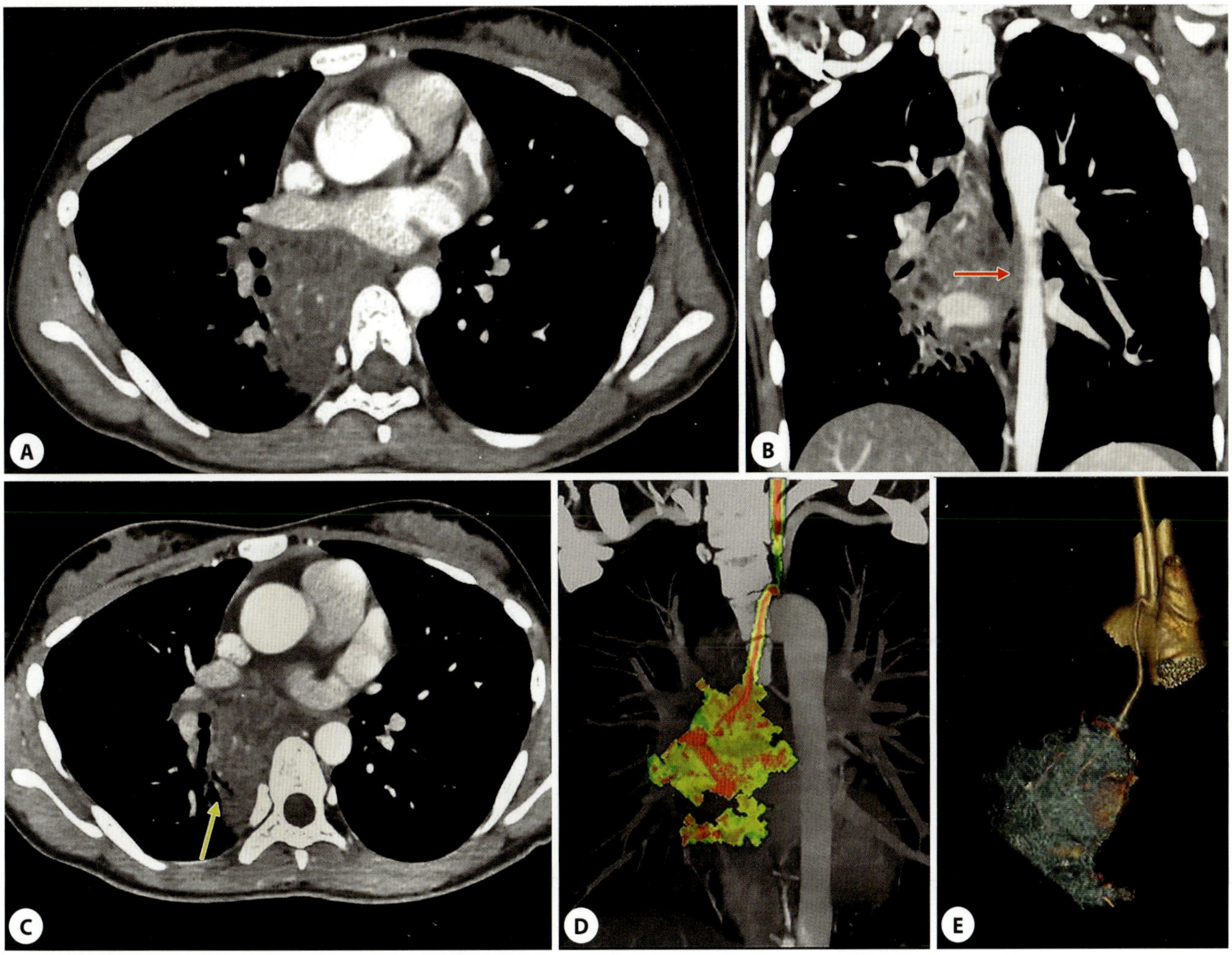

CLINICAL BACKGROUND

A 12-year-old girl came with repeated pulmonary infection.

IMAGING FINDINGS

Fairly defined heterogeneously enhancing soft tissue dense lesion, measuring approximately (5.7 × 3.9 cm) noted in posterior segment of right lower lobe/no evidence of cavitation or calcification within the lesion. Adjacent lung collapse noted in right lower lobe with "air bronchogram" sign (yellow arrow). The lesion causes compression and displacement of esophagus (red arrow). Left vertebral artery noted arising from the aortic arch/anomalous systemic arterial supply to the right lower lobe lesion, from a branch arising from left vertebral artery noted. No demonstrable systemic venous drainage. No significant mediastinal lymphadenopathy **(Figs. 1A to E)**.

DISCUSSION

The aortic arch typically gives rise to three primary vessels: The brachiocephalic trunk (BT), left common carotid artery (LCC), and left subclavian artery (LSA). The left vertebral artery (LVA) generally originates from the LSA, medial to the thyrocervical trunk. However, a variation known as Adachi type C occurs when a fourth vessel, an anomalous left vertebral artery, arises directly from the aortic arch. This variation has been reported in 0.68–5.8% of cases.[1]

Pulmonary sequestration (PS) is a rare congenital malformation of the lungs, characterized by a mass of abnormal lung tissue that is supplied by an anomalous systemic artery and disconnected from the normal bronchopulmonary tree. PS is classified into two subtypes: Intralobar and extralobar, based on the presence or absence of independent pleura. Intralobar sequestration (ILS), which is more common, shares the visceral pleura with the adjacent lung, whereas extralobar sequestration is surrounded by its own separate pleura.[2]

In most cases, PS is supplied by a single systemic artery, although there are instances where multiple arteries are involved. The arterial supply to PS most often originates from the thoracic aorta (reported in 46.1–86.1% of cases) and the abdominal aorta (in 6.9–31.6% of cases). Other possible sources of arterial supply include the intercostal artery, diaphragmatic artery, aortic arch, subclavian artery, anonyma artery, pulmonary artery, left gastric artery, coronary artery, arteria lienalis, celiac trunk, and renal artery.

PS is also associated with various congenital anomalies, such as congenital diaphragmatic hernia, vertebral anomalies, congenital heart disease, pulmonary hypoplasia, colonic duplication, and congenital pulmonary airway malformation (also referred to as hybrid lesions).[3]

To date, this is the first reported case of a pulmonary sequestration receiving systemic arterial supply from an anomalous left vertebral artery originating directly from the aortic arch.

REFERENCES

1. Einstein EH, Song LH, Villela NL, et al. Anomalous Origin of the Left Vertebral Artery from the Aortic Arch. Aorta (Stamford). 2016;4(2):64-7.
2. Qian X, Sun Y, Liu D, et al. Pulmonary sequestration: a case report and literature review. Int J Clin Exp Med. 2015;8(11):21822-5.
3. Majumdar U, Sen P, Sood A. Intralobar bronchopulmonary sequestration: A case and brief review. Southwest J Pulm Crit Care. 2018;16(6):343-9.

86 Giant Lipoma of Finger

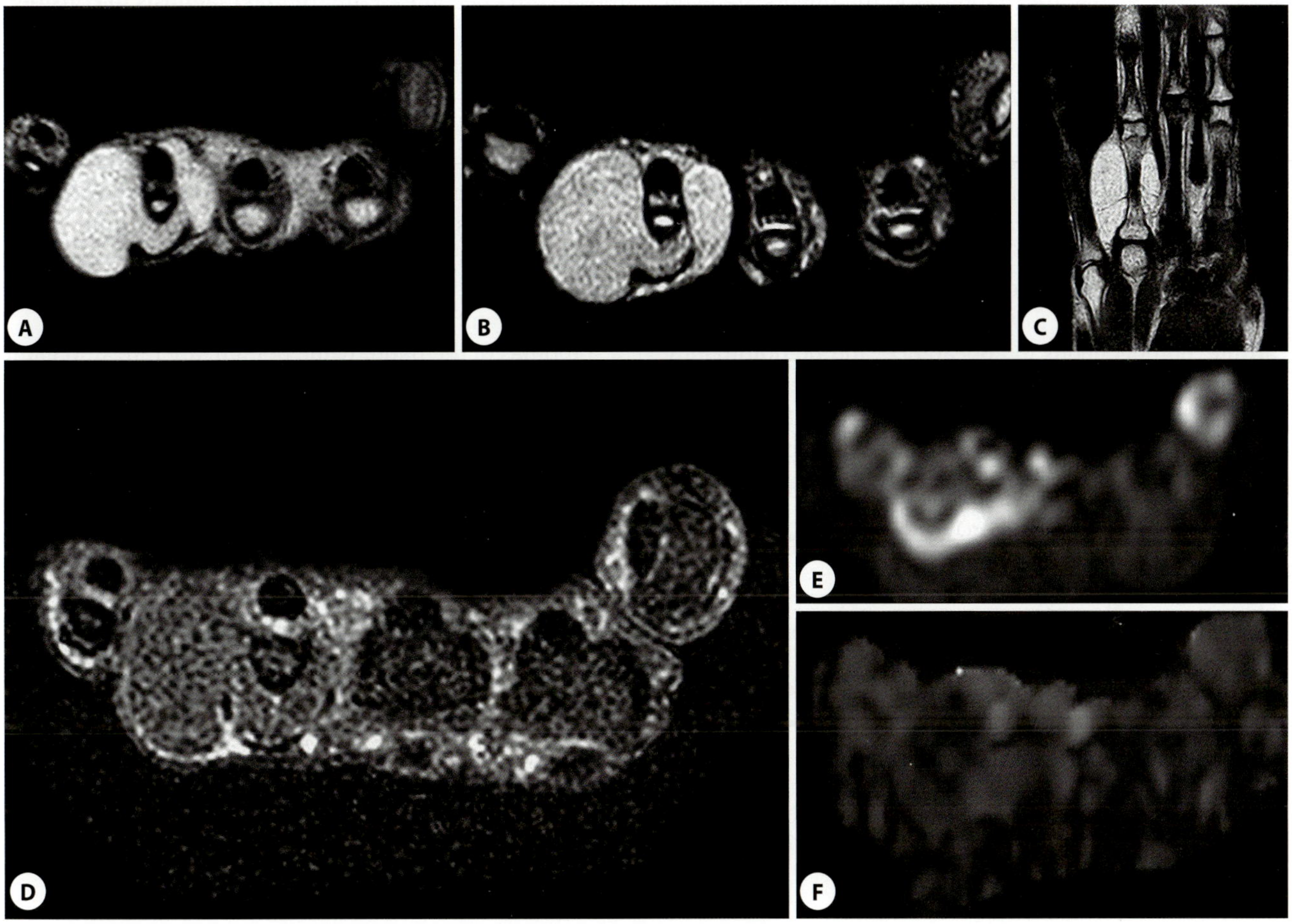

CLINICAL BACKGROUND

A 46-year-old female came with swelling in the right hand.

IMAGING FINDINGS

Well-defined T1/T2 hyperintense lesion with thin internal septations in proximal phalanx of ring finger. The lesion shows suppression of signal, on T1 fat sat sequence and noted deep to extensor digitorum in volar aspect causing tendon displacement/no diffusion restriction. No evidence of bony erosion or joint space involvement **(Figs. 1A to F)**.

DISCUSSION

Lipomas are the most common benign soft tissue tumors in humans, accounting for approximately 16% of mesenchymal tumors. They can develop anywhere in the body but are most frequently found in the upper body, with 15–20% of cases occurring in the head and neck region. Lipomas in the hand are rare, representing only 1–3.8% of all tumors in that area. Lipomas in the fingers are even more uncommon, with an incidence of just 1%.[1] A lipoma is considered "giant" if it exceeds 10 cm in size. Although the potential for malignant transformation in lipomas is uncertain, larger lipomas may have an increased risk of harboring malignant cells.[1]

On imaging, lipomas typically present as well-defined, homogeneous, and hyperechoic masses, with no posterior enhancement or Doppler signal. For giant lipomas (greater than 5 cm), MRI is often recommended for detailed evaluation. MRI typically reveals a well-defined lesion with its own capsule, homogeneous in appearance, and predominantly composed of fat. Lipomas appear hyperintense on T1- and T2-weighted images and hypointense on fat saturation sequences. MRI is especially helpful for preoperative planning. Lipomas in the wrist can sometimes cause carpal tunnel syndrome due to compression of the median nerve. Additionally, large lipomas in the palm can cause nerve elongation, neurological symptoms, or even tendon erosion, which may lead to spontaneous rupture of the flexor tendons of the fingers.[1]

When a mass is larger than 5 cm and is hypervascularized, liposarcoma becomes a differential diagnosis to consider. Liposarcoma is the most common soft tissue sarcoma in adults, with an incidence between 1.1 and 2.5 per million, and it is most frequently diagnosed between the ages of 50 and 70 years. MRI can help distinguish between lipoma and liposarcoma by assessing the fat content of the mass. Lipomas generally contain more than 75% pure fat, while liposarcomas contain less fat. Additionally, lipomas tend to have thin septa with minimal gadolinium enhancement, whereas liposarcomas have thickened septa with significant enhancement.[2]

Lipomas of the hand, while benign, are rare, and giant lipomas are exceedingly rare. Given their proximity to critical vascular and neural structures, careful surgical dissection is necessary to avoid complications.[1,2]

REFERENCES

1. Pertea M, Lunca S, Filip A, et al. Atypical Sites of the Lipoma on the Hand and Fingers: Clinical and Imaging Features and Surgical Outcomes. Diagnostics. 2022;12:2286.
2. Chedi Saadi, Khairi Saibi, Meriem Oumaya, et al. Giant Lipoma of the Hand: An Exceedingly Rare Condition! EAS J Orthop Physiother. 2023;5(4):45-8.

87 Cardiac Calcified Amorphous Tumor

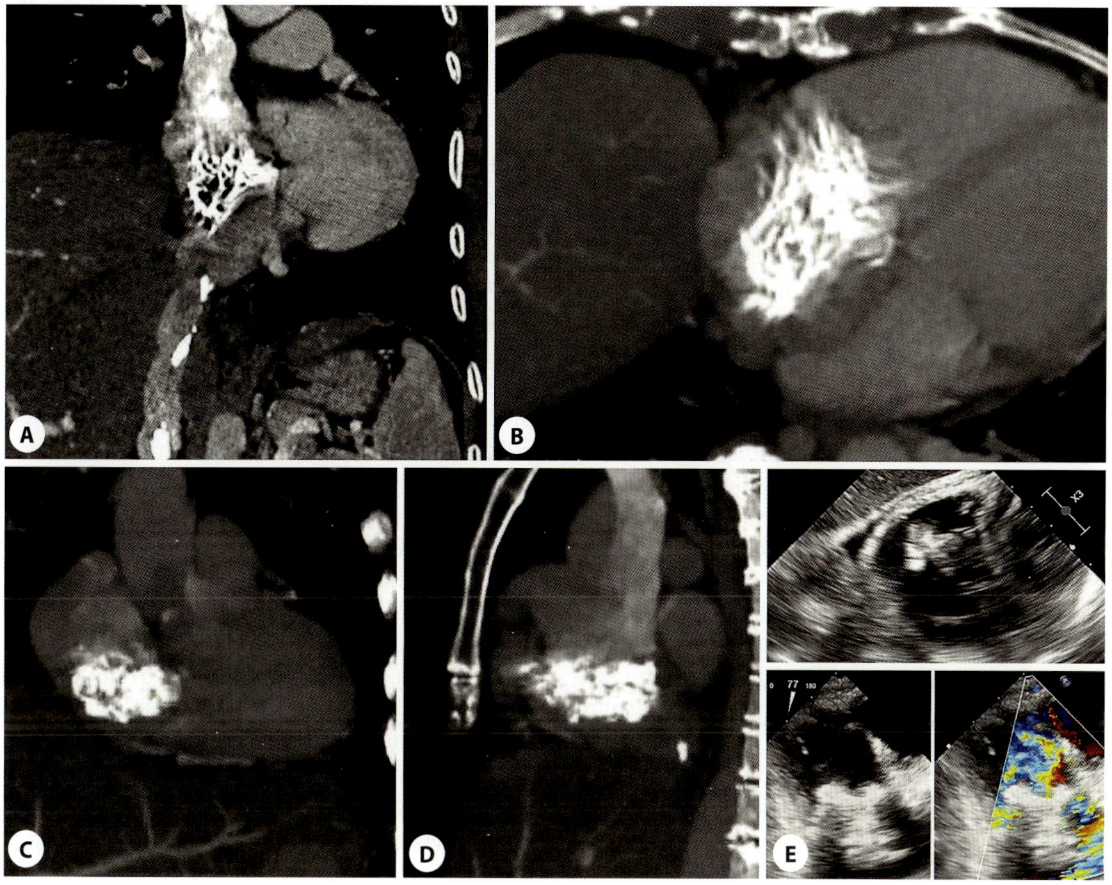

CLINICAL BACKGROUND

A 54-year-old female patient came with complaints of nonspecific chest pain.

IMAGING FINDINGS

Poorly defined, soft tissue dense mildly enhancing calcified lesion noted, in right atrium extending into IVC orifice and atrioventricular orifice **(Figs. 1A to E)**.

Dilated right atrium and right ventricle with early reflux of contrast into IVC. Peripheral calcifications in IVC.

DISCUSSION

Cardiac calcified amorphous tumors (CCATs) are uncommon benign lesions found within the heart. They are histologically characterized by nodular calcifications set against a backdrop of degenerated fibrous material. The term "CCAT" was introduced by Reynolds in 1997. These tumors can occur in any heart chamber, but they are predominantly located in the left ventricle, and most documented cases indicate that they tend to be pedunculated.[1]

When viewed on CT scans, CCATs typically manifest as irregular masses with partial or diffuse calcifications, particularly in the left ventricle. A distinctive feature of CCATs is their lack of enhancement on contrast-enhanced CT imaging. On MRI, these tumors generally appear homogeneous with low signal intensity on both unenhanced T1 and T2 weighted images; however, some cases might present with high or intermediate signal intensity on the same sequences.[1]

In differentiating CCATs from other conditions, a calcified thrombus must be considered. Ventricular thrombi are often seen in patients with myocardial scarring or significant left ventricular dysfunction and typically present as linear formations along the endocardial surface. The imaging characteristics of thrombi on MRI vary with their age; chronic organized left ventricular thrombi generally appear as low-signal-intensity masses, sometimes accompanied by calcifications, adjacent to a compromised left ventricular wall.[1]

Fibromas, another category of benign cardiac tumors, should also be part of the differential diagnosis when dealing with calcified cardiac masses. Unlike CCATs, fibromas are usually found with small foci of calcification at their center, while diffuse calcification is less common. On MRI, fibromas appear hypointense on T2-weighted images and isointense on T1-weighted images when compared to muscular tissue. Following the administration of intravenous contrast, they typically exhibit minimal or no early enhancement; however, intense delayed enhancement is a key feature that helps distinguish fibromas from other conditions.[1]

Cardiac myxomas represent the most prevalent primary cardiac tumors in adults, constituting about half of all primary benign cardiac tumors. These tumors are mostly located in the left atrium and are attached to the interatrial septum by a stalk, though they can occasionally be found in the ventricles. Myxomas may exhibit dystrophic calcifications from recurrent hemorrhagic events, which can be observed as hypointense regions on MRI. A critical distinguishing feature between myxomas and both thrombi and CCATs is the enhancement seen in myxomas post-gadolinium contrast administration on MRI.[1]

Primary cardiac osteosarcomas are infrequent yet aggressive heart tumors characterized by large and irregular calcified areas. On MRI, these tumors typically present as poorly defined masses with aggressive growth patterns and significant enhancement after the administration of gadolinium chelates. Additionally, they may be associated with lung or lymph node metastases.[1]

Valvular vegetations should also be considered in the differential diagnosis for CCATs, especially when they are located near heart valves. Caseous calcification of the mitral annulus (CCMA) is a rare condition marked by degenerative changes in the calcified mitral annulus. CCMA usually presents as a focal lesion adjacent to the posterior mitral leaflet. On MRI, CCMA often appears hypointense on T1 and T2-weighted images. On CT, it is typically observed as a well-defined, calcified mass near the mitral valve, exhibiting variable attenuation. Late gadolinium-enhanced MRI may reveal subtle peripheral enhancement.[1]

REFERENCE

1. Ufuk F, Kilic ID. Case 315: Cardiac Calcified Amorphous Tumor. Radiology. 2023;308(1).

88 Inflammatory Manubriosternal Arthritis

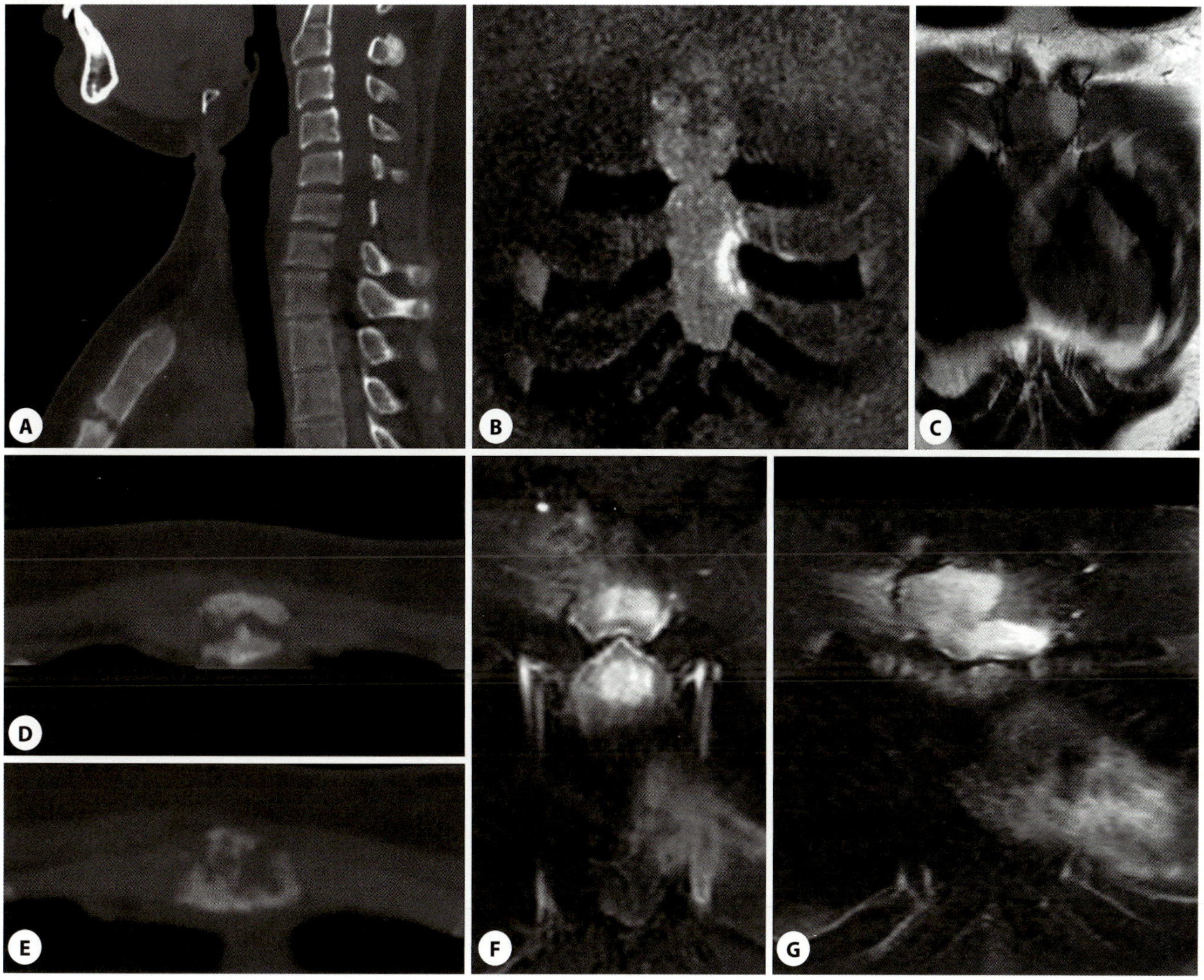

CLINICAL BACKGROUND

A 19-year-old male patient came with complaints of chest tenderness.

IMAGING FINDINGS

Erosions noted in the manubriosternal joint with bone sclerosis. MRI shows loss of normal T1 fat signals involving the right side, manubrium sternum and body of sternum with marrow edema/edema also noted in the left IV costosternal joint **(Figs. 1A to G)**.

DISCUSSION

Anterior chest wall pain is an often overlooked aspect of axial spondyloarthritis, a chronic inflammatory condition affecting various systems. Spondyloarthritis encompasses a range of chronic inflammatory disorders that primarily target the axial skeleton, peripheral joints, entheses, and additional organ systems. This spectrum is categorized based on the predominant clinical features, with axial spondyloarthritis (AxSpA) serving as the primary example of immune-mediated inflammatory rheumatic diseases, particularly characterized by axial involvement and sacroiliac joint engagement, which is closely associated with HLA-B27 positivity.[1]

AxSpA is a type of chronic inflammatory arthritis that impacts the axial skeleton and sacroiliac joints, affecting fewer than 1% of the population. The involvement of the manubriosternal joint, which can lead to anterior chest wall pain, is a rare initial symptom of AxSpA. It is crucial to maintain a high degree of clinical suspicion and consider a broad differential diagnosis in patients presenting with atypical, noncardiac anterior chest wall pain.[2]

To diagnose AxSpA, imaging must show evidence of sacroiliitis, along with inflammatory symptoms suggestive of spondyloarthritis. Some patients may also test positive for HLA-B27. MRI is particularly valuable in identifying early changes associated with spondyloarthritis, such as subtle erosions, bone edema, and inflammatory signs. Another well-documented characteristic of AxSpA includes structural lesions marked by new bone formation. It is worth noting that inflammatory markers are often not elevated in many patients with AxSpA. When standard X-ray imaging fails to provide conclusive results, MRI of the chest wall emerges as the most effective tool for evaluating signs of inflammatory arthritis.[1,2]

REFERENCES

1. Oye M, Ali AA, Wasserman PL, et al. Manubriosternal Joint Involvement as a Presenting Feature of Axial Spondyloarthritis. Cureus. 2021;13(12).
2. Elhai M, Paternotte S, Burki V, et al. Clinical characteristics of anterior chest wall pain in spondyloarthritis: an analysis of 275 patients. Joint Bone Spine. 2012;79:476-81.

89

Necrotizing Retroperitoneal Fasciitis

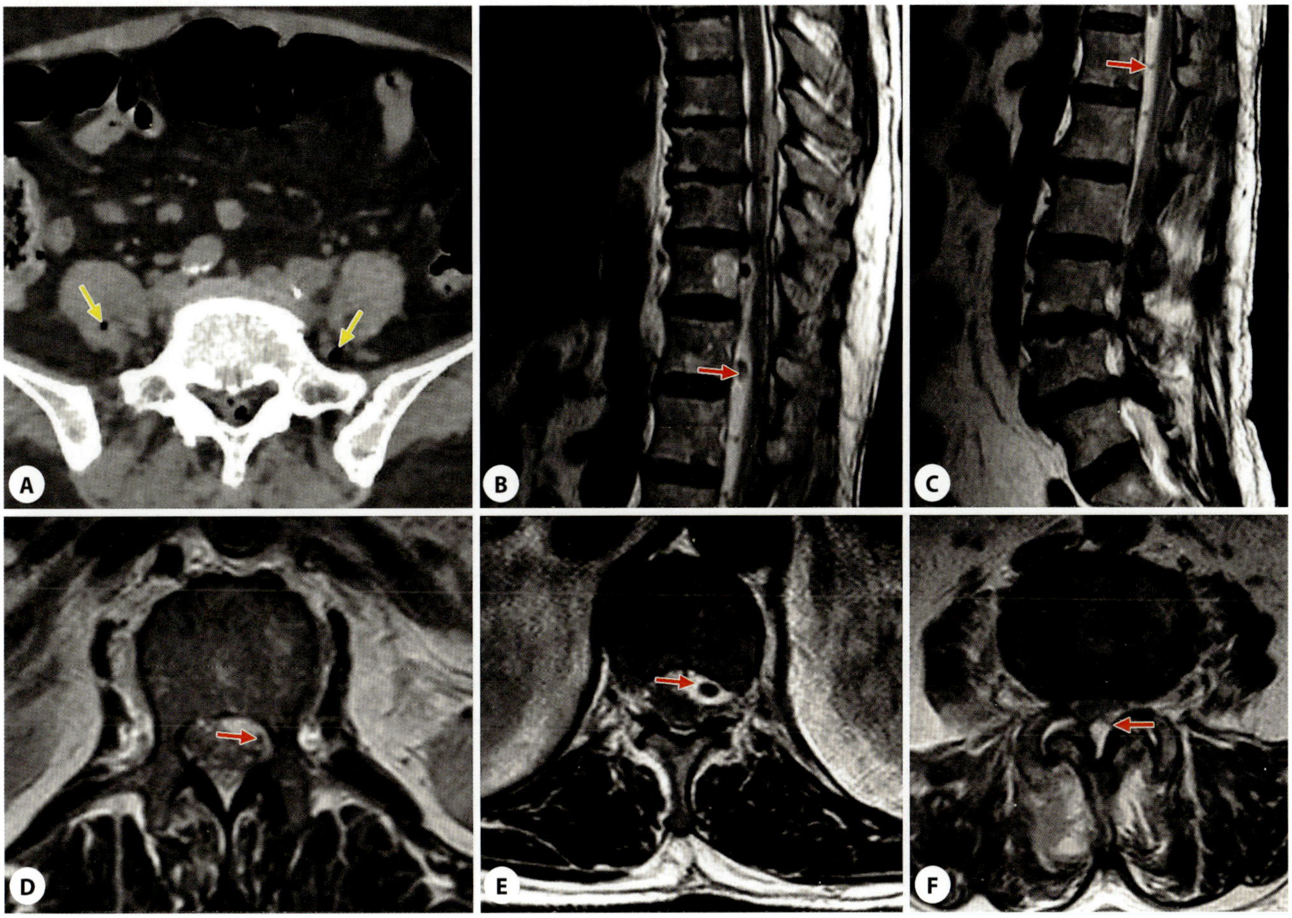

CLINICAL BACKGROUND

A 65-year-old female patient came with complaints of back pain.

IMAGING FINDINGS

- Air pockets noted in the retroperitoneum posterior to psoas and in intraspinal regions (Pneumorrhachis) (yellow arrow) **(Figs. 1A to F)**.
- Small T2/STIR hyperintense epidural collection with air foci in the left posterior and anterior epidural space extending from D8 to D12 vertebra (red arrow).
- Small epidural collection seen at L3-L4 level at posterior epidural space.
- STIR hyperintense area, suggestive of severe edema with multiple air foci seen in the bilateral paravertebral soft tissues and bilateral psoas muscles.

DISCUSSION

Retroperitoneal fasciitis is defined by the inflammation of deep soft tissues and fascial fat planes in the retroperitoneal space of the abdomen and pelvis, typically resulting from the spread of infection from primary sources such as appendicitis, diverticulitis, and pyelonephritis. The condition can either originate in the retroperitoneum itself or spread into it through direct or indirect pathways.[1]

Although rare, retroperitoneal fasciitis can be a serious and life-threatening complication of infection. Timely diagnosis is essential, often achieved through a combination of strong clinical suspicion and characteristic imaging findings that lead to prompt surgical intervention. Computed tomography (CT) is instrumental in revealing early signs of the condition, assessing the extent of the disease to guide surgical strategy, identifying the initial source of infection, and monitoring treatment efficacy. Clinicians should consider the possibility of retroperitoneal fasciitis in patients exhibiting symptoms of sepsis, particularly when they report pain that seems disproportionate to clinical findings.[1]

When there is a suspicion of retroperitoneal fasciitis, emergency CT scans can aid in rapid diagnosis and assessment of disease spread. Typical CT findings include fascial thickening and enhancement, muscle edema, fat stranding, fluid collections, and abscess formation. The presence of gas tracking along fascial planes in the retroperitoneum is a hallmark sign of this condition, although it may not be present in every case. Another significant diagnostic indicator is the asymmetric involvement of retroperitoneal fascial planes and deep tissues. The fasciitis may arise from infections in the retroperitoneal organs or may spread through direct or indirect pathways from other primary infection sites in the body. Signs of indirect tracking and transgression of fascial planes may suggest a more severe infection, characteristic of the necrotizing form of retroperitoneal fasciitis.[1]

A high level of suspicion is crucial; in our case, the patient initially presented with back pain, and the presence of air pockets in the retroperitoneum, along with pneumorrhachis, were key indicators that led to an MRI of the spine to investigate potential spinal pathology. It is important to note that even with aggressive antibiotic therapy, early and repeated surgical débridement may be necessary to excise necrotic tissue in cases of necrotizing retroperitoneal fasciitis.[1]

REFERENCE

1. Chingkoe CM, Jahed A, Loreto MP, et al. Retroperitoneal Fasciitis: Spectrum of CT Findings in the Abdomen and Pelvis. RadioGraphics. 2015;35(4):1095-107.

90 Septic Arthritis Shoulder

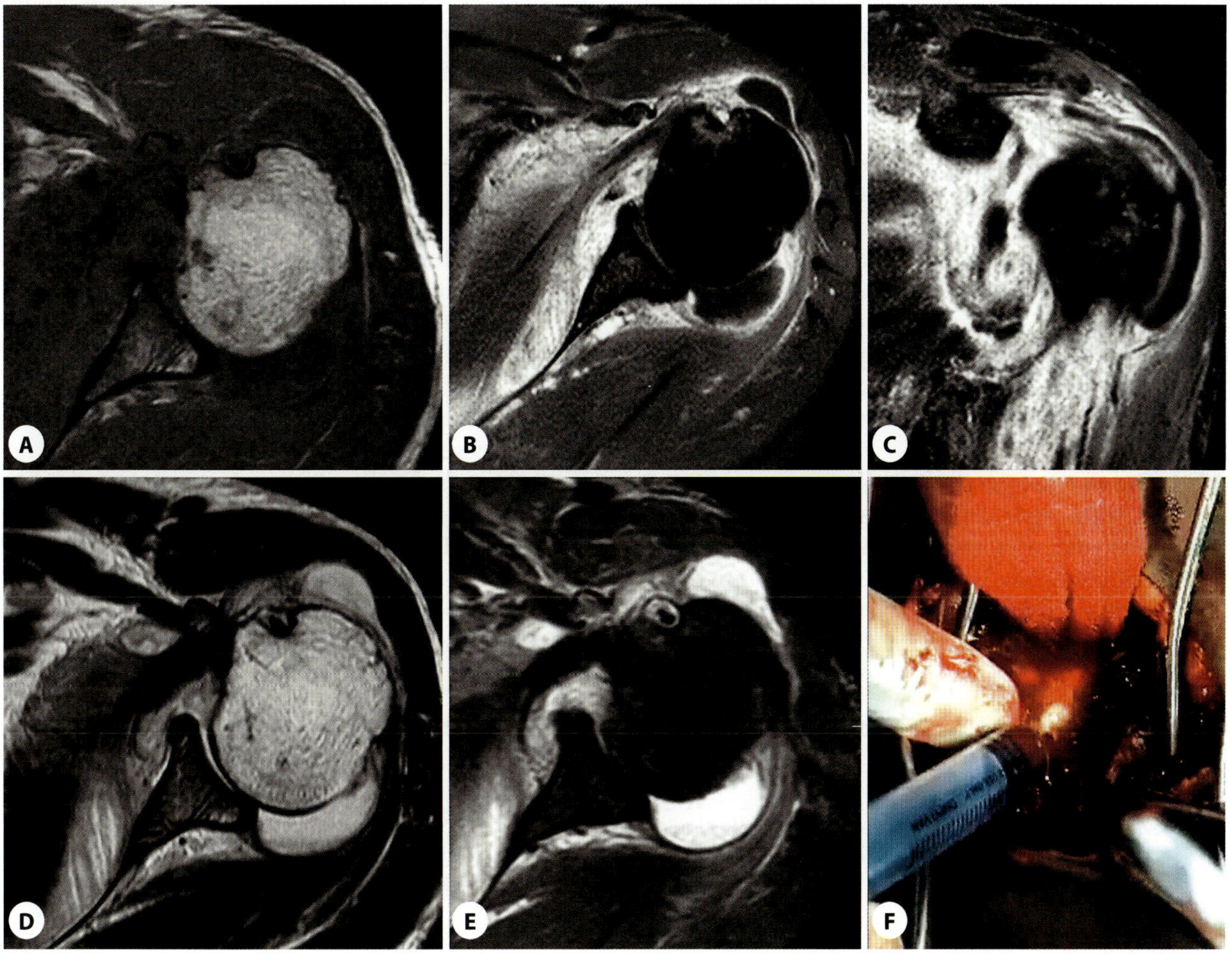

CLINICAL BACKGROUND

A 41-year-old male patient came with complaints of severe left shoulder pain.

IMAGING FINDINGS

Gross glenohumeral joint effusion seen subacromial/subdeltoid and subcoracoid bursal effusion seen. On post-contrast study, synovial thickening with enhancement seen. The effusion is seen to be tracking along the biceps tendon with associated biceps brachii muscle edema **(Figs. 1A to F)**.

Severe infraspinatus and subscapularis muscle edema seen, around the shoulder joint. The edema is seen to be extending to the upper biceps brachii and upper neck muscles. Above mentioned muscles shows moderate heterogenous enhancement on postcontrast study.

Thickened inferior glenohumeral ligament seen. Severe soft tissue edema seen surrounding the shoulder joint. Intraoperative image also shown.

DISCUSSION

Septic arthritis is a prevalent and often debilitating condition that necessitates prompt diagnosis for optimal outcomes. Early identification of septic arthritis is critical, as delays can lead to significant cartilage and joint damage due to the enzymes released by neutrophils, synovial cells, and bacteria. Any postponement in diagnosing septic arthritis can elevate morbidity and result in complications such as bone and cartilage destruction, osteonecrosis, secondary osteoarthritis, osteomyelitis, and ultimately ankylosis.[1]

Magnetic resonance imaging (MRI) has become increasingly valuable in assessing musculoskeletal infections, effectively evaluating bone marrow, soft tissues, and joints. MRI findings in patients with septic arthritis can be abnormal as soon as 24 hours after infection onset. The presence of joint effusions is a key indicator of septic arthritis. While the synovium is typically not well-defined on MRI, it becomes visibly thickened in cases of septic arthritis. Distinguishing the enhancement of the proliferating synovium from that of joint fluid can be challenging.[2]

MRI may also help detect coexisting osteomyelitis in individuals with septic arthritis. Reactive bone marrow edema associated with septic arthritis can sometimes be misinterpreted as osteomyelitis. In genuine bone infections, the marrow edema tends to be larger and more multifocal than in reactive edema.[2] Adjacent soft tissue edema and fluid collections can be identified, and contrast-enhanced images can be beneficial in differentiating these collections from myositis. As the disease progresses, articular cartilage and cortical bone destruction occurs, leading to the formation of bony erosions. Chronic stages may reveal joint space narrowing, subchondral cysts, and significant bony destruction, ultimately resulting in complete ankylosis.[3]

In imaging, the primary differential diagnosis for septic arthritis is inflammatory arthritis. The presence of bone erosions accompanied by marrow edema typically suggests a joint infection. Nevertheless, joint aspiration is the most critical step in definitively diagnosing septic arthritis. The presence of perisynovial edema supports a diagnosis of septic arthritis over rheumatoid arthritis (RA). Simultaneous involvement of the glenohumeral and acromioclavicular joints is more commonly observed in RA than in septic arthritis. Additionally, tuberculosis (TB) is a significant cause of septic arthritis. The hallmark features of tuberculous arthritis include osteoporosis, cartilage destruction, and marginal erosions (known as Phemister's triad), often associated with effusions, synovial thickening, and osteolysis. Thickened synovium may appear hypointense on T2-weighted images due to granuloma presence, with associated collections and sinus tracts also visible. Sclerosis and periostitis may occur, resembling chronic osteomyelitis.[3]

REFERENCES

1. Karchevsky M, Schweitzer ME, Morrison WB, et al. MRI Findings of Septic Arthritis and Associated Osteomyelitis in Adults. Am J Roentgenol. 2004;182:119-22.
2. Weishaupt D, Schweitzer ME, Alam F, et al. MR Imaging of Inflammatory Joint Diseases of the Foot and Ankle. Skeletal Radiol. 1999;28:663-9.
3. Kizildag B, Sener A, Komurcu E, et al. Glenohumeral Joint Tuberculosis with Multiple Cold Abscesses: An Uncommon Cause of Shoulder Pain. BMJ Case Rep. 2013:2013:bcr2013200592.

91 VALF: A Rare Cause of Cervical Radiculopathy

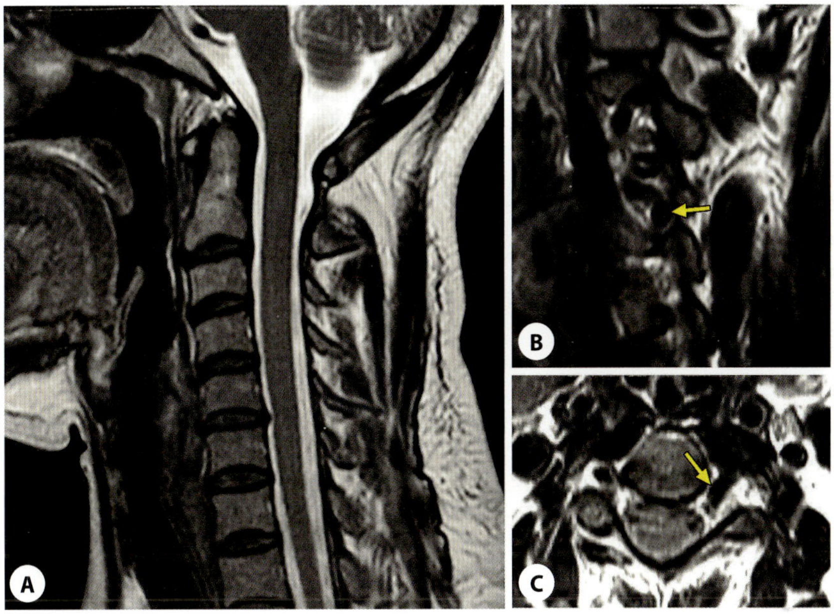

CLINICAL BACKGROUND

A 56-year-old female patient came with complaints of left shoulder and back pain.

IMAGING FINDINGS

Left vertebral artery loop at the level of C3-C4 with protrusion into left neural foramen, causing compression of exiting nerve roots at corresponding level (yellow arrow) **(Figs. 1A to C)**.

No significant disc bulge or nerve root compression at rest of the levels.

DISCUSSION

Vertebral artery loop formation causing encroachment on cervical neural foramen and canal is a rare cause of cervical radiculopathy. Hadley first described the bony erosion of cervical vertebrae caused by VALF and Paksoy et al. reported the incidence of the VALF as 7.51% in their 173 patients, presenting with symptoms of cervicobrachial pain. In most cases, the V2 segment contains the symptomatic VA loop (90.5%), compared with only 7.6% in the V1 and 1.9% in the V3 segment. The importance is that if we have mistaken his symptom as common radiculopathy due to disc herniation or spondylosis, it may have led to a possible VA injury casualty during the surgery.[1,2]

The mechanism of VALF is not clear. Oga et al. reported that VALF is developed in association with cervical spondylotic changes.[3] Hemodynamic stress such as hypertension and atherosclerosis were suggested as other possible causes. Some authors reported cases that cervical trauma might be a cause of VALF (as it is in our case). High pulsatile arterial pressure causes migration of VA and erosion of the adjacent bony structures. VALF may also be a rare cause of vertebrobasilar insufficiency.[1]

In plain radiograph, VALF may show erosion of adjacent bony structures with sharp and sclerotic margins. A common radiographic finding of this lesion is enlargement of the affected intervertebral neural foramen. CT may show VALF as a mass enlarging the intervertebral foramen or other adjacent bony structure. Additionally, CT or MR angiography should be performed to differentiate these vascular lesions and assess the morphology and tract of the vasculature.[1,2]

Cervicobrachial neuralgia produced by vascular compression presents with paresthesia and dysesthesia of the fingers without a triggering factor, the lack of nocturnal symptoms, and the rarity of neurologic deficits. Conservative treatment may include nonsteroidal anti-inflammatory treatments, physiotherapy or injection therapy and has been recognized as successful in several cases. When conservative treatment has failed, several surgical procedures, including decompressive laminectomy, foraminotomy with sectioning of the compressed rootlet, vascular reconstruction or microvascular decompression, have been considered as effective strategies.[1-3]

REFERENCES

1. Kim HS, Lee JH, Cheh G, et al. Cervical radiculopathy caused by vertebral artery loop formation: a case report and review of the literature. J Korean Neurosurg Soc. 2010;48(5):465-8.
2. Tack L, Linden P, Mortelé P, et al. Cervical radiculopathy caused by vertebral artery loop formation: a case report. Radiol Case Rep. 2021;16(7):1919-23.
3. Oga M, Yuge I, Terada K, et al. Tortuosity of the vertebral artery in patients with cervical spondylotic myelopathy. Risk factor for the vertebral artery injury during anterior cervical decompression. Spine (Phila Pa 1976). 1996;21:1085-9.

92 Ectopic Duodenal Varices

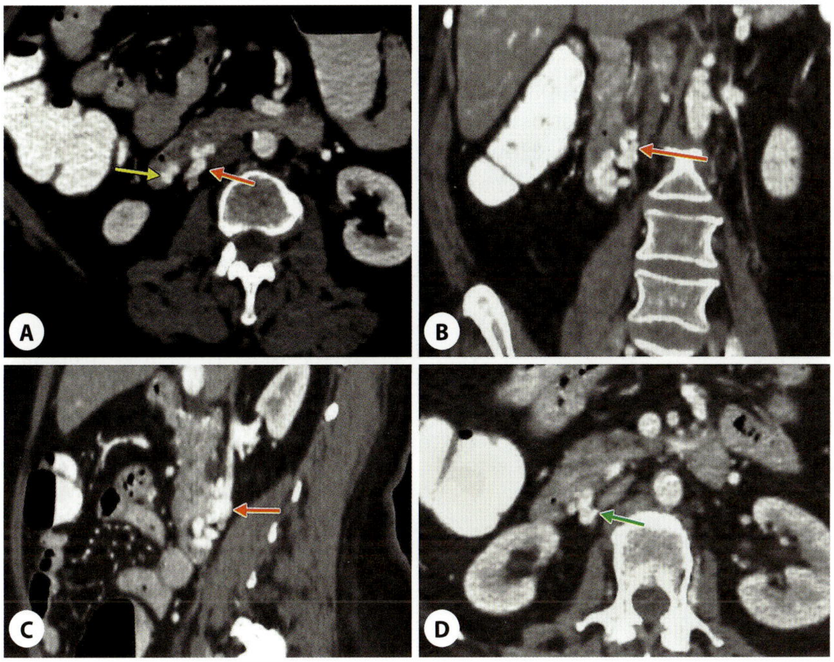

CLINICAL BACKGROUND

A 71-year-old female patient came with complaints of upper GI-bleed.

IMAGING FINDINGS

Dilated vascular channels seen in retroperitoneum, posterior to second and third part of duodenum (red arrow), connecting portal vein confluence and draining into right renal vein (green arrow). Multiple dilated intramural/ submucosal collaterals seen in second and third part of duodenum (yellow arrow) **(Figs. 1A to D)**.

DISCUSSION

Duodenal varices are a rare manifestation of portal hypertension that can lead to significant gastrointestinal bleeding, often with high mortality rates. Portal hypertension is a progressive complication of liver cirrhosis, resulting in the formation of portosystemic collaterals, which typically develop at the esophagogastric junction, abdominal wall, and rectum. Ectopic varices refer to the dilatation of veins at sites outside the esophagus and stomach, and these may appear individually or in conjunction with other varices.[1]

Approximately 17% of ectopic varices are found in the duodenum, which can be affected at any location along its length. The duodenal bulb is the most frequent site for these varices, followed by the descending duodenum. Hemorrhage from ectopic varices contributes to about 5% of cases of bleeding associated with portal hypertension, but the mortality rate can be as high as 40%.[2]

Computed tomography (CT) angiography can effectively identify bleeding duodenal varices when the hemorrhage is significant. Varices in the duodenum may develop following band ligation of esophageal varices, likely serving as alternative sites for spontaneous portosystemic shunting. These ectopic varices arise from collateral veins that originate from the portal vein trunk or the superior mesenteric vein, draining into the inferior vena cava via retroperitoneal veins of Retzius.[2,3]

Interventional radiologists begin by diagnosing the underlying causes of portal hypertension and evaluating both afferent and efferent veins of the ectopic varices through CT imaging. In cases of decompensated portal hypertension leading to the development of ectopic varices, placement of a transjugular intrahepatic portosystemic shunt (TIPS) is often the first-line treatment. However, TIPS alone may not be sufficient for controlling ectopic variceal bleeding, as it may not adequately address focal mesenteric venous obstruction. Consequently, additional variceal embolization is recommended following TIPS placement. Retrograde transvenous obliteration can be a definitive treatment when the efferent vein draining into the systemic vein is accessible. Conversely, antegrade transvenous obliteration is essential in managing ectopic varices, given their complex anatomy and the frequent absence of catheterizable portosystemic shunts. Superficial veins in the portal venous system, such as recanalized umbilical veins, may allow for safe access during antegrade procedures. Due to the lack of consensus and established guidelines, a multidisciplinary approach is crucial for tailored management of ectopic varices.[4]

REFERENCES

1. Liu M, Li W, Li P, et al. Ectopic duodenal variceal bleed successfully treated with TIPS and 2 years follow-up: A Case Report. Radiol Case Rep. 2020;15(9):1570-4.
2. Norton ID, Andrews JC, Kamath PS. Management of ectopic varices. Hepatology. 1998;28:1154-1158.
3. Wu WC, Wang LY, Yu FJ, et al. Bleeding duodenal varices after gastroesophageal varices ligation: a case report. Kaohsiung J Med Sci. 2002;18:578-81.
4. Kin HC, Miyayama S, Lee EW, et al. Interventional Radiology for Bleeding Ectopic Varices: Individualized Approach Based on Vascular Anatomy. RadioGraphics. 2024;44:8.

93 INH Induced Cerebellar Toxicity

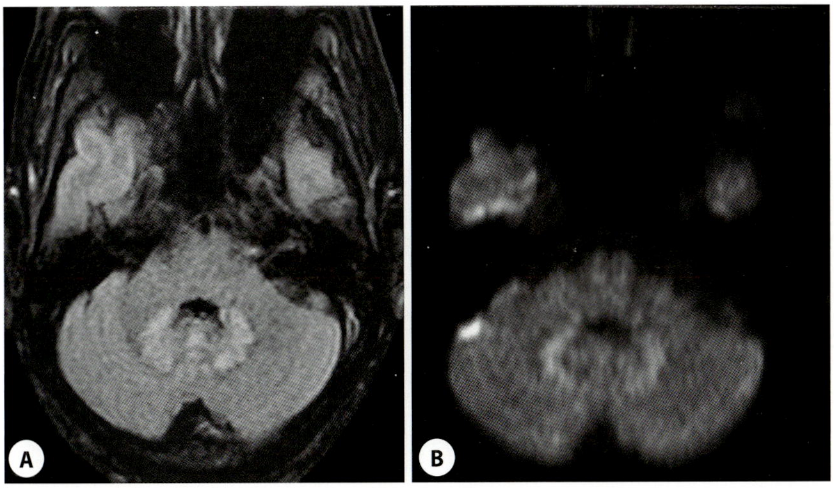

CLINICAL BACKGROUND

A 60-year-old male patient, known case of CKD and TB, on ATT came with complaints of dysarthria and gait disturbance.

IMAGING FINDINGS

Diffusion/FLAIR hyperintensity noted in bilateral dentate nucleus **(Figs. 1A and B)**.

DISCUSSION

Drug-induced cerebellitis involving dentate nuclei is classically seen with metronidazole toxicity. Rare association with INH (this is our second case—first one already published in IJRI.),[1] an antituberculous drug, has been documented in patients with renal function impairment. INH is both hepatotoxic and neurotoxic. The later often manifest in the form of peripheral neuropathy, due to its interference with pyridoxine metabolism resulting in vitamin deficiency.[2,3]

Central nervous system (CNS) involvement by its metabolite, known as isonicotinylhydrazide, can result in encephalopathy. Cerebellum involvement is rare, but do occur, involving the bilateral dentate nuclei with resultant edema due to reduced gamma-aminobutyric acid (GABA) levels and down regulation of N-methyl-D-aspartate (NMDA) receptors. INH is primarily excreted through kidneys and hence reduced clearance in CKD patients is responsible for neurotoxicity. Hence, patients with CKD are prone to INH-induced cerebellitis.[2,3]

MRI findings include classical bilateral and symmetrical T2/FLAIR hyperintensity involving the dentate nuclei, suggestive of edema. Differential diagnosis includes methyl bromide toxicity, enteroviral infections, maple syrup urine disease, and metronidazole toxicity. Atypical Wernicke's encephalopathy can be considered in the differential diagnosis if the involvement of the dentate nuclei is not an isolated finding.[1-3]

The meticulous medical history and clinical investigations is important to exclude other possible differential diagnoses. Early diagnosis and treatment in the form of INH withdrawal and pyridoxine supplementation can potentially reverse the edema and cause dramatic improvement in the patient's symptoms.[1,3]

REFERENCES

1. Kumar SSR, Jayanthan SS, Rupesh G. Isoniazid: A rare drug-induced cause for bilateral dentate nuclei hyperintensity. Indian J Radiol Imaging. 2020;30(2):218-21.
2. Deepesh A, Pendharkar HS. Isoniazid toxicity presenting as bilateral dentate hyperintensities. Neurol India. 2017;65:1193.
3. Binwal VK, Syed T, Ahir D. Isoniazid-Induced cerebellitis and psychosis in chronic kidney disease patient with tubercular pleural effusion. J Integr Nephrol Androl. 2016;3:60-1.

94 Myocardial Bridging: Left Anterior Descending

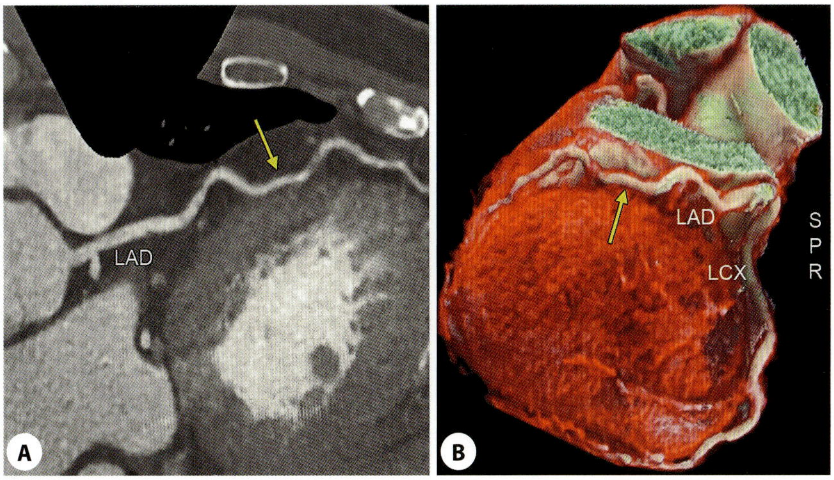

CLINICAL BACKGROUND

A 56-year-old male patient came with complaints nonspecific chest pain.

IMAGING FINDINGS

Short segment, superficial, partial encasement of mid portion of LAD in the left ventricular wall noted, for a length of (1.6 cm). No significant compression of tunneled segment **(Figs. 1A and B)**.

DISCUSSION

Myocardial bridging is a congenital anomaly characterized by myocardial encasement of a coronary artery segment, which normally courses epicardially. This is also called tunneled artery. Despite the fact that it is a congenital anomaly, symptoms usually do not develop before the third decade of life. Although myocardial bridging is considered a benign variation, it is clinically important because of its association with myocardial ischemia and secondary complications. MDCT is evolving rapidly as a noninvasive method in the diagnosis of myocardial bridging.[1]

Myocardial bridging was first defined at autopsy by Reyman in 1737. Later, Portmann and Iwig angiographic ally described temporary occlusion in a segment of the left anterior descending artery (LAD) during the systolic phase. In 1976, Noble et al. detected this temporary occlusion in selective coronary angiography in 27 (0.5%) of 5,250 patients and named it the "milking effect." In their studies of autopsies, Ferreira et al. distinguished between two types of bridging: Superficial bridges (75% of cases) and deep bridges (25% of cases). However, there are no certain depth criteria set to classify myocardial bridges.[1]

This anomaly is more frequently seen in patients with hypertrophic cardiomyopathy; the prevalence rating is up to 30% on coronary angiography. The anomaly is also seen with increased prevalence in patients who have undergone heart transplantation.

Myocardial bridges are mostly seen on the LAD mid segment. Multiplanar reconstruction images assessed from MDCT angiography provide information about the lumen and walls of the coronary arteries and the myocardium in any plane requested. Therefore, myocardial bridging can be shown on MDCT regardless of the thickness and direction of muscle bundles within the myocardial bridging. Carrascosa et al. evaluated the diameter in the systolic and diastolic phases and the percentage and length of stenosis due to myocardial bridging on both MDCT and conventional angiography, and the results were correlated which was found to be consistent. In that study, it was concluded that MDCT is an alternative fast, noninvasive diagnostic technique that accurately allows the evaluation of myocardial bridging. MDCT is also efficient in showing the presence of other coronary artery, myocardial, epicardial, and neighbouring thoracic abnormalities, which are important in treatment planning.[1]

REFERENCE

1. T Hazirolan, M Canyigit, M Karcaaltincaba, et al. Myocardial bridging on MDCT. Am J Roentgenol. 2007;188:1074-80.

95 Prolapsed Submucosal Leiomyoma—Cellular Variant

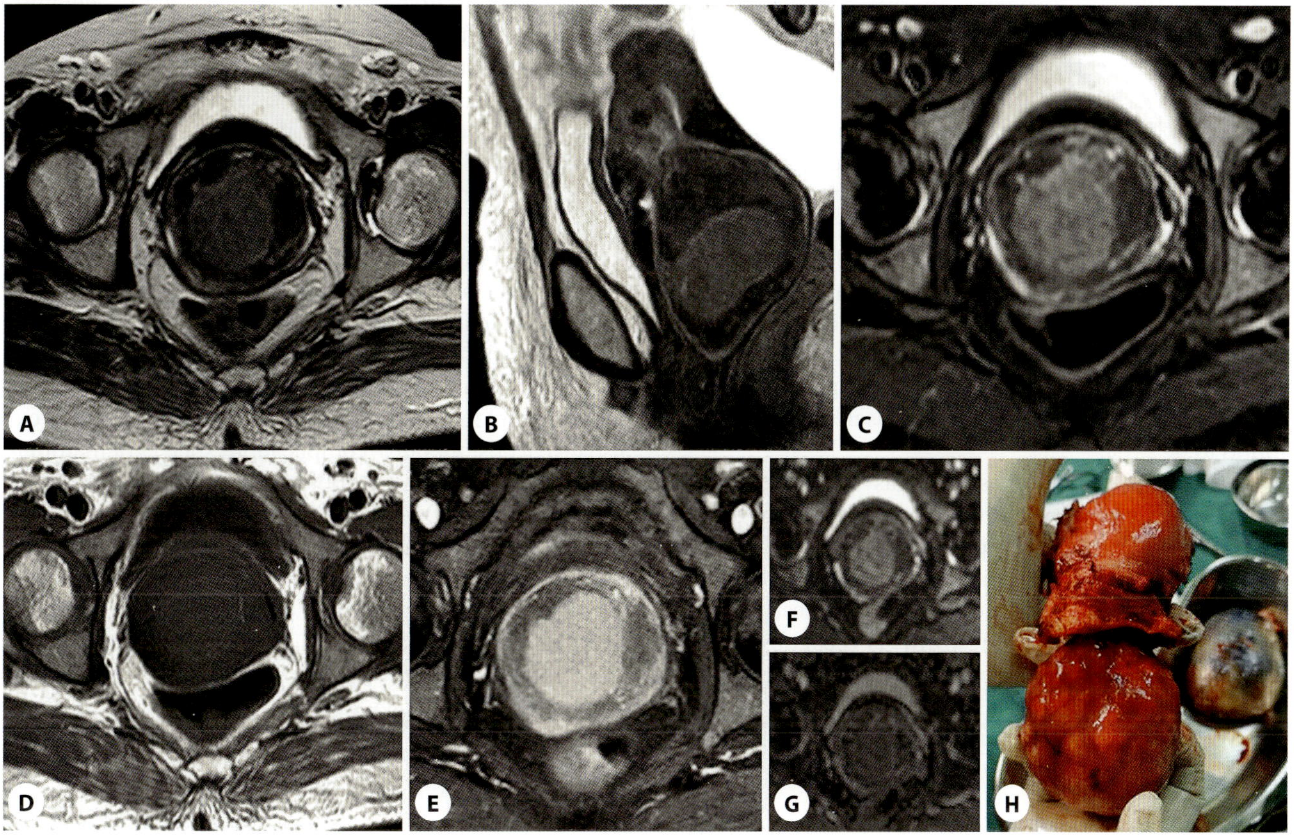

CLINICAL BACKGROUND

A 48-year-old female patient came with complaints of lower abdominal pain.

IMAGING FINDINGS

Large T1/T2 and STIR heterointense lesion seen arising from the submucosal surface of anterior myometrium prolapsing into cervical canal the lesion shows internal T2/STIR hyperintense areas. The lesion shows mild homogeneous postcontrast enhancement. The lesion shows mild diffusion restriction. Postoperative image also shown **(Figs. 1A to H)**.

DISCUSSION

Uterine leiomyomas, commonly referred to as fibroids, are benign tumors that represent the most prevalent type of solid tumor found in the uterus. They are primarily composed of smooth muscle tissue and varying amounts of fibrous connective elements. These tumors are hormone-dependent and typically develop during the reproductive years, affecting approximately 20–30% of women. They may experience rapid growth during pregnancy or when hormonal contraceptives are used and usually regress after menopause. As leiomyomas enlarge, they may outstrip their blood supply, leading to different forms of degeneration, including hyaline, myxoid, cystic, and red degeneration.[1]

These tumors can present as single or multiple lesions and are classified based on their location within the uterus: Submucosal, intramural, or subserosal. Submucosal leiomyomas account for about 5% of all uterine leiomyomas. They may be pedunculated and can prolapse into the uterine cavity. In a study of 1,785 women undergoing abdominal surgery for uterine leiomyomas, the prevalence of prolapsing submucosal leiomyomas was found to be 2.5%.[1]

Submucosal leiomyomas can be asymptomatic or may present with various symptoms, including menorrhagia, dysmenorrhea, infertility, pelvic pressure, or palpable masses. Although transvaginal ultrasound is commonly used to diagnose and characterize these tumors, magnetic resonance imaging (MRI) is recognized as the most accurate technique for the detection, localization, and characterization of leiomyomas. Specifically, MRI outperforms ultrasound in assessing the presence of prolapse, its extent, and the location of the stalk in submucosal leiomyomas.[1,2]

Typically, nondegenerated uterine leiomyomas appear as well-defined masses with homogeneous hypointense signals compared to adjacent myometrium on both T1- and T2-weighted images. Conversely, cellular leiomyomas, which contain densely packed smooth muscle cells, may exhibit relatively higher signals on T2-weighted images and show enhancement on contrast-enhanced scans. These tumors are often bordered by a low-signal intensity margin. Occasionally, a high-intensity rim may be observed on T2-weighted images, indicating dilated lymphatics, veins, or edema. Areas of increased signal intensity can also be present in certain degenerative types, such as cystic or myxoid degeneration.[2]

Beyond diagnosis and characterization, MRI plays a crucial role in pretreatment planning by identifying lesions that are amenable to various treatment approaches, such as hysteroscopic resection for submucosal-intramural leiomyomas or myomectomy (transabdominal or laparoscopic) for intramural and subserosal types. MRI can also reveal postoperative complications such as hematomas, abscesses, fistulas, uterine ruptures, and peritoneal inclusion cysts. Additionally, MRI facilitates monitoring changes in the size of individual leiomyomas and the uterus during therapy with GnRH analogues. Three-dimensional contrast-enhanced MRI angiography can visualize the uterine arteries, providing vital information for planning leiomyoma embolization. After embolization, MRI can be used to assess the degree of shrinkage and loss of enhancement of the leiomyomas.[1-3]

REFERENCES

1. Panageas E, Kier R, McCauley TR, et al. Submucosal uterine leiomyomas: diagnosis of prolapse into the cervix and vagina based on MR imaging. AJR Am J Roentgenol. 1992;159(3):555-8.
2. Murase E, Siegelman ES, Outwater EK, et al. Uterine leiomyomas: histopathologic features, MR imaging findings, differential diagnosis, and treatment. Radiographics. 1999;19(5):1179-97.
3. Spies JB, Roth AR, Jha RC, et al. Leiomyomata treated with uterine artery embolization: factors associated with successful symptom and imaging outcomes. Radiology. 2002;222(1): 45-52.

96 Malignant Colonic Stricture

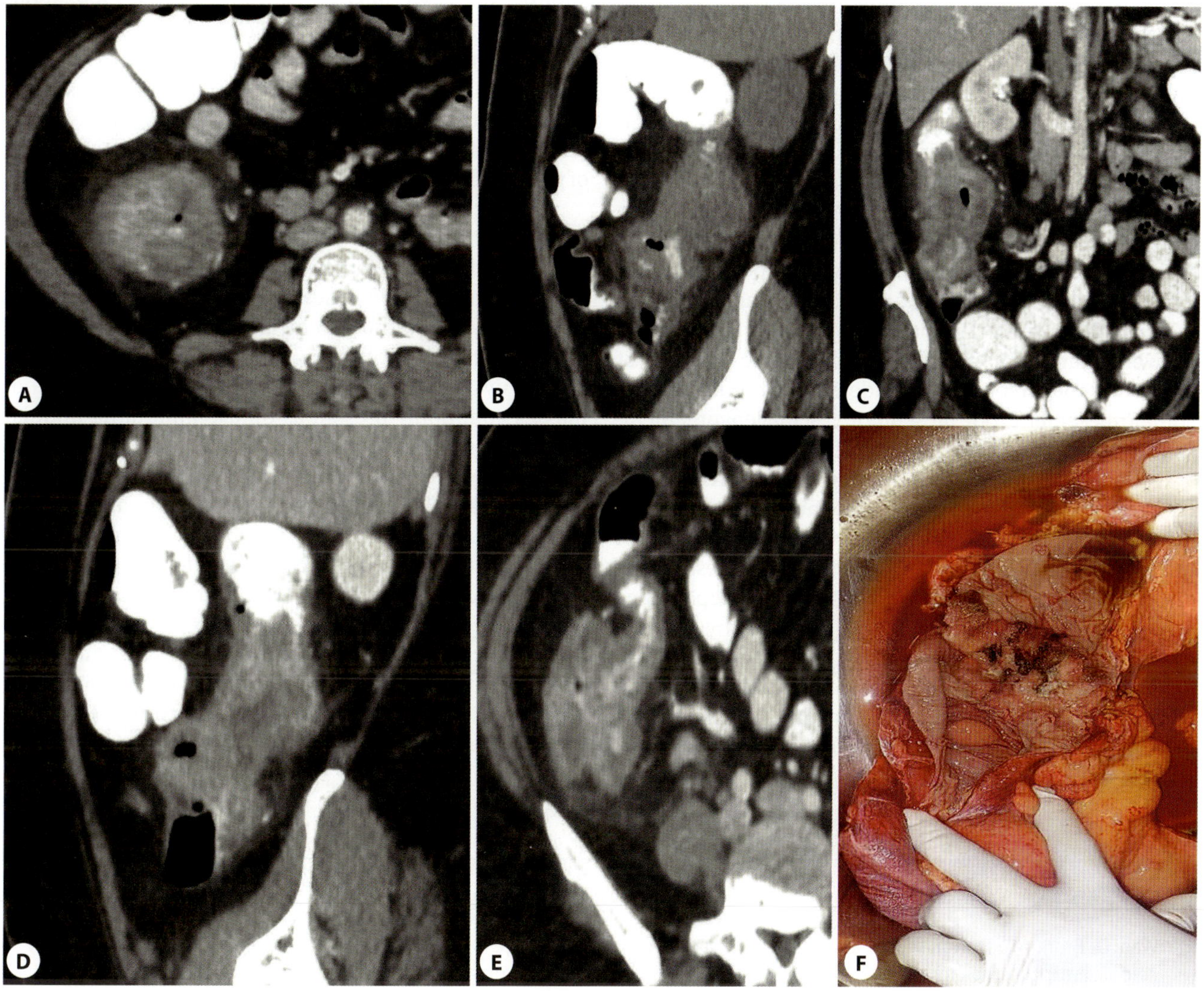

CLINICAL BACKGROUND

A 42-year-old female patient came with complaint of altered bowel habits and constipation.

IMAGING FINDINGS

Long segment irregular wall thickening noted in cecum, ascending colon and ileocecal junction, for a length of 10.0 cm (maximum thickness 2.0 cm), causing luminal narrowing. Thickening of terminal ileum seen, maximum thickness ~7–8 mm for a length of (3.0–4.0 cm). Adjacent mesenteric fat stranding and multiple enlarged mesenteric lymph nodes in RIF. Postoperative image also shown **(Figs. 1A to F)**.

DISCUSSION

Colonic strictures can arise from various etiologies, broadly classified into benign lesions, malignant lesions, or pseudostrictures. Endoscopic evaluation remains the standard approach for assessing colonic pathology; however, 5-15% of endoscopic procedures may not be able to traverse stenotic regions in the colon. Noninvasive imaging techniques like computed tomography (CT) are increasingly utilized to evaluate colonic conditions and provide additional extraluminal information that may inform treatment decisions and prognosis.[1]

One common etiology is diverticular stricture, which typically affects the descending and sigmoid colon. These strictures are often elongated, usually measuring at least 5 cm in length, and exhibit concentric narrowing of the colonic lumen. In about 10% of cases, the ends of chronic strictures may present with shouldered or tapered margins, which can resemble features of a stenosing neoplasm, making differentiation challenging. The diagnosis of a diverticular stricture is more likely in the absence of associated pericolonic lymphadenopathy, fluid at the colonic mesenteric root, mesenteric vascular engorgement, extraluminal air, and pericolonic inflammation.[1,2]

Strictures resulting from chronic Crohn's disease are characterized by a persistent transmural inflammatory process that leads to fibrosis, affecting any part of the gastrointestinal tract. This condition presents as discontinuous lesions (noncontiguous, with skip lesions separated by intervening islands of healthy tissue), asymmetric disease, and shows a strong preference for the terminal ileum and proximal colon, while the rectum is often spared. The asymmetric nature of involvement can result in eccentric loss of haustration and pseudosacculation.[3]

Ischemic injury can lead to smooth, fibrotic, tubular strictures of varying lengths, particularly when segmental colonic involvement occurs, and these strictures typically have tapering margins. Infectious strictures often show nonspecific features on CT, frequently mimicking findings associated with Crohn's disease; however, the presence of fibrofatty proliferation in adjacent mesenteric regions is almost exclusively linked to Crohn's disease. Radiation-induced strictures typically develop 6-24 months after treatment initiation, with the rectosigmoid junction being the most commonly affected site. The CT findings resemble those of chronic ischemic colitis, featuring nonspecific uniform wall thickening, increased pelvic fat, and thickening of perirectal fibrous tissue.[1,3]

Colonic strictures due to primary carcinoma account for approximately 60% of large bowel obstructions, with the sigmoid colon being the most frequently involved site. These strictures are often described as "apple-core" lesions, typically short (around 3-4 cm) and characterized by severe luminal narrowing with abrupt shouldering of the margins. On CT, dysplasia-associated nonadenomatous lesions or masses commonly present as diffuse infiltrating nodular lesions or sessile polypoid abnormalities. These lesions tend to be elongated (2-6 cm) with rigid, tapering margins. The associated mural thickening is usually asymmetric, and the mucosa may appear irregular with localized loss of stratification. A mural thickness greater than 1.5 cm is a strong indicator of carcinoma, especially in the context of ulcerative colitis. Carcinomas arising from Crohn's disease often occur in the proximal colon and areas that mirror the distribution of Crohn's rather than typical locations for de novo cancers. Typical malignant features on CT include mucosal destruction, mass effect, and infiltration through the colonic wall.[1,4]

REFERENCES

1. Wan D, Bruni SG, Dufton JA, et al. Differential diagnosis of colonic strictures: pictorial review with illustrations from computed tomography colonography. Can Assoc Radiol J. 2015;66(3):259-71.
2. Chintapalli KN, Chopra S, Ghiatas AA, et al. Differentiation of diverticulitis versus colon cancer using helical CT findings. Radiology. 1999;210:429-35.
3. Regge D, Neri E, Turini F, et al. Role of CT colonography in inflammatory bowel disease. Eur J Radiol. 2009;69:404-8.
4. Xie J, Itzkowitz S. Cancer in inflammatory bowel disease. World J Gastroenterol. 2008;14:378-89.

97

CT Cisternography in CSF Rhinorrhea

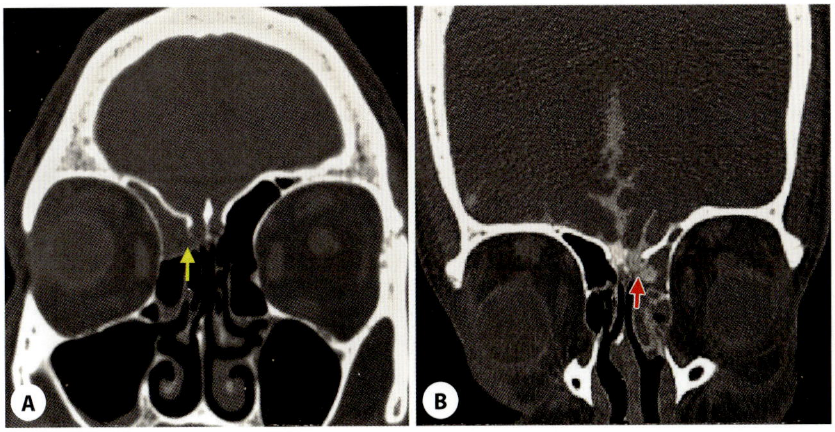

CLINICAL BACKGROUND

A 55-year-old male RTA with head injury patient came with complaints of rhinorrhea.

IMAGING FINDINGS

Bony dehiscence noted in lateral lamella and cribriform plate on right side, measuring (4 × 6 mm), (yellow arrow) with demonstrable active contrast leakage, following intrathecal injection of contrast into right fronto-ethmoid sinus (red arrow). (Cisternography image in prone position) **(Figs. 1A and B)**.

DISCUSSION

Cerebrospinal fluid (CSF) rhinorrhea refers to the leakage of CSF from the subarachnoid space through defects in the osseous and dural structures at the skull base into the nasal cavity. The causes of CSF rhinorrhea can be broadly categorized into traumatic (including iatrogenic) and nontraumatic origins; the latter includes tumors and spontaneous leaks. CSF rhinorrhea can further be classified into active, characterized by continuous dripping, or inactive, where the dripping is intermittent. Various imaging modalities, such as isotope scans, computed tomography (CT), and magnetic resonance (MR) imaging, are utilized to localize and characterize the skull base defects suspected of causing CSF leakage.[1]

High-resolution computed tomography (HRCT) is effective for visualizing bony details, but it may struggle to differentiate between paranasal sinus secretions and leaked CSF. In contrast, contrast-enhanced CT cisternography offers critical confirmation of a CSF leak alongside precise anatomical localization of the osseous defect; however, it may come with significant side effects, including headaches, meningeal irritation, and seizures. Unlike CT cisternography, MR cisternography does not require an active CSF leak to identify the leak site. As a result, inactive leaks may often go undiagnosed with CT cisternography, though CT remains superior for assessing bony anatomy.[2]

CT cisternography is performed in two phases: First, a noncontrast high-resolution CT scan is obtained in the supine position, spanning from the skull vault to the mandible. This is followed by the intrathecal administration of 20 mL of omnipaque (300 mg/mL) via lumbar puncture. Patients are then positioned prone for 10 minutes to facilitate the opacification of the cisterns before undergoing another CT scan in the prone position. Noncontrast CT findings are evaluated independently to identify any bony defects, and the contrast-enhanced CT cisternography results are compared with the noncontrast images.[3]

Although there is no universally accepted gold standard for diagnosing CSF leaks, Hablas et al. demonstrated that the combination of noncontrast CT and contrast-enhanced CT cisternography offers a sensitivity of 95% and a specificity of 100%, surpassing the accuracy of either technique used alone. Therefore, CT cisternography proves to be highly beneficial for assessing patients with CSF leaks, as the combination of noncontrast and contrast images enhances the detection of leakage sites, especially when the leaks are small, thus aiding in effective treatment planning.[3]

REFERENCES

1. Scoffings DJ. Imaging of acquired skull base cerebrospinal fluid leaks. Neuroimaging Clin N Am. 2021;31(4):509-22.
2. Vemuri NV, Karanam LS, Manchikanti V, et al. Imaging review of cerebrospinal fluid leaks. Indian J Radiol Imaging. 2017;27(4): 441-6.
3. Hablas LT, Ammar AM, Elnagar RM. CSF rhinorrhea: non-contrast CT, contrast-enhanced CT cisternography or combined? Egypt J Radiol Nucl Med. 2022;53:201.

98 Takayasu Arteritis

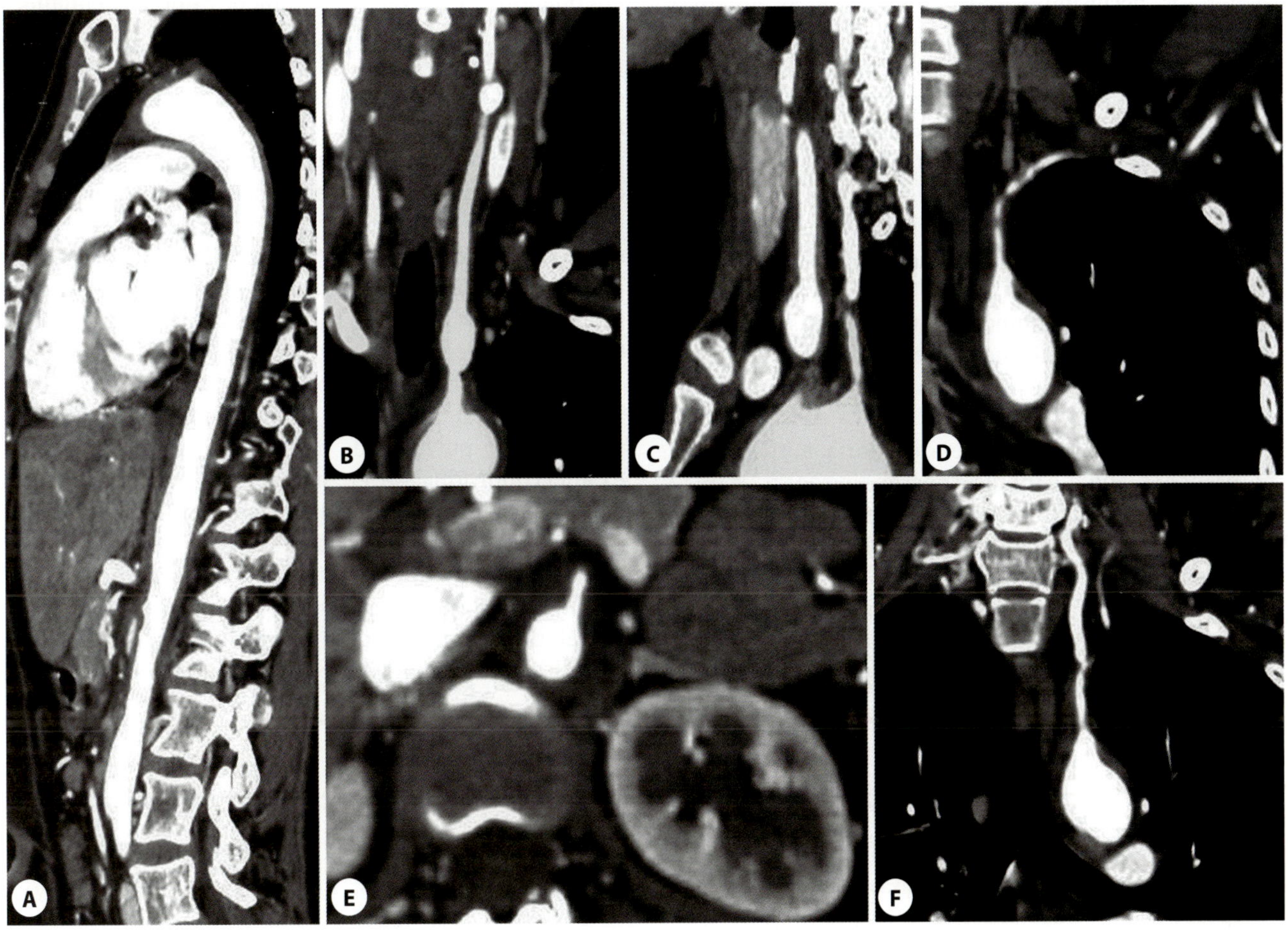

CLINICAL BACKGROUND

A 31-year-old female came with complaints of easy fatigue and weight loss.

IMAGING FINDINGS

Diffuse concentric wall thickening involving arch, thoracic and abdominal aorta and its main branches includes brachiocephalic trunk, left subclavian, left axillary, SMA, right/left common carotid and left vertebral arteries **(Figs. 1A to F)**.

DISCUSSION

Takayasu arteritis (TA) is a chronic inflammatory condition characterized by idiopathic inflammation of large vessels, particularly affecting the aorta and its major branches, as well as the coronary and pulmonary arteries. The inflammation can lead to significant changes in the vessel walls, including concentric thickening, fibrosis, and thrombosis, resulting in stenosis, occlusion, vascular remodeling, or aneurysm formation. The classification of Takayasu arteritis is based on the affected arteries, with six distinct types documented.[1]

Historically, conventional angiography has been considered the definitive method for diagnosing TA. However, multidetector CT angiography (CTA) has emerged as a valuable noninvasive imaging technique that effectively reveals both luminal and mural lesions in the aorta and its branches, thus aiding in the early identification of vasculitis related to TA.[2]

The proposed angiographic classification is as follows:

- *Type I:* Involves only the branches of the aortic arch.
- *Type IIa:* Affects the ascending aorta, aortic arch, and its branches.
- Type IIb: Involves the ascending aorta, aortic arch, its branches, and the thoracic descending aorta.
- *Type III:* Affects the descending thoracic aorta, abdominal aorta, and/or renal arteries, without involvement of the ascending aorta or aortic arch.
- *Type IV:* Exclusively involves the abdominal aorta and/or renal arteries.
- *Type V:* Combines characteristics of type IIb and type IV.

Additionally, involvement of the coronary and pulmonary arteries is indicated with C (+) or P (+), respectively, with type V being the most frequently observed variant.[1]

On CT imaging, one of the characteristic features of TA is the concentric thickening of the vessel walls. Another important sign is calcification within these thickened walls. On precontrast CT scans, this thickening appears with high attenuation compared to the lumen, while postenhanced CTA images typically show a double ring enhancement pattern in the venous phase. Stenosis is frequently observed, affecting around 90% of patients, while ectasia and aneurysms are less common.[1] Stenotic lesions often present as concentric narrowing of the arterial lumen, and in some cases, proximal vessels may appear normal or dilated while exhibiting tapered narrowing in distal segments, giving rise to a "rat tail"-like configuration.[1,3] The identification of collateral vessels may also occur with luminal narrowing, which can be instrumental in planning treatment strategies.

In the differential diagnosis, several conditions should be considered, including atherosclerosis, giant cell arteritis, and polyarteritis nodosa. Atherosclerosis tends to affect individuals over the age of 45 years and is not typically associated with long segment luminal stenosis. Giant cell arteritis usually occurs in patients over 50 years, most commonly affecting the branches of the external and internal carotid arteries. Polyarteritis nodosa is more prevalent in adults aged 30–50, with a greater incidence in males, and primarily affects gastrointestinal and renal arteries.[1]

REFERENCES

1. Zhu FP, Luo S, Wang ZJ, et al. Takayasu arteritis: Imaging spectrum at multidetector CT angiography. Br J Radiol. 2012;85(1020):e1282-92.
2. Brunner J, Feldman BM, Tyrrell PN, et al. Takayasu arteritis in children and adolescents. Rheumatology. 2010;49:1806-14.
3. Matsunaga N, Hayashi K, Sakamoto I, et al. Takayasu arteritis: protean radiologic manifestations and diagnosis. Radiographics. 1997;17:579-94.

99 Urinary Bladder Rupture

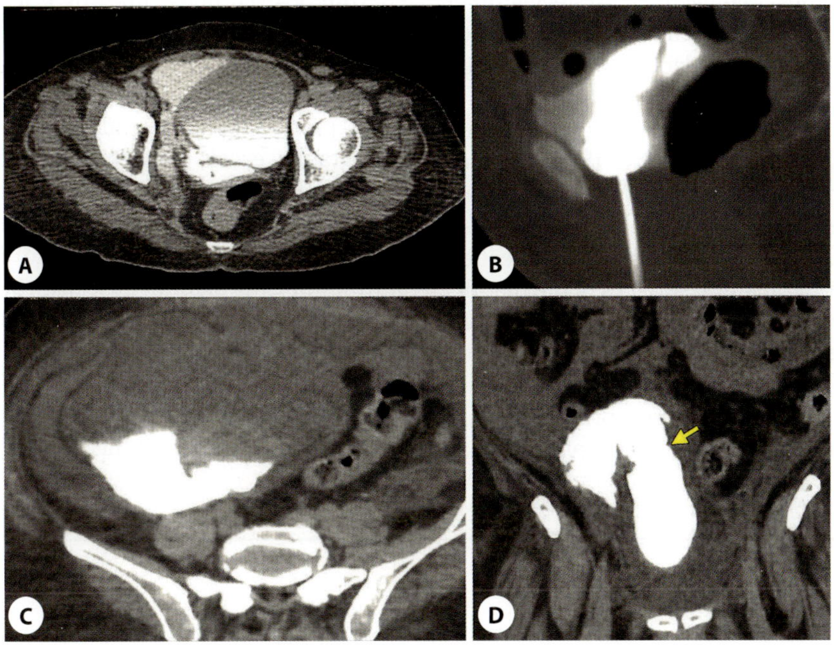

CLINICAL BACKGROUND

A 56-year-old female and 55-year-old male, RTA patients came with complaints lower abdominal pain.

IMAGING FINDINGS

Delayed imaging (first patient) shows (15 minutes) extravasation of contrast into perivesical region (extra-peritoneal). Cystogram shows a rent in right posterior aspect of urinary bladder close to right UV-junction (blue arrow) with contrast leak **(Figs. 1A to D)**.

Delayed imaging (second patient) shows (30 minutes) extravasation of contrast into intra-peritoneal cavity. Cystogram shows a rent in superior wall/dome of urinary bladder (yellow arrow) with contrast leak.

DISCUSSION

Bladder injuries are categorized into extraperitoneal (EP) and intraperitoneal (IP) injuries. Generally, EP bladder injuries are associated with pelvic fractures, while IP injuries often result from high-energy impacts to an overdistended bladder. Approximately 60% of bladder traumas are classified as extraperitoneal, 30% as intraperitoneal, and 10% as combined injuries. Management strategies differ: EP injuries are typically treated with an indwelling catheter, whereas definitive repair is required for intraperitoneal and complex bladder injuries.[1]

The bladder dome is covered by peritoneum, and the bladder neck is anchored to the pelvis through fascia and ligaments. Intraperitoneal bladder ruptures occur at the dome and above the peritoneal reflection, whereas extraperitoneal ruptures happen below this reflection, primarily on the anterior or lateral surfaces of the bladder. If left untreated, bladder ruptures can result in severe complications, including peritonitis, sepsis, and fistula formation. Effective management necessitates prompt evaluation, accurate diagnosis, and appropriate treatment tailored to the rupture's location and severity. Most patients can expect a return to normal bladder function after appropriate intervention.[1,2]

For hemodynamically stable patients presenting with gross hematuria, retrograde cystography—either computed tomography (CT) or conventional X-ray—is indicated. Both methods have similar sensitivity and specificity in detecting bladder injuries, though intravenous contrast CT with delayed phase imaging is less effective compared to retrograde cystography. According to the European Association of Urology guidelines, CT cystography is preferred over traditional X-ray cystography due to its rapid processing time and convenience. Moreover, CT cystography excels at identifying other intra-abdominal issues and bony fragments within the bladder.

Imaging characteristics of EP bladder trauma include contrast extravasation confined to the perivesical space surrounding the bladder base, with potential extravasation into adjacent areas such as the thighs, penis, perineum, or anterior abdominal wall if the urogenital fascia is compromised. In contrast, IP bladder trauma shows contrast extravasation into the peritoneal cavity, which outlines bowel loops and fills paracolic gutters.[2,3]

REFERENCES

1. Chan DP, Abujudeh HH, Cushing GL, et al. CT cystography with multiplanar reformation for suspected bladder rupture: experience in 234 cases. AJR Am J Roentgenol. 2006;187(5): 1296-302.
2. Coccolini F, Moore EE, Kluger Y, et al. Kidney and urogenital trauma: WSES-AAST guidelines. World J Emerg Surg. 2019;14:54.
3. Bryk DJ, Zhao LC. Guideline of guidelines: A review of urological trauma guidelines. BJU Int. 2016;117(2):226-34.

100 Calcifying Epithelioma of Malherbe

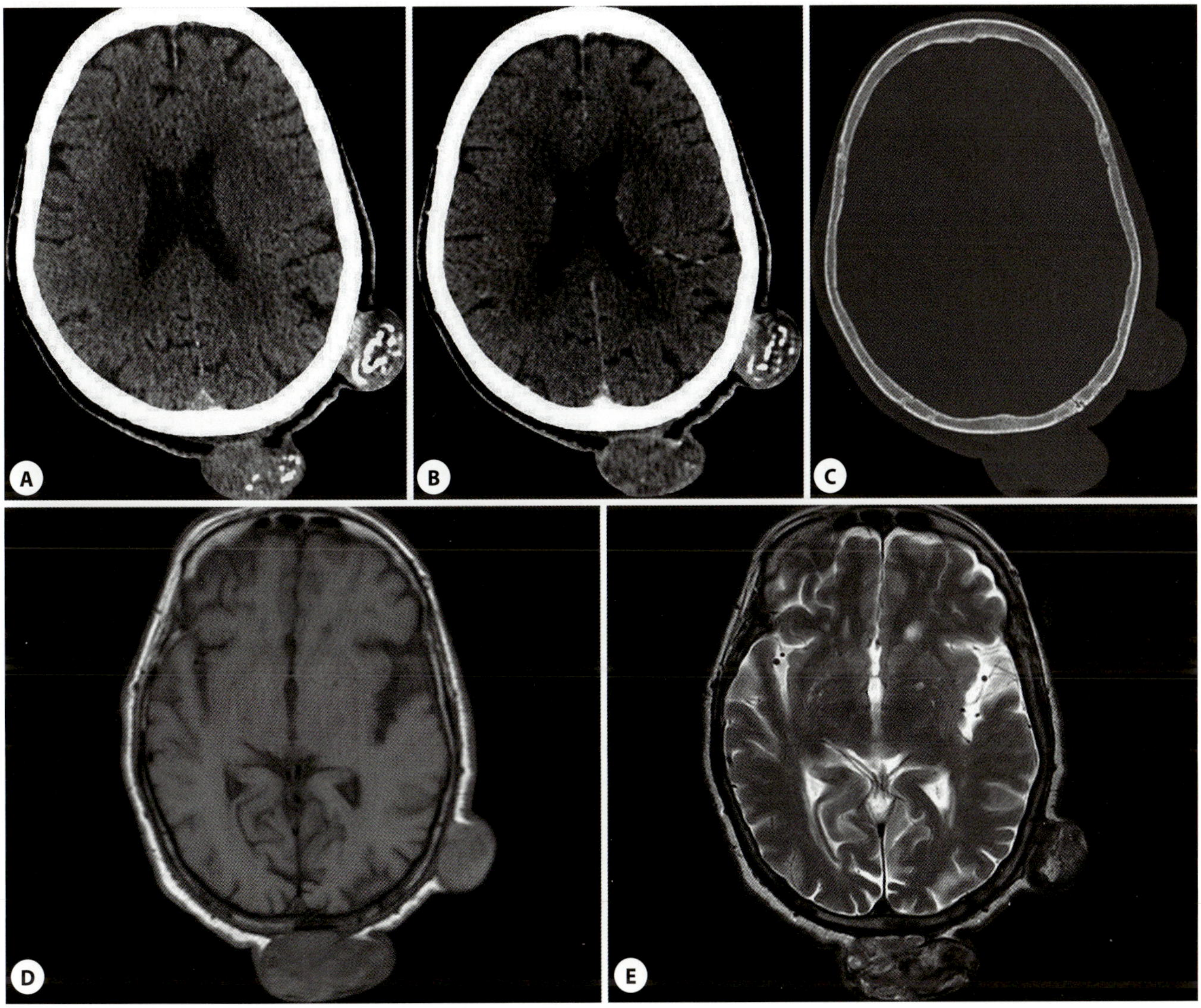

CLINICAL BACKGROUND

A 79-year-old female came with complaints of multiple scalp swelling.

IMAGING FINDINGS

Multiple well defined heterodense lesions with calcifications seen in scalp. The lesions show thin peripheral postcontrast enhancement/underlying bony calvarium appears normal. No evidence of intracranial extension.

MR screening shows T1 iso-hyper-intense and T2 heterointense subcutaneous lesions in scalp **(Figs. 1A to E)**.

DISCUSSION

Pilomatrixoma, also known as calcifying epithelioma of Malherbe, is a benign tumor originating from the hair follicle matrix. In 1880, Malherbe and Chenantais first referred to this calcifying lesion as "epithelioma," believing it originated from sebaceous glands. However, in 1961, Forbis and Helwing introduced the term pilomatrixoma after research clarified its true origin in the hair follicle matrix. Although these tumors are typically solitary, they can occur in multiples and are associated with various syndromes, including myotonic dystrophy, familial adenomatous polyposis, Gardner syndrome, Turner syndrome, xeroderma pigmentosum, Rubinstein-Taybi syndrome, Sotos syndrome, and basal cell nevus syndrome.[1]

Ultrasound is the primary imaging modality used to evaluate pilomatrixomas, often providing sufficient information for diagnosis. Characteristic imaging features include a hypoechoic rim, internal reticulations, and dense calcifications, as well as peripheral or central vascularity noted during Doppler examination. In cases where the diagnosis remains unclear, both MRI and CT can serve as valuable alternatives.[2]

CT imaging is becoming more prevalent for these tumors, particularly in assessing head and neck pilomatrixomas. A critical aspect of evaluation is the confinement of lesions to the skin and subcutaneous fat, with the surrounding fat typically appearing intact without any stranding or edema. More than 80% of these tumors display microscopic calcification or ossification. While the exact incidence of radiographically visible calcifications is unknown, heavily calcified tumors are notable for their distinctive radiographic appearance. On T1-weighted MRI images, pilomatrixomas often present as isointense or slightly hyperintense compared to adjacent skeletal muscle, with both peripheral and central areas exhibiting heterogeneous enhancement. The presence of heterogeneous enhancement and the absence of restricted diffusion can help distinguish pilomatrixomas from dermoid cysts.[2]

Surgical excision is the preferred treatment when necessary. The recurrence rate for pilomatrixomas ranges from 2 to 6%, often attributed to incomplete excision. Additionally, there have been 125 documented cases of malignant pilomatrixomas, referred to as "pilomatrix carcinomas".[1]

REFERENCES

1. Le C, Bedocs PM. Calcifying Epithelioma of Malherbe. 2023 Jun 12. In: StatPearls [Internet]. Treasure Island (FL): StatPearls Publishing; 2024 Jan.
2. Bulman JC, Ulualp SO, Rajaram V, et al. Pilomatricoma of childhood: A common pathologic diagnosis yet a rare radiologic one. AJR Am J Roentgenol. 2016;206(1):182-8.

Index

D

E

F

G

H

I

O

P

R

S

T

U